PALS

Pediatric Advanced Life Support

Study Guide

THIRD EDITION

Barbara Aehlert, RN, BSPA
Southwest EMS Education, Inc.
Phoenix, Arizona/Pursley, Texas

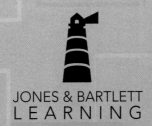

JONES & BARTLETT
LEARNING

World Headquarters
Jones & Bartlett Learning
5 Wall Street
Burlington, MA 01803
978-443-5000
info@jblearning.com
www.jblearning.com

Jones & Bartlett Learning books and products are available through most bookstores and online booksellers. To contact Jones & Bartlett Learning directly, call 800-832-0034, fax 978-443-8000, or visit our website, www.jblearning.com.

Substantial discounts on bulk quantities of Jones & Bartlett Learning publications are available to corporations, professional associations, and other qualified organizations. For details and specific discount information, contact the special sales department at Jones & Bartlett Learning via the above contact information or send an email to specialsales@jblearning.com.

Production Credits
Chief Executive Officer: Ty Field
President: James Homer
SVP, Editor-in-Chief: Michael Johnson
SVP, Chief Marketing Officer: Alison M. Pendergast
Executive Publisher: Kimberly Brophy
Executive Acquisitions Editor—EMS: Christine Emerton
Vice President of Sales, Public Safety Group: Matthew Maniscalco
Director of Sales, Public Safety Group: Patricia Einstein
Production Editor: Tina Chen
Director of Marketing: Alisha Weisman
VP, Manufacturing and Inventory Control: Therese Connell
Director of Photo Research and Permissions: Amy Wrynn
Printing and Binding: Courier Companies
Cover Printing: Courier Companies

ISBN: 978-1-284-03808-8

6048

Printed in the United States of America
16 15 14   10 9 8 7 6 5 4 3 2

To

My daughters, Andrea and Sherri
For the beautiful young women you have become

About the Author

Barbara Aehlert is the President of Southwest EMS Education, Inc. in Phoenix, Arizona, and Pursley, Texas. She has been a registered nurse for more than 35 years with clinical experience in medical/surgical and critical care nursing and, for the past 25 years, in prehospital education. Barbara is an active ACLS, BLS, and PALS instructor.

Preface

This book is designed for use by healthcare professionals including Pediatricians, Family Practice Physicians, Anesthesiologists, Emergency Physicians, Nurses, and Respiratory Therapists preparing for a Pediatric Advanced Life Support (PALS) Student Course.

Each chapter contains learning objectives that are followed by a review of the critical elements related to the subject. A fifty-question pretest and posttest are provided, in addition to short quizzes at the conclusion of each chapter. Answers and rationales are provided for all questions in this text.

With the assistance of the text reviewers, every effort has been made to provide information that is consistent with current research and resuscitation guidelines. However, the reader is advised to consult expert opinion articles and guidelines for more authoritative advice. In clinical practice, it is essential to confirm all medication doses, indications, and contraindications before use. The author and publisher assume no responsibility or liability for loss or damage resulting from the use of information contained within.

Barbara Aehlert, RN, BSPA

Acknowledgments

I would like to thank the following individuals for their assistance with this text:

The many reviewers of this book who devoted countless hours to intensive review; their comments were invaluable in helping develop and fine-tune the manuscript in this or the previous editions.

Laura Bayless and Gayle May for their oversight of this project.

Sean Newton, CEP for his assistance with the photos in the first edition of this text.

Ed and Pat Tirone for graciously providing photos of their daughters, Kimberly and Sarah.

Contents

Pretest

Questions

1. Which of the following lists conditions that affect the upper airway?
   A) Bacterial tracheitis, epiglottitis, bronchiolitis
   B) Bronchiolitis, croup, asthma
   C) Asthma, bronchiolitis, pneumonia
   D) Croup, epiglottitis, bacterial tracheitis

2. Systemic complications of vascular access include:
   A) Phlebitis
   B) Cellulitis
   C) Hematoma formation
   D) Catheter-fragment embolism

3. A child with signs of cyanosis, diminished breath sounds with minimal chest excursion, and an inadequate ventilatory rate is exhibiting signs of:
   A) Hyperthermia
   B) Hypovolemia
   C) Respiratory failure
   D) Early respiratory distress

4. In the pediatric patient, cardiac arrest is most often due to:
   A) Hypothermia
   B) Acid-base imbalance
   C) Respiratory failure
   D) Sepsis

5. Which of the following statements is correct regarding the laryngeal mask airway (LMA)?
   A) The LMA is available in only one size.
   B) Direct visualization of the oropharynx is required for LMA insertion.
   C) The inflatable mask of the LMA ensures an airtight seal to protect the lower airway from aspiration.
   D) LMA insertion should be considered in the case of unsuccessful bag-mask ventilation or failed tracheal intubation.

6. The intravenous dose of epinephrine for an infant or child is:
   A) 0.1 mg/kg (0.1 mL/kg) of 1:1000 solution
   B) 0.01 mg/kg (0.1 mL/kg) of 1:10,000 solution
   C) 0.02 mg/kg of 1:1000 solution
   D) 0.04 mg/kg of 1:10,000 solution

7. Suctioning of the newly born infant should be limited to _____ per attempt.
   A) 3 to 5 seconds
   B) 5 to 10 seconds
   C) 10 to 15 seconds
   D) 15 to 30 seconds

8. Which of the following statements regarding vagal maneuvers is correct?
   A) Carotid sinus massage is recommended for infants and young children.
   B) Application of pressure to the eye is safe if performed in older children.
   C) Vagal maneuvers should be attempted only after administration of adenosine.
   D) Vagal maneuvers may be tried in the stable but symptomatic child in supraventricular tachycardia.

9. You are a paramedic called to a private residence for a 6-month-old infant with difficulty breathing. Upon your arrival, the infant's mother is frantic. Mom states she went to check on the napping infant and found him blue and not breathing. She picked up the infant and ran to the phone to call 9-1-1. The infant began spontaneously breathing while she was on the phone. You find the infant awake and alert with normal color and vital signs for age. Mom is uncertain if her baby requires transport to the hospital. Your best course of action will be to:
   A) Allow the mother to refuse further care. The infant is in no obvious distress at this time.
   B) Contact Child Protective Services.
   C) Explain your concerns regarding the infant's reported color change and apneic episode and encourage the mother to permit transport for physician evaluation.
   D) Remain on the scene until the mother has made a follow-up appointment with the infant's pediatrician.

10. Procainamide:
    A) May cause narrowing of the QRS width and hypertension.
    B) Is most effective when infused rapidly over 5 to 10 minutes.
    C) Is the drug of choice in the management of symptomatic bradycardia.
    D) Is used for a wide range of atrial and ventricular dysrhythmias, including supraventricular and ventricular tachycardia.

Questions 11-18 refer to the following scenario:

An apneic and pulseless 6-year-old boy is brought by ambulance to the emergency department. Emergency Medical Technicians report the child was the front-seat passenger of a vehicle involved in a rollover crash. The child was not restrained. Examination confirms that the child is apneic and pulseless, with contusions noted on the anterior chest and open fractures of both femurs. Chest compressions are being performed and the child is being ventilated with 100% oxygen with a bag-mask device.

11. Positive-pressure ventilation should be provided at a rate of:
    A) 8 to 12 breaths/minute
    B) 10 to 14 breaths/minute
    C) 14 to 30 breaths/minute
    D) 12 to 20 breaths/minute

12. The cardiac monitor has been applied and reveals the following rhythm.

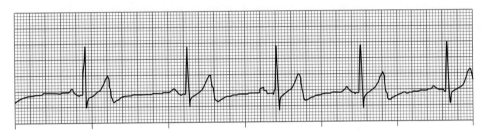

    The rhythm displayed is:
    A) Sinus bradycardia
    B) Ventricular fibrillation
    C) Complete AV block
    D) Supraventricular tachycardia

13. Despite the rhythm observed on the cardiac monitor, the child is unresponsive, apneic, and pulseless. This clinical situation is called:
    A) Asystole
    B) Ventricular fibrillation
    C) Pulseless electrical activity
    D) Pulseless ventricular tachycardia

14. List four possible reversible causes of this clinical situation.
    A)
    B)
    C)
    D)

15. In addition to other injuries, physical examination of this child revealed anterior chest contusions. Select the correct statement regarding thoracic trauma and the pediatric patient.
   A) Children are more likely to sustain rib fractures than adults are.
   B) Pneumothorax and hemothorax are among the most common thoracic injuries seen in children.
   C) Thoracic trauma in children is associated with a low mortality rate.
   D) A pulmonary contusion is a life-threatening injury that is readily recognized in the pediatric trauma patient.

16. A first-line medication used in the management of this clinical situation is:
   A) Atropine
   B) Dopamine
   C) Epinephrine
   D) Sodium bicarbonate

17. The first-line medication given in the management of this clinical situation is used to:
   A) Decrease myocardial contractility
   B) Increase systemic vascular resistance
   C) Decrease heart rate
   D) Increase myocardial consumption

18. Despite the interventions performed thus far, the child's cardiac rhythm remains unchanged. A pulse is not present. Should defibrillation be performed?

19. Which of the following statements is true regarding the use of the Glasgow Coma Scale (GCS)?
   A) The GCS is used to assess the patient's verbal response, motor response, and pupillary reactivity.
   B) When assigning a score using the GCS, the maximum possible score is 13.
   C) When using the GCS, the minimum possible score is 3.
   D) The GCS is used to assess the patient's verbal response, motor response, and capillary refill.

20. Pediatric rhythm disturbances can be categorized as normal for age, fast, slow, or absent/pulseless. List three examples of rhythm disturbances found in the absent/pulseless rhythm category.
   A)
   B)
   C)

21. Which of the following formulas may be used to approximate the correct uncuffed tracheal tube size in a child?
   A) Age in years/2 + 12
   B) 70 + (2 × age in years)
   C) (4 + age in years)/4
   D) 90 + (2 × age in years)

22. A 5-year-old girl is unresponsive, apneic, and pulseless. Cardiopulmonary resuscitation is being performed. The cardiac monitor reveals ventricular fibrillation. Which of the following interventions should be performed next?
    A) Establish vascular access and administer epinephrine 0.01 mg/kg.
    B) Defibrillate with 2 J/kg.
    C) Perform synchronized cardioversion with 1 J/kg.
    D) Establish vascular access and administer amiodarone 5 mg/kg.

23. Which of the following statements is correct regarding pediatric defibrillation?
    A) Use of an automated external defibrillator (AED) in infants is not recommended.
    B) Remove oxygen sources from the area of the patient before delivering electrical therapy.
    C) The initial recommended energy level for pulseless VT or VF is 4 to 10 J/kg.
    D) If defibrillation of an infant is indicated, use of an AED with a pediatric attenuator is essential.

24. Administration of magnesium sulfate is appropriate for which of the following dysrhythmias?
    A) Sinus bradycardia
    B) Atrial fibrillation
    C) Torsades de pointes
    D) Complete atrioventricular block

25. Which of the following statements is correct?
    A) Sodium bicarbonate should be routinely administered in cardiac arrest.
    B) Assessment of blood glucose concentration is unnecessary during a resuscitation effort.
    C) Family members should be given the option of being present during resuscitation of an infant or child.
    D) Central venous access is recommended as the initial route of vascular access in cardiac arrest.

26. Select the **incorrect** statement regarding sinus tachycardia.
    A) Sinus tachycardia is a normal compensatory response to the need for increased cardiac output or oxygen delivery.
    B) In sinus tachycardia, the heart rate is usually more than 220 beats per minute in infants or 200 beats per minute in children.
    C) The onset of a sinus tachycardia occurs gradually.
    D) Patient management includes treatment of the underlying cause that precipitated the rhythm.

27. A 2-year-old boy appears to be choking. You find the child responsive, but cyanotic. He is unable to cough or speak. Initial interventions in this situation should include:
    A) Performing a blind finger sweep to remove the obstruction
    B) Alternating 5 back slaps with 5 chest thrusts
    C) Performing direct laryngoscopy to visualize the obstruction
    D) Informing the child that you are going to help him, and then performing abdominal thrusts

28. An adult bag-mask used with supplemental oxygen set at a flow rate of 15 L/min (but with no reservoir) will deliver approximately _____ oxygen to the patient.
    A) 16% to 21%
    B) 35% to 40%
    C) 40% to 60%
    D) 65% to 90%

29. The drug of choice for a stable but symptomatic child in supraventricular tachycardia is:
    A) Atropine
    B) Adenosine
    C) Albuterol
    D) Amiodarone

30. A 44-pound child presents with fever, irritability, mottled color, cool extremities, and a prolonged capillary refill time. The appropriate initial fluid bolus for administration to this child is:
    A) 100 mL of normal saline over 30 to 60 minutes
    B) 200 mL of 5% dextrose in water in less than 20 minutes
    C) 400 mL of normal saline or Ringer's lactate in less than 20 minutes
    D) 800 mL of normal saline or Ringer's lactate infused over 30 to 60 minutes

31. Select the **incorrect** statement regarding the use of cricoid pressure.
    A) Cricoid pressure is used to minimize the risk of choking in a conscious infant or child.
    B) Cricoid pressure may be considered to minimize gastric inflation in an unresponsive patient.
    C) Cricoid pressure is applied using one fingertip in infants and the thumb and index finger in children.
    D) Cricoid pressure may result in tracheal obstruction in infants if excessive pressure is used.

32. Which of the following is correct regarding bradycardia in a newborn?
    A) Bradycardia should initially be treated with a fluid bolus of 20 mL/kg.
    B) Ensuring adequate oxygenation and ventilation are the initial steps in treating bradycardia in a newborn.
    C) Administration of epinephrine is the first action to perform when treating bradycardia in a newborn.
    D) Transcutaneous pacing should be used as the initial step in treating bradycardia in a newborn.

Questions 33-36 pertain to the following scenario:

You are called to see an 18-month-old child with difficulty breathing. Mom reports the child has had a "barking" cough and cold for the past 2 days and appears worse today. You note the child is cyanotic and appears limp in his mother's arms. His ventilatory rate is rapid and shallow. Moderate intercostal retractions are visible.

33. Your initial assessment reveals a patent airway. The child's ventilatory rate is 60/min. Auscultation of the chest reveals wheezes bilaterally. A weak brachial pulse is present at a rate of 194 beats/min. The skin is cyanotic. Capillary refill is 2 to 3 seconds; temperature is 101.8° F; and the pulse oximeter reveals a SpO_2 of 80%. This child's presentation is most consistent with:
    A) Respiratory distress
    B) Respiratory failure
    C) Respiratory arrest
    D) Cardiopulmonary arrest

34. Your next course of action should be to:
    A) Begin chest compressions
    B) Administer supplemental oxygen by nasal cannula
    C) Administer supplemental oxygen using a nonrebreather mask
    D) Assist ventilations with supplemental oxygen and a bag-mask device

35. Suspecting that this child has croup, a physician orders nebulized epinephrine. What is the rationale for the use of epinephrine in this situation?
    A) Epinephrine is being ordered to slow heart rate.
    B) Epinephrine is being ordered to decrease secretions.
    C) Epinephrine administration will reduce mucosal edema and relax bronchial smooth muscle.
    D) Epinephrine administration will improve mental status and decrease myocardial oxygen demand.

36. You should anticipate orders for which of the following medications?
    A) Dexamethasone
    B) Diphenhydramine
    C) A sedative
    D) An opiate

37. Exhaled carbon dioxide (CO_2) monitoring:
    A) Exhaled CO_2 monitoring provides essential information regarding patient oxygenation.
    B) Exhaled CO_2 can be measured using a disposable colorimetric device or a capnometer.
    C) Exhaled CO_2 monitoring should be performed to monitor tracheal tube position during the transport of an intubated patient of any age.
    D) Exhaled CO_2 monitoring is recommended as confirmation of tracheal tube position for patients of all ages with a perfusing cardiac rhythm.

38. The presence of compensated shock can be identified by:
    A) Assessment of heart rate, ECG rhythm, and skin temperature
    B) Assessment of the presence and strength of peripheral pulses, mental status, and pupil response to light
    C) Assessment of heart rate, presence and strength of peripheral pulses, and the adequacy of end-organ perfusion
    D) Assessment of end-organ perfusion, ECG rhythm, and pupil response to light

Questions 39–45 refer to the following scenario:

A 3-year-old is found barely responsive by her babysitter. The babysitter was distracted "for just a minute" by a telephone call and lost track of the child. The child was found on the ground just outside the garage door. The patient's skin looks flushed and she is laboring to breathe. You note that secretions are draining from the patient's mouth and she has been incontinent of urine. The child is unaware of your presence.

39. From the information provided, complete the following documentation regarding the Pediatric Assessment Triangle.
    A) Appearance:
    B) Breathing:
    C) Circulation:

40. Based on the information provided, your **FIRST** intervention should be to:
    A) Establish vascular access
    B) Suction the airway
    C) Administer nebulized albuterol
    D) Insert an advanced airway

41. For each of the following, record the estimated values for a 3-year-old child.
    A) Weight: _____
    B) Ventilatory rate: _____
    C) Heart rate: _____
    D) Blood pressure: _____

42. Your assessment reveals that the child will open her eyes and withdraw in response to a painful stimulus but makes incomprehensible sounds. Her Glasgow Coma Scale score is:
    A) 6
    B) 8
    C) 10
    D) 12

43. The child's ventilatory rate is 44/min, heart rate is 158/min, and blood pressure is 80/60. Her skin is warm and moist. Her pupils are equal and reactive at 2 mm. Auscultation of her lungs reveals bilateral diffuse wheezes. Excessive oral secretions are present. These findings are most consistent with the _____ toxidrome.

44. Further questioning of the babysitter reveals that the child may have been out of sight for 20 to 30 minutes before she was found. The babysitter recalls having seen an open bottle of white liquid on the floor of the garage. As you continue interviewing the babysitter, a coworker tells you that he smells garlic on the child's breath. This child was most likely exposed to:
    A) An organophosphate
    B) Camphor
    C) Ethylene glycol
    D) Gasoline

45. You are instructed to administer atropine to this patient. Which of the following statements is correct?
    A) Question the order. Atropine is indicated for symptomatic bradycardias. This patient is not bradycardic.
    B) Administer the atropine as instructed. Atropine is being ordered in this situation to increase the patient's blood pressure.
    C) Question the order. Although atropine may be used in situations such as this, the patient is tachycardic. Atropine is contraindicated if a tachycardia is present.
    D) Administer the atropine as instructed. In this situation, atropine is being given to dry the patient's airway of secretions.

46. Which of the following statements is correct regarding newborn resuscitation?
    A) Most cardiac arrests in newborns are cardiac in origin.
    B) The recommended compression to ventilation ratio is 15:2.
    C) Most newborns require some assistance with ventilation at birth.
    D) Heart rate may be assessed by auscultating the apical pulse or palpating the base of the umbilical cord.

47. Medications used to maintain cardiac output include:
    A) Midazolam, epinephrine, and naloxone
    B) Lorazepam, midazolam, and naloxone
    C) Diazepam, dopamine, and dobutamine
    D) Dopamine, epinephrine, and dobutamine

48. In a perfusing patient, oxygen saturation should be monitored and oxygen administered, if necessary, to maintain a saturation of __ or higher.
    A) 90%
    B) 94%
    C) 98%
    D) 100%

49. Amiodarone:
    A) Should be administered over 20 to 60 minutes in cardiac arrest.
    B) Should be administered IV push in a patient with a perfusing rhythm.
    C) May cause hypotension, bradycardia, and prolongation of the QT interval.
    D) Is most effective when administered simultaneously with procainamide.

50. Synchronized cardioversion may be warranted in an unstable patient with which of the following dysrhythmias?
    A) Torsades de pointes or atrial tachycardia
    B) Atrial fibrillation or monomorphic ventricular tachycardia
    C) Complete atrioventricular block or atrial flutter
    D) Ventricular fibrillation or supraventricular tachycardia

Pretest Answers

1. D. Pneumonia, asthma, and bronchiolitis are conditions that affect the lower airway. Croup, epiglottitis, and bacterial tracheitis are conditions that affect the upper airway.

2. D. Systemic complications of vascular access include sepsis, fluid overload/electrolyte imbalance, hypersensitivity reactions, air embolism, catheter-fragment embolism, and pulmonary thromboembolism. Local complications include pain and irritation, cellulitis, phlebitis, thrombosis, bleeding, hematoma formation, inadvertent arterial puncture, infiltration and extravasation, and nerve, tendon, ligament, and/or limb damage.

3. C. A child with signs of cyanosis, diminished breath sounds with minimal chest excursion, and an inadequate ventilatory rate is exhibiting signs of respiratory failure. Signs of respiratory failure include the findings of respiratory distress with any of the following additions or modifications: sleepy, intermittently combative, or agitated; increased ventilatory effort at sternal notch, absent or significantly decreased breath sounds, marked use of accessory muscles, retractions; head bobbing, grunting, gasping; central cyanosis despite oxygen administration; poor peripheral perfusion; mottling; marked tachycardia (bradycardia is a late sign), decreased muscle tone, decreased level of consciousness or response to pain; inadequate ventilatory rate, effort, or chest excursion, or tachypnea with periods of bradypnea; slowing to bradypnea/agonal breathing.

4. C. In adults, sudden nontraumatic cardiopulmonary arrests are usually the result of underlying cardiac disease. In children, cardiac arrests are usually the result of respiratory failure (asphyxia precipitated by acute hypoxia or hypercarbia) or circulatory shock (ischemia from hypovolemia, sepsis, or myocardial dysfunction [cardiogenic shock]).

5. D. The LMA is available in sizes for neonates, infants, young children, older children, and small, normal, and large adults. The LMA is inserted through the mouth into the pharynx without visualization. The inflatable LMA mask does not ensure an airtight seal to protect the airway against gastric regurgitation. Leakage of the mask may allow aspiration of emesis and gastric distention may occur with misplacement. When used by appropriately trained professionals, use of an LMA should be considered during resuscitation, especially in the case of unsuccessful bag-mask ventilation or failed tracheal intubation.

6. B. Because epinephrine is supplied in different dilutions, it is important to ensure selection of the correct concentration before administering this medication. The intravenous dosage of epinephrine for an infant or child is 0.01 mg/kg [0.1 mL/kg] of 1:10,000 solution.

7. A. Suctioning of the newly born infant should be limited to 3 to 5 seconds per attempt.

8. D. Vagal maneuvers may be tried in the stable but symptomatic child in supraventricular tachycardia. When indicated, vagal maneuvers should be tried before administration of adenosine. Application of pressure to the eye should not be performed in a patient of any age because this can damage the retina. Carotid sinus massage may be used in older children.

9. C. The infant has experienced an Apparent Life-Threatening Event (ALTE). These events can involve any of the following: apnea, color change (cyanosis, pallor, or erythema), marked change in muscle tone (limpness), choking or gagging. The infant should be transported and evaluated by a physician.

10. D. Procainamide is used for a wide range of atrial and ventricular dysrhythmias, including supraventricular and ventricular tachycardia. Procainamide must be infused slowly (over 30 to 60 minutes) while continuously monitoring the patient's electrocardiogram and blood pressure. Epinephrine (not procainamide) is the drug of choice in the management of symptomatic bradycardia. The infusion of procainamide should be stopped or slowed if the QRS lengthens more than 50% of its original width or hypotension occurs.

11. D. Positive-pressure ventilation for this child should be provided at a rate of 12 to 20 breaths/minute (1 breath every 3 to 5 seconds). Each breath should be given over 1 second.

12. A. The rhythm shown is a sinus bradycardia.

13. C. Despite the presence of an organized rhythm on the monitor that you would expect to produce a pulse, the child is pulseless. This situation is called pulseless electrical activity (PEA). Many conditions may cause PEA. PEA has a poor prognosis unless the underlying cause can be rapidly identified and appropriately managed.

14. Possible reversible causes of PEA include hypovolemia (replace volume), hypoxia (give oxygen), hydrogen ion (correct acidosis), hypo-/hyperkalemia (correct electrolyte disturbances), hypoglycemia (give dextrose if indicated), hypothermia (use rewarming measures), toxins/poisons/drugs (give antidote/specific therapy), cardiac tamponade (pericardiocentesis), tension pneumothorax (needle decompression, chest tube insertion) and thrombosis (coronary or pulmonary).

15. B. The most common thoracic injuries seen in children are pneumothorax, hemothorax, pulmonary contusion, fractures, and damage to major blood vessels, the heart, and diaphragm. In children, thoracic trauma is associated with a high mortality rate. The greater elasticity and resilience of the chest wall in children makes rib and sternum fractures less common than in adults however, force is more easily transmitted to the underlying lung tissues, resulting in pulmonary contusion, pneumothorax, or hemothorax. A pulmonary contusion is a potentially life-threatening injury that is frequently missed due to the presence of other associated injuries.

16. C. Epinephrine is a first-line medication used in the management of PEA.

17. B. Epinephrine stimulates alpha, beta-1, and beta-2 receptors. Effects of alpha receptor stimulation results in constriction of the arterioles in the skin, mucosa, kidneys, and viscera → increased systemic vascular resistance. These effects are beneficial in cardiac arrest because blood is shunted to the heart and brain. Effects of beta-1 receptor stimulation include increased force of contraction (+ inotropic effect) and increased heart rate (+ chronotropic effect). These effects result in increased myocardial workload and oxygen requirements. Stimulation of beta-2 receptors results in relaxation of bronchial smooth muscle.

18. No. Although the patient has no pulse, *organized* electrical activity is visible on the cardiac monitor. Defibrillation is used to terminate *disorganized* cardiac rhythms, such as ventricular fibrillation. The shock attempts to deliver a uniform electrical current of sufficient intensity to simultaneously depolarize ventricular cells, including fibrillating cells, briefly "stunning" the heart. This provides an opportunity for the heart's natural pacemakers to resume normal activity.

19. C. The Glasgow Coma Scale is used to assess a patient's level of responsiveness by evaluating best verbal response, best motor response, and eye opening. The minimum possible score is 3, maximum possible score 15. When caring for an infant or child, use the GCS that has been modified for pediatric use.

20. Absent/pulseless rhythms include (A) pulseless ventricular tachycardia, in which the ECG displays a wide QRS complex at a rate faster than 120 beats/min, (B) ventricular fibrillation, in which irregular chaotic deflections that vary in shape and amplitude are observed on the ECG but there is no coordinated ventricular contraction, (C) asystole, in which no cardiac electrical activity is present, and (D) pulseless electrical activity (PEA), in which electrical activity is visible on the ECG but central pulses are absent.

21. C. If an uncuffed tracheal tube is used for intubation, use of a 3.5-mm ID tube for infants up to one year of age and a 4-mm ID tube for patients between 1 and 2 years of age is considered reasonable.[1] After age 2, the following formula can be used to estimate uncuffed tracheal tube size: Uncuffed tracheal tube ID (mm) = 4 + (age in years/4).

22. B. The definitive treatment for ventricular fibrillation (VF) or pulseless ventricular tachycardia (VT) is defibrillation. When pulseless VT or VF is present, defibrillation takes priority over attempts to establish vascular access or administration of medications. Synchronized cardioversion is not indicated for VF.

23. B. To reduce the risk of fire, remove supplemental oxygen sources (masks, nasal cannulae, resuscitation bags, and ventilator tubing) from the area of the patient's bed before defibrillation and cardioversion attempts and place them at least 3 1/2 to 4 feet away from the patient's chest. If defibrillation of an infant is indicated, use of a manual defibrillator is preferred. If a manual defibrillator is not available, an AED equipped with a pediatric attenuator is desirable. If neither is available, use a standard AED. It is acceptable to use an initial energy dose for pulseless VT or VF of 2 to 4 J/kg. If the dysrhythmia persists, it is reasonable to increase the dose to 4 J/kg. If the dysrhythmia persists, subsequent energy levels should be at least 4 J/kg. Higher energy levels may be considered but should not exceed 10 J/kg or the adult maximum dose.

24. C. Administration of magnesium sulfate is indicated for the treatment of documented hypomagnesemia or for torsades de pointes (polymorphic VT associated with a long QT interval).

25. C. When possible, family members should be given the option of being present during resuscitation of an infant or child. When energy requirements rise, infants and children may become hypoglycemic because of rapidly depleted carbohydrate stores. Check the blood glucose concentration during the resuscitation and treat hypoglycemia promptly. Routine administration of sodium bicarbonate is not recommended in cardiac arrest. Because insertion takes time and specially trained personnel to perform, central venous access is not recommended as the initial route of vascular access during an emergency.

26. B. Sinus tachycardia is a normal compensatory response to the need for increased cardiac output or oxygen delivery. In sinus tachycardia, the heart rate is usually less than 220 beats per minute in infants or 180 beats per minute in children. Onset of the rhythm occurs gradually. The ECG shows a regular, narrow QRS complex rhythm that often varies in response to activity or stimulation. P waves are present before each QRS complex. The history given typically explains the rapid heart rate (i.e., pain, fever, volume loss due to trauma, vomiting, or diarrhea). Patient management includes treatment of the underlying cause that precipitated the rhythm (e.g., administering medications to relieve pain, administration of fluids to correct hypovolemia due to diarrhea).

27. D. Inform the child that you are going to help him, then administer abdominal thrusts until the object is expelled or the child becomes unresponsive. A blind finger sweep should not be performed in an infant or child, and is never appropriate in a responsive choking victim. A blind finger sweep may push the foreign body into the airway, causing further obstruction. Back slaps and chest thrusts are appropriate maneuvers to relieve foreign body airway obstruction in infants, not children. Although direct laryngoscopy may ultimately be necessary, it is not performed before attempting less invasive methods of relieving the obstruction.

28. C. An adult bag-mask used with supplemental oxygen set at a flow rate of 15 L/min (but with no reservoir) will deliver approximately 40% to 60% oxygen to the patient.

29. B. In stable patients with SVT, adenosine is the drug of choice because of its rapid onset of action and minimal effects on cardiac contractility.

30. C. Administer a bolus of 20 mL/kg of isotonic crystalloid solution (NS or LR) over 5 to 20 minutes. 44 pounds = 20 kilograms. For this child, the appropriate initial fluid bolus is 400 mL of normal saline or Ringer's lactate.

31. A. Cricoid pressure (also called the Sellick maneuver) may be considered to minimize gastric inflation in an unresponsive patient but may require a third rescuer if cricoid pressure cannot be applied by the rescuer who is securing the mask (of a bag-mask device) to the face.

32. B. Bradycardia in the newborn is usually secondary to inadequate lung inflation and hypoxia, so ensuring adequate oxygenation and ventilation are essential steps in correcting a low heart rate. However, epinephrine administration or volume expansion, or both, may be necessary if the heart rate remains slower than 60 beats per minute despite adequate ventilation with 100% oxygen and chest compressions.

33. B. This child's presentation is most consistent with respiratory failure. The presence of tachypnea and tachycardia reflects compensatory mechanisms that are attempting to increase cardiac output. However, these mechanisms will fail (signifying the onset of cardiopulmonary failure) as oxygen demand increases and the child tires. Aggressive treatment is essential.

34. D. When a patient demonstrates signs of respiratory failure or respiratory arrest, assist ventilation using a bag-mask device with supplemental oxygen.

35. C. Epinephrine has been used for many years to treat croup. The alpha-adrenergic effect of epinephrine is beneficial by reducing mucosal edema. Smooth muscle relaxation due to beta-adrenergic effects may benefit those children with croup who are also wheezing. After nebulized therapy (using racemic or levo-epinephrine), these effects are noted within 10 to 30 minutes and last for about one hour. Epinephrine use is typically reserved for patients who have moderate to severe respiratory distress because of the potential for adverse effects including agitation, tachycardia, and hypertension.

36. A. Systemic steroids (such as dexamethasone) are often used for mild to severe croup because of their anti-inflammatory effects and can be administered by way of nebulization and oral or intravenous routes. Generally, sedatives should not be used in the child with croup because (a) they can depress the respiratory drive and (b) restlessness is used as one means of evaluating the severity of airway obstruction and the need for intubation. Opiates should not be used because they may depress ventilations and dry secretions.

37. A. The patient's exhaled CO_2 values should correlate with his vital signs and assessment findings. Exhaled CO_2 can be measured using a disposable colorimetric device or a capnometer. Exhaled CO_2 monitoring is recommended as confirmation of tracheal tube position for patients of all ages with a perfusing cardiac rhythm; however, it should not be used as the *only* means of assessing tracheal tube placement. A pulse oximeter provides information about oxygenation. It does not reflect the adequacy of ventilation. Capnography provides information about ventilation but does not reflect the adequacy of oxygenation. Exhaled CO_2 monitoring should be routinely used to monitor tracheal tube position during the transport of an intubated patient of any age.

38. C. The presence of compensated shock can be identified by evaluation of heart rate, the presence and volume (strength) of peripheral pulses, and the adequacy of end-organ perfusion (Brain – assess mental status, skin – assess capillary refill, skin temperature, and kidneys – assess urine output).

39. Pediatric Assessment Triangle (general impression) findings:
    Appearance: barely responsive, incontinent of urine, unaware of your presence
    Breathing: increased work of breathing evident
    Circulation: skin is flushed; no evidence of bleeding

40. B. The presence of secretions draining from the mouth of a child that is unaware of your presence requires **immediate** intervention. Clear the airway with suctioning.

41. "Normal" values for a 3-year-old child:
    A) Weight: 14 kg (31 lb.)
    B) Ventilatory rate: 24 to 40
    C) Heart rate: 90 to 150
    D) Blood pressure: BP 70 mm Hg or higher

42. B. The patient's Glasgow Coma Scale score is 8.
    Eyes: To pain   2
    Verbal: Incomprehensible sounds   2
    Motor: Withdraws from pain   4

43. This patient's physical findings are most consistent with the cholinergic toxidrome.

44. A. The patient's physical findings and additional information regarding the events surrounding the exposure strongly suggests organophosphate exposure.

45. D. Atropine is the antidote for the muscarinic effects of organophosphate exposure. The goal of atropine administration in this situation is drying of airway secretions to maintain oxygenation and ventilation. Tachycardia is NOT a contraindication to its use.

46. D. Heart rate in the newborn may be evaluated by listening to the apical beat with a stethoscope or feeling the pulse by lightly grasping the base of the umbilical cord. It is estimated that about 10% of newborns require some assistance to begin breathing at birth. The recommended compression to ventilation ratio is 3:1. Most newborns who require cardiac compressions are asphyxiated. Consider using a compression to ventilation ratio of 15:2 if the arrest is believed to be of cardiac origin.

47. D. Dopamine, epinephrine, and dobutamine are medications used to maintain cardiac output. Midazolam (Versed), lorazepam (Ativan), and diazepam (Valium) are benzodiazepines used for sedation. Naloxone (Narcan) is an opioid (narcotic) antagonist.

48. B. In a perfusing patient, oxygen saturation should be monitored and oxygen administered, if necessary, to maintain a saturation of 94% or higher.

49. C. Amiodarone may cause hypotension, bradycardia, and prolongation of the QT interval. Amiodarone should be administered IV push during cardiac arrest and over 20 to 60 minutes in a patient with a perfusing rhythm. Amiodarone should not be administered with procainamide without first seeking expert consultation because each drug may cause QT prolongation.

50. B. Synchronized cardioversion may be warranted in an unstable patient with supraventricular tachycardia due to reentry, atrial fibrillation, atrial flutter, atrial tachycardia, or monomorphic ventricular tachycardia with a pulse.

References

1. Kleinman ME, Chameides L, Schexnayder SM, et al. Part 14: Pediatric advanced life support: 2010 American Heart Association Guidelines for Cardiopulmonary Resuscitation and Emergency Cardiovascular Care. *Circulation.* 2010;122(suppl 3):S876 –S908.

Chain of Survival and Emergency Medical Services for Children

1

Case Study

A 3-year-old is found floating face down in the family pool. The child's distraught mother says she last saw the child about 15 minutes ago. Mom removed the child from the pool and then called 9-1-1. She is performing cardiopulmonary resuscitation (CPR) per the emergency medical services (EMS) dispatcher's instructions via the telephone. Police officers are the first to arrive on the scene. They begin CPR after confirming that the child is unresponsive, apneic, and pulseless.

What prevention measures could have been implemented to prevent this tragic situation?

Objectives

1. Identify the links in the Pediatric Chain of Survival.
2. Explain the purpose of the emergency medical services for children (EMSC) program.
3. Define the terms *primary prevention*, *secondary prevention*, and *tertiary prevention* as they relate to injury prevention.

Pediatric Chain of Survival

In adults, sudden nontraumatic cardiopulmonary arrests are usually the result of underlying cardiac disease. In children, causes of nontraumatic cardiopulmonary arrest include bronchospasm, congenital cardiac abnormalities, dysrhythmias, foreign body aspiration, gastroenteritis, seizures, sepsis, drowning, sudden infant death syndrome (SIDS), and upper and lower respiratory tract infection, among other causes.

The importance of prevention is reflected in the links of the Pediatric Chain of Survival.

The Pediatric Chain of Survival represents a sequential series of events to assess, support, or restore effective ventilation and circulation to the infant or child experiencing a respiratory or cardiorespiratory arrest. The sequence consists of five important steps:

- Prevention of illness and injury
- Early CPR
- Early EMS activation
- Rapid Advanced Life Support (ALS)
- Integration of post-cardiac arrest care

Note that activating EMS is delayed until after a trial of early CPR. This is based on the higher likelihood of respiratory conditions and lower likelihood of ventricular fibrillation as the cause of cardiopulmonary arrest in the pediatric patient.

It is estimated that about 6% of the children who experience an out-of-hospital cardiac arrest and 8% of those who receive prehospital resuscitation survive.[1] Survival rates can be improved with prompt bystander CPR.

The Role of Emergency Care Professionals in Caring for the Ill or Injured Child

Emergency care of children and families requires specific knowledge, equipment, skills, and resources. A child's physiologic response to a critical illness or injury differs from an adult's for such conditions as shock and prolonged respiratory distress. The etiologies of catastrophic events, such as cardiopulmonary arrest, are different from those in adults. In children, the signs and symptoms of distress may be subtle.

The impact of an injured or acutely ill child is devastating not only for the child, but also for the child's family and the emergency care provider. When treating the child, we must remember to treat the family. Psychological and emotional management of the family is important at this critical time.

Emergency Medical Services for Children

History and Legislation

Early EMS systems (mid to late 1960s and early 1970s) focused on providing rapid intervention for sudden cardiac arrest in adults and rapid transport for motor vehicle crash victims. Because these systems focused on adult care, outcomes for adults in emergencies improved dramatically, whereas the specialized needs of children experiencing a medical emergency went largely unrecognized. As a result, the equipment, training, experience, and expertise of prehospital personnel were often less developed to meet the needs of children.

In the mid-1970s, this weakness in the EMS system began to be recognized. Healthcare professionals including pediatric surgeons, pediatricians, emergency physicians, and other concerned groups worked to ensure that the special needs of children were integrated into the EMS system. Their efforts remained unfunded until Congress enacted legislation in 1984 (Public Law 98-555) authorizing the use of federal funds for EMSC.

EMSC efforts have improved the availability of child-size equipment in ambulances and emergency departments (EDs). EMSC has initiated hundreds of programs to prevent injuries and has provided thousands of hours of training to emergency medicine technicians (EMTs), paramedics, and other emergency medical care providers.

Purpose

The federal EMSC program defines the population of children to include those from birth to 21 years of age.

The EMSC program is designed to reduce child and youth mortality and morbidity sustained due to severe illness or trauma. It aims to:

- Ensure state-of-the-art emergency medical care for the ill or injured child and adolescent
- Ensure that pediatric service is well integrated into an EMS system backed by optimal resources
- Ensure that the entire spectrum of emergency services, including primary prevention of illness and injury, acute care, and rehabilitation, is provided to children, adolescents, and adults.

Scope

The EMSC program is responsible for a broad spectrum of services including prevention, early recognition of problems, initial stabilization of infants and children, and rehabilitative care.

EMSC encompasses seven phases of child and family services:

1. Prevention
2. System access
3. Field treatment (prehospital response)
4. Transport
5. Emergency department (ED) (stabilization) care

6. Inpatient services (definitive care)
7. Rehabilitation (physical therapy, occupational therapy, social services)

Prevention Programs

Pediatric injuries are a major public health concern. Toddlers are at greatest risk for burns, drowning, falls, and poisonings. Young school-aged children are at risk for pedestrian injuries, bicycle-related injuries, motor vehicle occupant injuries, burns, and drowning. Teenagers are at risk for motor vehicle occupant trauma, drowning, burns, and intentional trauma.

Two criteria by which the significance of childhood injuries can be measured are death and **morbidity**. Although death is the worst possible outcome, injuries cause widespread morbidity, which results in the need for medical care and an inability to perform normal daily activities.

The type, number, and severity of pediatric injuries in a given area depend partly on regional characteristics.

- Geography (type of terrain, average response times for emergency care)
- Climate and weather conditions (temperature extremes, violent storms)
- Population density (crime rates, 9-1-1 coverage, availability of medical services)
- Population traits (ethnic backgrounds, education levels)
- Age also influences injury rates and patterns

Successful injury prevention requires an approach that incorporates the "Four E's": education, enforcement, environmental modification, and engineering.

- Education attempts to bring about positive behavioral changes by informing various groups about the existence of hazards and explaining ways to reduce or prevent the injuries these hazards may cause.
- Enforcement attempts to reduce dangerous behaviors through legislation that requires individuals, manufacturers, and local governments to comply with certain safety practices. Examples include mandatory seat belt and helmet laws, handgun control, zoning codes that require fences around private swimming pools, and safety regulations governing the manufacture of children's toys.
- Environmental modifications target social issues and physical features within a community that contribute to injury patterns. Examples include providing free smoke detectors or bike helmets to low-income families.
- Engineering involves technological changes that make products or the environment safer. Examples include childproof caps for medications and household solvents.

Epidemiology of Pediatric Illness and Injury

Use of the term *accident*, which implies an unpredictable or unavoidable event, is being replaced with the term *injury* to more accurately reflect the nature of the problem.

Unintentional injuries are the leading killer of children ages 14 and under.

Understanding Injury Prevention

Enforcement is viewed by some as interference with individual rights, which may result in resistance to new legislation.

The most effective prevention strategies combine methods from multiple categories from the "Four E's." For example, a legislative change might combine environmental modification, enforcement, and education strategies to increase public acceptance.

Pediatric Equipment

When caring for the pediatric patient, treatment interventions are usually based on the weight of the child. As a result, a range of age-appropriate and size-appropriate equipment (including bags and masks, tracheal tubes, and intravenous catheters) must be readily available for use in pediatric emergencies. The equipment and supplies must be logically organized, routinely checked, and readily available.

Studies have documented unreliability at estimating children's weights, a high rate of errors made when performing drug calculations, and a loss of valuable resuscitation time secondary to computing drug dosages and selecting equipment.

Length-based resuscitation tapes (Figure 1-1) are one example of a system that may be used to estimate weight by length and simplify selection of the medications and supplies needed during the emergency care of children. In the example shown, the tape assigns children to a color zone on the basis of their length. Appropriate resuscitation medication doses and equipment sizes are listed on the tape, as well as abnormal vital signs, fluid calculations, and energy levels recommended for defibrillation. If the child is taller than the tape, standard adult equipment and medication dosages are used.

Treatment Protocols and Practice Guidelines

Treatment protocols and procedures specific to the pediatric patient are essential and should be developed to guide and maintain consistency in the delivery of emergency care. As protocols are developed, prevention, access, prehospital care, ED care, inpatient services, and rehabilitation must be considered.

Prehospital

Prehospital management of the pediatric patient necessitates the development and implementation of protocols for pediatric triage, transport, and treatment. Medical direction guidelines for the management of pediatric patients should exist for basic life support (BLS) and ALS prehospital providers. These guidelines may exist in off-line protocols or online

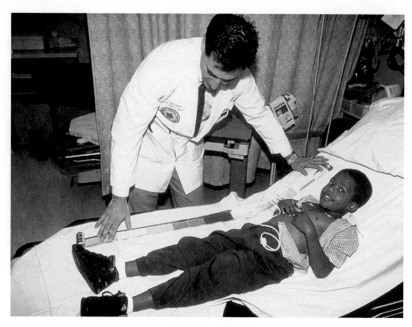

Figure 1-1 A length-based resuscitation tape is used to quickly estimate a child's height and determine equipment needs and medication doses.

medical direction.

Appropriate prehospital triage of the pediatric patient requires knowledge of community levels of pediatric care, available transport methods, and skill in pediatric assessment. Pediatric triage protocols should include hospital bypass criteria. The National Association of EMS Physicians has developed pediatric field treatment protocols for prehospital professionals. These protocols are available online at www.naemsp.org.

Because caregivers often take an ill or injured child directly to the ED, it is essential that EDs and hospitals provide treatment that conforms to the recognized level of care with appropriate equipment, trained personnel, patient care guidelines, and an organized system of care response.

Emergency Departments

Minimum voluntary requirements endorsed by the American College of Emergency Physicians (ACEP), the American Academy of Pediatrics, and a task force sponsored by the federal EMSC program have been published. These guidelines outline necessary resources for pediatric emergency care in all EDs, and address stabilization and transfer of selected patients to specialized pediatric centers (e.g., pediatric trauma centers, pediatric critical care centers).

When a child requires specialized care, agreements should exist between hospitals to facilitate transfer of the child and ensure a smooth and rapid transition. Children who experience a major complication or disability because of their illness or injury should be linked to rehabilitation services as early as possible.

Primary Care Providers

Children should have a designated primary care provider for preventive health services and management of healthcare conditions before they become emergencies. These primary care providers should be prepared to manage potential emergencies in their office setting until prehospital professionals are able to respond.

Identifying the Ill or Injured Child

Public Information and Education

Parents and other guardians, such as childcare providers, day care workers, and babysitters need to know how to do the following:

- Distinguish emergent and nonemergent events
- Perform emergency first aid procedures
- Contact the child's physician
- Access the emergency care system
- Authorize emergency care and provide essential information to emergency care professionals

Emergency Care Professionals

Emergency care professionals:

- Must be trained and competent in the care of pediatric patients. Support personnel from respiratory therapy, radiology, laboratory, and other departments should be oriented to the care of the pediatric patient.
- Must be able to recognize the signs that indicate a child's condition is becoming potentially life-threatening. This requires understanding that there are differences in anatomic and physiologic characteristics, as well as cognitive, emotional, and psychosocial responses, in pediatric age groups.

Essential knowledge for emergency care professionals includes growth and development, pediatric triage and acuity level identification, pediatric assessment and intervention techniques, common pediatric disease and injury processes, and prevention strategies as they relate to the infant, child, and adolescent.[2]

Children account for a small percentage of the total patients treated by emergency care professionals. Therefore, there are frequently insufficient opportunities to use pediatric assessment and life-saving skills. Because skill decay is rapid, frequent practice sessions and refresher training are extremely important to maintaining preparedness.

Case Study Resolution

Primary prevention measures applicable in this situation include the use of a pool fence and a self-latching and locking gate surrounding the entire pool area, and ensuring that the caregivers know how to swim. Parents, other relatives, and neighbors should be taught CPR. These individuals should also be taught that **constant** supervision of children is necessary, particularly around water.

As a healthcare professional, you play a vital role in the Chain of Survival. By working together, we can increase the pediatric patient's chance of survival.

Web Resources

- *www.aap.org* (American Academy of Pediatrics)
- *http://bolivia.hrsa.gov/emsc/* (Emergency Medical Services for Children)
- *www.naemsp.org* (National Association of EMS Physicians)

References

1. Berg MD, Schexnayder SM, Chameiders L, et al. Part 13: Pediatric basic life support: 2010 American Heart Association Guidelines for Cardiopulmonary Resuscitation and Emergency Cardiovascular Care. Circulation. 2010; 122 (suppl 3) S862–S875.
2. Emergency Nurses Association. ENPC provider manual. Park Ridge, IL: Emergency Nurses Association, 1998.

Chapter Quiz

1. The efforts of the _____ _____ _____ _____
   _____ program have improved the availability of child-size equipment in ambulances and
   emergency departments, initiated hundreds of programs to prevent injuries, and provided thousands of
   hours of training to emergency medical care providers.

2. True or False: The upper age limit of a child, as defined by the federal EMSC program, is 14 years of age.

3. List the seven phases of child and family services encompassed by the EMSC program:
   1. _____
   2. _____
   3. _____
   4. _____
   5. _____
   6. _____
   7. _____

4. Which of the following correctly reflects the sequential steps in the pediatric Chain of Survival?
   A) Early EMS activation, early ALS, prevention of illness or injury, early CPR, post-cardiac arrest care
   B) Early CPR, prevention of illness or injury, early ALS, early EMS activation
   C) Early ALS, early EMS activation, early CPR, prevention of illness or injury
   D) Prevention of illness or injury, early CPR, early EMS activation, early ALS, post-cardiac arrest care

5. _____ prevention involves measures that can be applied in advance to reduce the
   likelihood that an injury will occur. _____ prevention includes interventions that will help
   prevent or minimize an injury while it happens. _____ prevention includes measures to
   lessen the severity of an injury and improve the patient's outcome *after* the injury has occurred.

6. List the "Four E's" required for successful injury prevention:
   1. _____
   2. _____
   3. _____
   4. _____

Chapter Quiz Answers

1. The efforts of the *Emergency Medical Services for Children* (EMSC) program have improved the availability of child-size equipment in ambulances and emergency departments, initiated hundreds of programs to prevent injuries, and provided thousands of hours of training to emergency medical care providers.

2. False. The federal EMSC program defines the population of children to include those from birth to 21 years of age.

3. The seven phases of child and family services encompassed by the EMSC program are:
    * Prevention
    * System access
    * Field treatment (prehospital response)
    * Transport
    * Emergency department (stabilization) care
    * Inpatient services (definitive care)
    * Rehabilitation (physical therapy, occupational therapy, social services)

4. D. The pediatric Chain of Survival represents a sequential series of events to assess, support, or restore effective ventilation and circulation to the child experiencing a respiratory or cardiorespiratory arrest. The sequence consists of five important steps: 1) Prevention of illness or injury, 2) Early CPR, 3) Early EMS activation, 4) Early ALS, and 5) Integration of post-cardiac arrest care.

5. *Primary* prevention involves measures that can be applied in advance to reduce the likelihood that an injury will occur. *Secondary* prevention includes interventions that will help prevent or minimize an injury while it happens. *Tertiary* prevention includes measures to lessen the severity of an injury and improve the patient's outcome *after* the injury has occurred.

6. Successful injury prevention requires an approach that incorporates the "Four E's": Education, Enforcement, Environmental modification, and Engineering.

Patient Assessment

2

Case Study

Your patient is a 4-year-old boy with a fever. The boy clings to his father as Dad explains that the child has been sick with a fever for the past 2 days and has been crying frequently.

Using the Pediatric Assessment Triangle (PAT), your general impression of the child is that he is awake and aware of your presence. His ventilatory rate is within normal limits for his age with no evidence of increased breathing effort. Chest expansion appears symmetric. His nose is running and his skin appears flushed.

Based on the information provided, is this child "sick" or "not sick"? How should you proceed?

Objectives

1. Discuss the components of a pediatric assessment.
2. Describe techniques for successful assessment of infants and children.
3. Identify key anatomic and physiologic characteristics of infants and children and their implications.
4. Identify normal age group–related vital signs.
5. Discuss the appropriate equipment used to obtain pediatric vital signs.
6. Identify the components of pediatric triage.

Initial Evaluation of the Acutely Ill or Injured Child

Scene Survey

- Hazards
  - Note any hazards or potential hazards and any visible mechanism or injury or illness.
  - Presence of pills, medicine bottles, or household chemicals may indicate a possible toxic ingestion.
  - Injury and history that does not coincide with the mechanism of injury may indicate child abuse.
- Relationships/interaction
  - Observe the interaction between the caregiver and the child and determine the appropriateness of their interaction. Does the interaction demonstrate concern, or is it angry or indifferent?

- Other important assessments that can be made during the scene survey include the following:
  ○ Orderliness, cleanliness, and safety of the home.
  ○ General appearance of other children in the family.
  ○ Presence of any medical devices used for the child (e.g., ventilator).
  ○ Indications of parental substance abuse. Parental substance abuse is associated with a more than twofold increase in the risk of exposure to childhood physical and sexual abuse.[1]
- Determine if additional resources are necessary including law enforcement, fire equipment, extrication equipment, special rescue services, additional medical personnel, or special transport services (aeromedical transport).

Pediatric Assessment: Components

The steps used to perform a pediatric assessment are described here as a linear process for clarity. In practice, some steps may be performed simultaneously, particularly if additional healthcare professionals are available to assist.

- Initial assessment
  - Pediatric Assessment triangle (PAT) (general impression)
  - Primary survey (ABCDE assessment)
  - Secondary survey
    ○ Vital signs
    ○ Focused history
    ○ Detailed physical examination
- Reassessment

Pediatric Assessment Triangle

Initial Assessment

- General impression/"across-the-room" assessment (Figure 2-1)
  - Because approaching an ill or injured child can increase agitation, possibly worsening the child's condition, the PAT is performed **before** approaching or touching the child.
- Pause a short distance from the patient and, using your senses of sight and hearing (look and listen), quickly determine if a life-threatening problem exists that requires immediate intervention.
- Can be completed in 60 seconds or less.
- No equipment (cardiac monitor, blood pressure cuff, stethoscope) required. The PAT and primary survey are used to quickly determine if a child is "sick" or "not sick." Remember that your patient's condition can change at any time. A patient that initially appears "not sick" may rapidly deteriorate and appear "sick." Reassess frequently.
- Establishes severity of illness or injury [sick (unstable) or not sick (stable)]

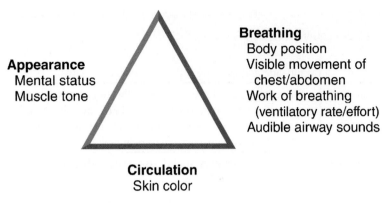

Figure 2-1   Pediatric Assessment Triangle.

- Identifies general category of physiologic abnormality (e.g., cardio-pulmonary, neurologic, metabolic, toxicologic, trauma)
- Determines urgency of further assessment and intervention

Appearance

- Reflects the adequacy of oxygenation, ventilation, brain perfusion, homeostasis, and central nervous system function
- Assessment areas
  - **T**one (muscle tone)
  - **I**nteractivity/mental status
    - Level of responsiveness
    - Interaction with caregiver
    - Response to you or other healthcare professionals
  - **C**onsolability
  - **L**ook or gaze
  - **S**peech or cry
- Normal findings: normal muscle tone, child responds to name (if older than 6 to 8 months of age), equal movement of all extremities, eyes open, normal speech or cry.
- Abnormal findings:
  - Agitation, marked irritability, reduced responsiveness, drooling (beyond infancy), limp or rigid muscle tone, inconsolable crying, failure to recognize caregiver, paradoxical irritability (irritable when held and lethargic when left alone; may be seen in infants and small children with neurologic infections).
  - If the child exhibits abnormal findings, proceed immediately to the primary survey.

(Work of) Breathing

- Reflects the adequacy of airway, oxygenation, and ventilation (Table 2-1).
- Assessment areas:

TICLS (pronounced tickles) is a mnemonic used to recall the areas to be assessed related to the child's appearance.

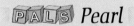 *Pearl*

The TICLS Assessment Tool

Tone: Is the child moving vigorously, or is the child limp, listless, or flaccid?
Interactivity: Is the child alert and attentive to his or her surroundings, or uninterested/apathetic?
Consolability: Can the child be comforted by the caregiver or healthcare professional?
Look/Gaze: Do the child's eyes follow your movement, or is there a vacant stare?
Speech/cry: Is the child's speech or cry strong, or is it weak or hoarse?

From the American Academy of Pediatrics. *Textbook of pediatric education for prehospital professionals.* Sudbury, MA: Jones & Bartlett, 2000.

TABLE 2-1 *Abnormal Airway Sounds*

Gasping	Inhaling and exhaling with quick, difficult breaths
Grunting	Short, low-pitched sound heard at the end of exhalation that represents an attempt to generate positive end-expiratory pressure (PEEP) by exhaling against a closed glottis, prolonging the period of oxygen and carbon dioxide exchange across the alveolar-capillary membrane; a compensatory mechanism to help maintain patency of small airways and prevent atelectasis
Gurgling	Abnormal respiratory sound associated with collection of liquid or semi-solid material in the patient's upper airway
Snoring	Noisy breathing through the mouth and nose during sleep, caused by air passing through a narrowed upper airway
Stridor	Harsh, high-pitched sound heard on inspiration associated with upper airway obstruction; frequently described as a high-pitched crowing or "seal-bark" sound
Wheezing	High-pitched "whistling" sounds produced by air moving through narrowed airway passages

- Body position
- Visible movement (chest/abdomen)
- Ventilatory rate
- Ventilatory effort
- Audible airway sounds
- Normal findings: quiet, nonlabored breathing; equal chest rise and fall; ventilatory rate within normal range.
- Abnormal findings:
  - Abnormal body position (e.g., **sniffing position**, **tripod position**, **head bobbing**), **nasal flaring**, retractions, muffled or hoarse speech, **stridor**, **grunting**, **gasping**, **gurgling**, **wheezing**, ventilatory rate outside normal range, accessory muscle use.
  - If the child exhibits abnormal findings, proceed immediately to the primary survey.

Circulation

- Reflects the adequacy of cardiac output and perfusion of vital organs (i.e., core perfusion)
- Assessment areas: skin color.
- Normal findings: color appears normal for child's ethnic group.
- Abnormal findings:
  - Pallor, mottling, cyanosis.
  - If the child exhibits abnormal findings, proceed immediately to the primary survey.

On the basis of your general impression, decide if the child is sick (unstable) or not sick (stable).

- If the child's condition is urgent, proceed immediately with rapid assess-

---

PALS *Pearl*

- In a sniffing position, the child sits upright and leans forward with the chin slightly raised. In this position, the axes of the mouth, pharynx, and trachea are aligned and open the airway, increasing airflow.
- In a tripod position, the child sits upright and leans forward, supported by his or her arms, with the neck slightly extended, chin projected, and mouth open. This position is used to maintain airway patency.
- Head bobbing is an indicator of increased work of breathing in infants. The head falls forward with exhalation and comes up with expansion of the chest on inhalation.

ment of airway, breathing, and circulation. If a problem is identified, perform necessary interventions: "Treat as you find."

- If the child's condition is not urgent, proceed systematically:
  - Primary survey
  - Secondary survey
    ◦ Vital signs
    ◦ Focused history
    ◦ Physical examination
  - Reassessment

Primary Survey

The ABCDE sequence of the primary survey is taught to physicians, nurses, and prehospital personnel in many types of educational courses. In programs other than cardiac-related courses, the primary survey sequence stands for Airway, Breathing, Circulation, Disability (referring to a brief neurological exam), and Exposure/environment. In cardiac-related courses, the "D" stands for Defibrillation (if necessary).

The primary survey is also called the ABCDE assessment. During the primary survey, assessment and management occur simultaneously. The primary survey should be periodically repeated, particularly after any major intervention or when a change in the patient's condition is detected.

The primary survey focuses on basic life support (BLS) patient assessment and management. It usually requires less than 60 seconds to complete but may take longer if intervention is needed at any point.

- Systematic hands-on assessment.
- Purpose: determine if life-threatening conditions exist.
- Components: ABCDE
  - *A*irway, level of responsiveness, and cervical spine protection
  - *B*reathing (ventilation)
  - *C*irculation (perfusion)
  - *D*isability (mini-neurlogic exam)
  - *E*xpose/environment

Airway

The responsive child may have assumed a position to maximize his or her ability to maintain an open airway. Allow the child to maintain this position as you continue your assessment.

- Assessment
  - Goals:
    ◦ Open airway/absence of signs or symptoms of airway obstruction (e.g., stridor, dyspnea, hoarse voice)
    ◦ Able to handle oral secretions independently
    ◦ Patient speaks or makes appropriate sounds for age
  - Determine if the airway is open, maintainable, or unmaintainable:
    ◦ Open: able to be maintained independently
    ◦ Maintainable with positioning, suctioning
    ◦ Unmaintainable, requires assistance (e.g., tracheal intubation, cricothyrotomy, foreign body removal)
  - At this stage of your patient assessment, simultaneously establish the patient's mental status and his ability to maintain an open airway. Determine level of responsiveness using AVPU:
    ◦ A=*A*lert
    ◦ V=Responds to *v*erbal stimuli

- ○ P=Responds to *p*ainful stimuli
- ○ U=*U*nresponsive
- If cervical spine injury is suspected (by examination, history, or mechanism of injury), ask an assistant to manually stabilize the head and neck in a neutral, in-line position or maintain spinal stabilization if already completed.
- If the child is responsive and the airway is open (patent), move on to evaluation of the patient's breathing. If the child is responsive but cannot talk, cry, or cough forcefully, evaluate for possible airway obstruction.
- If the child is unresponsive, quickly check to see if he is breathing. If normal breathing is present, continue the primary survey. If the child is not breathing (or only gasping), check for a pulse for up to 10 seconds. If there is no pulse or you are unsure if there is a pulse, begin chest compressions (see Chapter 6).
- If the child is unresponsive and a pulse is present, use manual maneuvers such as a head tilt-chin lift or jaw thrust without head tilt to open the airway (see Chapter 4). If trauma is suspected, use the jaw-thrust without head tilt to open the airway. If the airway is not patent (clear of debris and obstruction), assess for sounds of airway compromise (snoring, gurgling, or stridor). Gurgling is an indication for immediate suctioning. Look in the mouth for blood, broken teeth, gastric contents, and foreign objects (e.g., loose teeth, gum, small toys). If present, position the patient to facilitate drainage and suction the mouth. If solid material is visualized, remove it with a gloved finger covered in gauze. If a foreign body obstruction is suspected but not visualized, clear the obstruction by performing abdominal thrusts (if the patient is 1 year of age or older) or chest thrusts (if the patient is younger than 1 year of age).
- Signs of distress may include the following:
  - ○ Preferred posture (e.g., tripod position, holding head to maintain an open airway)
  - ○ Drooling
  - ○ Difficulty swallowing
  - ○ Swelling of the lips and/or tissues of the mouth
  - ○ Inadequate air movement
  - ○ Obstruction by the tongue, blood, vomitus, foreign body
  - ○ Abnormal airway sounds
- Interventions
  - Spinal stabilization as needed for trauma
  - Jaw thrust without head tilt

The head tilt-chin lift should *not* be used to open the airway if trauma is suspected.

The assessment sequence described here assumes the patient is responsive or that a pulse is present if he is unresponsive. If a patient is unresponsive and not breathing (or only gasping), current cardiopulmonary resuscitation guidelines recommend a change in assessment sequence to Circulation-Airway-Breathing (C-A-B).

In the responsive patient (and in an unresponsive patient with a pulse), look, listen, feel: inspect, auscultate, palpate. In these patient situations, evaluation of breathing during the primary survey should take no more than 10 seconds.

- Head tilt-chin lift
- Suction
- Reposition
- Removal of foreign body
- Airway adjuncts (see Chapter 4)

Breathing

- Assessment
  - Goals:
    - Adequate gas exchange with no signs of hypoxia
      - Awake and alert
      - Maintain oxygen saturation of at least 94%
      - Skin color normal; warm and dry
      - Breathing is spontaneous, unlabored, and at a normal rate for age
      - Chest expansion is equal bilaterally
      - Breath sounds are present, clear, and equal bilaterally
    - Absence of dyspnea, stridor, and signs of increased work of breathing (e.g., retractions, grunting, tracheal tugging, accessory muscle use, nasal flaring, head bobbing).
- Confirm that the child *is* breathing and note significant abnormalities in the work of breathing. If the patient is breathing, determine if breathing is adequate or inadequate. If breathing is adequate, move on to assessment of circulation.
- **Look**
  - Assess the chest and abdomen for ventilatory movement. Evaluate the depth (tidal volume) and symmetry of movement with each breath.
    - **Tidal volume** is the volume of air moved into or out of the lungs during a normal breath. Tidal volume can be indirectly evaluated by observing the rise and fall of the patient's chest and abdomen.
    - **Minute volume** is the amount of air moved in and out of the lungs in one minute and is determined by multiplying the tidal volume by the ventilatory rate. Thus, a change in either the tidal volume *or* ventilatory rate will affect minute volume.
  - Determine the ventilatory rate.
    - The patient with breathing difficulty often has a ventilatory rate outside the normal limits for his or her age (Table 2-2). Count the ventilatory rate for 30 seconds and then double this figure to find the rate per minute.

TABLE 2-2 *Normal Ventilatory Rates by Age*

Age	Breaths/Min (At Rest)
Infant (1 to 12 mo)	30 to 60
Toddler (1 to 3 y)	24 to 40
Preschooler (4 to 5 y)	22 to 34
School-age (6 to 12 y)	18 to 30
Adolescent (13 to 18 y)	12 to 16

Respiratory distress is increased work of breathing (ventilatory effort). **Respiratory failure** is a clinical condition in which there is inadequate blood oxygenation and/or ventilation to meet the metabolic demands of body tissues.

- **Tachypnea** is a rapid rate of breathing. It may be an abnormal finding because of a disease process or a compensatory response (and outside the normal resting ventilatory rate ranges) secondary to excitement, anxiety, fever, and pain, among other causes. In the newly born, exposure to cold can increase the respiratory rate and may cause ventilatory distress.
  - At any age, a ventilatory rate greater than 60 per minute is abnormal.
  - As fatigue begins and hypoxia worsens, the child progresses to respiratory failure with slowing (and possible cessation) of the ventilatory rate.
- **Bradypnea** (abnormally slow rate of breathing) is an ominous sign in an acutely ill infant or child and may be caused by fatigue, hypothermia, or central nervous system depression, among other causes.
- Assess for the presence of respiratory distress/failure (Table 2-3). If respiratory distress is observed, *potential* ventilatory failure is present.
  - Note signs of increased work of breathing (ventilatory effort).
    - Anxious appearance, concentration on breathing
    - Use of accessory muscles: muscles of the neck, chest, and abdomen that become active during labored breathing
    - Leaning forward to inhale
    - Nasal flaring: widening of the nostrils on inhalation; an attempt to increase the size of the airway and increase the amount of available oxygen (Figure 2-2)
    - Retractions: sinking in of the soft tissues above the sternum (suprasternal) or clavicle (supraclavicular), or between (intercostal) or below (subcostal) the ribs during inhalation (Figures 2-3 and 2-4)

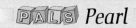 *Pearl*

Ventilations in infants and children younger than 6 or 7 years are primarily abdominal (diaphragmatic) because the intercostal muscles of the chest wall are not well developed and fatigue easily from the work of breathing. Effective ventilation may be jeopardized when diaphragmatic movement is compromised (e.g., gastric or abdominal distension) because the chest wall cannot compensate. As the child grows older, the chest muscles strengthen, and chest expansion becomes more noticeable.

The transition from abdominal (diaphragmatic) breathing to intercostal breathing begins between 2 and 4 years of age and is complete by 7 to 8 years of age.

TABLE 2-3 *Signs of Respiratory Distress and Respiratory Failure*

Respiratory Distress

- Nasal flaring
- Inspiratory retractions
- Increased breathing rate (tachypnea)
- Increased depth of breathing (hyperpnea)
- Head-bobbing
- Seesaw ventilations (abdominal breathing)
- Restlessness
- Tachycardia
- Grunting
- Stridor

Respiratory Failure

- Cyanosis
- Diminished breath sounds
- Decreased level of responsiveness or response to pain
- Poor skeletal muscle tone
- Inadequate ventilatory rate, effort, or chest excursion
- Tachycardia
- Use of accessory muscles of breathing

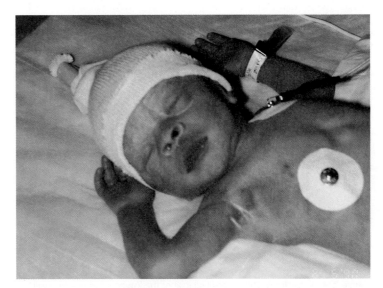

Figure 2-2 Nasal flaring. Widening of the nares may be seen in infants with respiratory distress.

- Indicate increased work of breathing
- In cases of severe obstruction, retractions may extend to the suprasternal notch and supraclavicular areas.
- Seesaw (chest/abdominal) movement
  - Increased ventilatory effort draws the chest in while thrusting the abdomen out
  - Indicator of severe respiratory distress
- Note the rhythm of breathing (regular, irregular, periodic)
  - Prolonged inspiration suggests an upper airway obstruction.
  - Prolonged expiration suggests a lower airway obstruction.

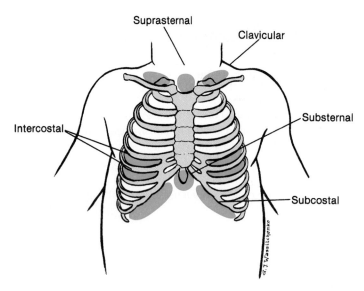

Figure 2-3 Location of retractions.

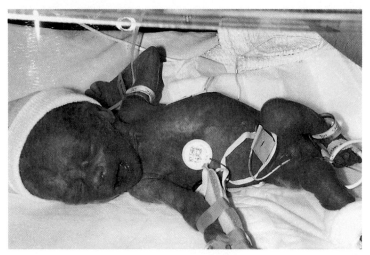

Figure 2-4 Retractions. The inward collapse of the lower anterior chest wall can be seen in this premature infant with respiratory distress syndrome.

- ○ **Listen**
  - ▪ Listen for air movement at the nose and mouth. Note if breathing is quiet, absent, or noisy (e.g., stridor, wheezing, snoring, crowing, gurgling). Wheezing may be heard through-out the lungs or, in the case of a foreign body obstruction, may be localized.
  - ▪ Listen for the presence and quality of bilateral breath sounds and briefly listen to heart sounds.
    - • Breath sounds are normally quiet. Because the chest of a child is small and the chest wall is thin, breath sounds are easily transmitted from one side of the chest to the other.

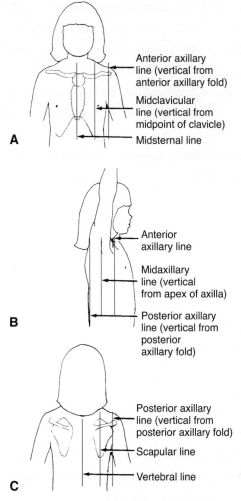

Anterior axillary line (vertical from anterior axillary fold)

Midclavicular line (vertical from midpoint of clavicle)

Midsternal line

A

Anterior axillary line

Midaxillary line (vertical from apex of axilla)

Posterior axillary line (vertical from posterior axillary fold)

B

Posterior axillary line (vertical from posterior axillary fold)

Scapular line

Vertebral line

C

Figure 2-5 Landmarks of the chest. **A,** Anterior. **B,** Right lateral. **C,** Posterior.

As a result, breath sounds may be heard despite the presence of a pneumothorax, hemothorax, or atelectasis. To minimize the possibility of sound transmission from one side of the chest to the other, listen along the midaxillary line (under each armpit) and in the midclavicular line under each clavicle (Figure 2-5). Alternate from side to side and compare your findings.

- Briefly listen to heart sounds to establish a baseline from which to compare (e.g., development of muffled heart sounds, a murmur, or rub).

- **Feel**
  ○ Feel for air movement from the nose or mouth against your chin, face, or palm. Palpate the chest for tenderness, instability, and crepitation.

The patient with inadequate breathing requires positive-pressure ventilation with supplemental oxygen.

- If the unresponsive patient is breathing adequately and there are no signs of trauma, place the patient in the recovery (lateral recumbent) position and administer supplemental oxygen if indicated.
- If breathing is difficult and the rate is too slow or too fast, provide supplemental oxygen and, if necessary, positive-pressure ventilation.
- If breathing is absent, insert an airway adjunct (if not previously done) and deliver two breaths with a pocket mask or bag-mask with supplemental oxygen. Give each breath over 1 second. Ensure that the patient's chest wall gently rises with each ventilation. Continue the primary survey.

- Interventions
  - Suction
  - Oxygen
  - Airway adjuncts
  - Positive-pressure ventilation

Circulation

- Goals
  - Adequate cardiovascular function and tissue perfusion
    - Awake and alert
    - Central and peripheral pulses are strong and regular
    - Heart rate and blood pressure are within normal range for age
    - Skin color normal; warm and dry
    - Capillary refill time is less than 2 seconds (assess in children younger than 6 years)
    - Adequate oral intake and hydration
    - Adequate urine output for age and weight
  - Effective circulating fluid volume
    - No evidence of external bleeding
    - Vital signs within normal limits for age
    - Moist mucous membranes
    - Urine output of 1 to 2 mL/kg/hr
    - Hemoglobin and hematocrit values within normal range
    - Normal skin turgor
  - Normal core body temperature
- Control of bleeding
  - Look for visible external hemorrhage. Control major bleeding, if present, by applying direct pressure over the bleeding site.
  - Consider possible areas of major internal hemorrhage.
    - Significant internal hemorrhage may occur in the chest, abdomen, pelvis, retroperitoneum, and femoral areas.

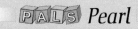
PALS *Pearl*

If the chest wall does not rise during positive-pressure ventilation, ventilation is inadequate or the airway is obstructed.

Assessment

PALS Pearl

The location for assessment of a central pulse varies according to the age of the child. In the newly born, assess the strength and quality of a central pulse by palpating the base of the umbilical cord between your thumb and index finger. In an infant, assess the brachial pulse. Assess the carotid or femoral pulse in any child over age one.

Assess a peripheral pulse while keeping one hand on the central pulse location. For example, if you are assessing a central pulse using the brachial artery, keep one hand on the brachial pulse and use your other hand to assess the peripheral (radial) pulse in the same extremity. Compare the strength and quality of the central and peripheral pulses. Although a peripheral pulse is not quite as strong as a central pulse, the rate and strength should be similar.

Hypotension often occurs well before the loss of central pulses.

Decreased skin perfusion is an early sign of shock.

TABLE 2-4 *Grading of Pulses*

Description	Grade
Full, bounding, not obliterated with pressure	+4
Normal—easily palpated, not easily obliterated with pressure	+3
Difficult to palpate, obliterated with pressure	+2
Weak, thready, difficult to palpate	+1
Absent pulse	0

- ◦ Pain or swelling in any of these areas may signal possible internal hemorrhage.
- Compare the strength and quality of central and peripheral pulses.
  - Palpation of pulses can be used to estimate heart rate, blood pressure, cardiac output, and systemic vascular resistance.
  - Pulse quality reflects the adequacy of peripheral perfusion (Table 2-4).
    - ◦ A weak central pulse may indicate decompensated shock.
    - ◦ A peripheral pulse that is difficult to find, weak, or irregular suggests poor peripheral perfusion and may be a sign of shock or hemorrhage.
  - Determine if the patient's heart rate is within normal limits for the child's age. Normal heart rates by age are listed in Table 2-5.
- Evaluate skin color, temperature, and moisture.
  - Skin color: pink, pale, cyanotic, mottled
    - ◦ Pink = normal perfusion
      - The hands and feet are normally warm, dry, and pink.
      - A newborn often has acrocyanosis (cyanotic hands and feet, while the rest of the body is pink) (Figure 2-6).
    - ◦ Pale
      - May be observed in respiratory failure.
      - Cool, pale extremities are associated with decreased cardiac output, as seen in shock and hypothermia.
    - ◦ Blue (cyanosis)
      - Suggests hypoxemia or inadequate perfusion.
      - In dark skin, cyanosis may observed as ashen gray lips and tongue.
    - ◦ Mottled: suggests decreased cardiac output, ischemia, hypoxia (Figure 2-7) but can be normal in an infant exposed to a cool environment.

TABLE 2-5 *Normal Heart Rates by Age*

Age	Beats/Min*
Infant (1 to 12 mo)	100 to 160
Toddler (1 to 3 y)	90 to 150
Preschooler (4 to 5 y)	80 to 140
School-age (6 to 12 y)	70 to 120
Adolescent (13 to 18 y)	60 to 100

*Pulse rates for a sleeping child may be 10% lower than the low rate listed in age group.

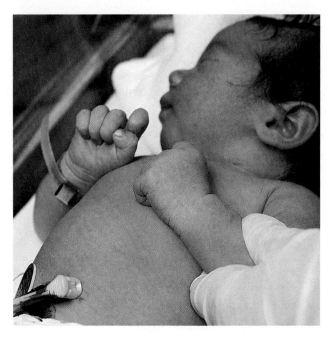

Figure 2-6 Acrocyanosis of the hands in a newborn.

- Skin temperature: hot, warm, cool
  - The skin surface is normally warm and equal bilaterally.
  - Use the dorsal surfaces of your hands and fingers to assess skin temperature.
  - As cardiac output decreases, coolness will begin in the hands and feet and ascend toward the trunk.
- Skin moisture: dry, moist, diaphoretic
  - The skin is normally dry with a minimum of perspiration.
  - Use the dorsal surfaces of your hands and fingers to assess the moisture of the skin.
- Skin turgor
  - To assess skin turgor (elasticity), grasp the skin on the abdomen between your thumb and index finger (Figure 2-8). Pull the skin

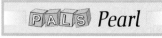 *Pearl*

Skin color is most reliably evaluated in the sclera, conjunctiva, nail beds, tongue, oral mucosa, palms, and soles.

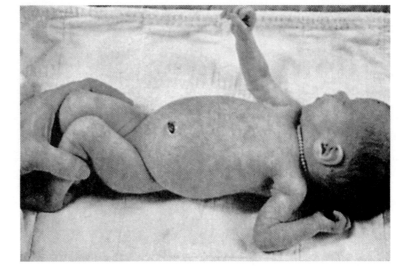

Figure 2-7 Mottling.

PALS Pearl

If capillary refill is initially assessed in the hand or fingers and it is delayed, recheck it in a more central location, such as the chest.

taut and then release quickly. Observe the speed with which the skin returns to its original contour when released.

- ○ The skin should resume its shape immediately with no tenting or wrinkling. Good skin turgor indicates adequate hydration.
- ○ Decreased skin turgor (a sign of dehydration and/or malnutrition) is present when the skin is released and it remains pinched (tented) and then slowly returns to its normal shape (Table 2-6).
- Evaluate capillary refill.
  - To assess capillary refill, firmly press the skin over the warmest point on the child's body and release. Observe the time it takes for the blanched tissue to return to its original color.
    - ○ If the ambient temperature is warm, color should return within 2 seconds.
    - ○ Capillary refill time of 3 to 5 seconds is delayed and may indicate poor perfusion or exposure to cool ambient temperatures.
    - ○ Capillary refill time longer than 5 seconds is markedly delayed and suggests shock (Figure 2-9).
  - Alternate sites for assessment of capillary refill include the forehead, chest, abdomen, or fleshy part of the palm.
- Oxygen
- Position
- Chest compressions
- Bleeding control
- Fluid replacement
- Defibrillation

A positive finding is more helpful than a negative one. Never assume a child is well hydrated based on good skin turgor.

A positive finding is more helpful than a negative one. Never assume a child is well perfused based on a good capillary refill time.

Interventions

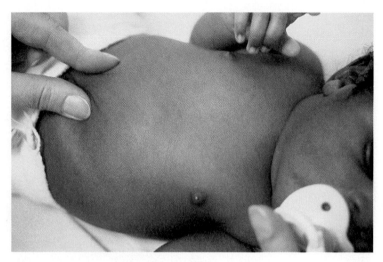

Figure 2-8 Assessing skin turgor in an infant.

TABLE 2-6 *Evaluating Skin Turgor and Estimating Dehydration*

Elapsed Time for Skin to Return to Normal	Approximate Degree of Dehydration
Less than 2 sec	Less than 5% of the child's body weight
2 to 3 sec	5% to 8% of the child's body weight
3 to 4 sec	9% to 10% of the child's body weight
More than 4 sec	More than 10% of the child's body weight

From Seidel HM, Ball JW, Dains JE, et al. *Mosby's guide to physical examination*, 5th ed. St. Louis: Mosby, 2003.

Disability

Assessment

- Goal: awake and alert
- A version of the Glasgow Coma Scale (GCS) modified for pediatric use is used during this phase of the primary survey to establish a baseline and for comparison in later, serial observations (Table 2-7).
- A GCS score that falls two points suggests significant deterioration; urgent patient reassessment is required.
  - To avoid confusion with spinal reflexes, assess the patient's motor response by applying a stimulus above the neck.
    - Question the parent/caregiver about the child's normal mood, activity level, attention span, and willingness and ability to cooperate.

Interventions

- Oxygen
- Ventilation
- Position
- Spinal stabilization

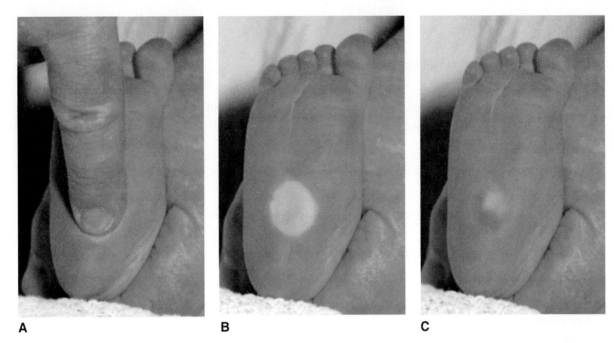

A   B   C

Figure 2-9 Capillary refill in a child in shock.

TABLE 2-7 *Adult, Child, and Infant Glasgow Coma Scale*

Glasgow Coma Scale	Adult / Child	Score	Infant
Eye opening	Spontaneous	4	Spontaneous
	To verbal	3	To verbal
	To pain	2	To pain
	No response	1	No response
Best **V**erbal response	Oriented	5	Coos, babbles
	Disoriented	4	Irritable cry
	Inappropriate words	3	Cries only to pain
	Incomprehensible sounds	2	Moans to pain
	No response	1	No response
Best **M**otor response	Obeys commands	6	Spontaneous
	Localizes pain	5	Withdraws from touch
	Withdraws from pain	4	Withdraws from pain
	Abnormal flexion (decorticate)	3	Abnormal flexion (decorticate)
	Abnormal extension (decerebrate)	2	Abnormal extension (decerebrate)
	No response	1	No response
	Total = E + V + M	3 to 15	

Expose/Environment

- Undress the patient
- Preserve body heat/maintain appropriate temperature
  - Respect modesty.
  - Keep the child covered if possible and replace clothing promptly after examining each body area.

Secondary Survey

The Secondary Survey focuses on advanced life support (ALS) interventions and management.

- Obtain vital signs, attach pulse oximeter, electrocardiogram (ECG), and blood pressure monitor.
- Obtain focused SAMPLE or CIAMPEDS history (See pages 46–47).
- (Advanced) *A*irway
- *B*reathing
- *C*irculation
- *D*etailed (or focused) examination, *D*ifferential diagnosis, *D*iagnostic procedures
- *E*valuate interventions, pain management
- *F*acilitate family presence for invasive and resuscitative procedures

Vital Signs

- Temperature
  - Obtain the child's temperature by an appropriate route (e.g., oral, axillary, rectal, tympanic) considering the child's age and clinical condition.
  - Temperature varies with exercise, crying, stress, and clothing.
  - Common signs of increased body temperature include flushed face and skin, malaise, low energy level, increased ventilatory and heart rates, and a "glassy look" to the eyes.
  - Infants and children may lose heat rapidly. Keep the child covered. It is particularly important to keep the head of an infant covered.
- Blood pressure
  - Blood pressure should be measured only after assessing pulse and ventilation. Children often become agitated during this procedure, which increases their pulse and ventilatory rate. To decrease children's anxiety about blood pressure measurement, tell them you are going to give their arm "a hug."
  - Measure blood pressure in children older than 3 years. In children younger than 3 years, a strong central pulse is considered an acceptable sign of adequate blood pressure. Table 2-8 shows the lower limit of normal systolic blood pressure by age.
  - The blood pressure should be measured with a cuff, with the

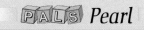
PALS Pearl

Maintaining appropriate temperature is particularly important in the pediatric patient because children have a large body surface area to weight ratio, providing a greater area for heat loss.

The Initial Assessment Algorithm is shown in Figure 2-10.

See Tables 2-2 and 2-5 for normal values for ventilatory rates and heart rates by age.

Blood pressure is one of the *least* sensitive indicators of adequate circulation in children.

The cuff should be at heart level and the arm should be fully supported by the rescuer.

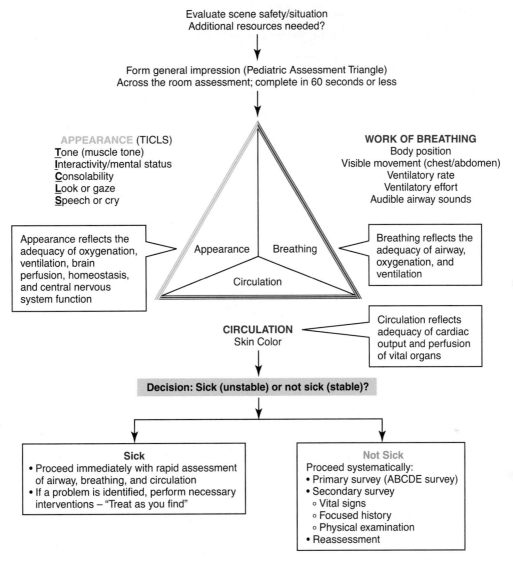

PEDIATRIC INITIAL ASSESSMENT ALGORITHM
GENERAL IMPRESSION

Evaluate scene safety/situation
Additional resources needed?

Form general impression (Pediatric Assessment Triangle)
Across the room assessment; complete in 60 seconds or less

APPEARANCE (TICLS)
Tone (muscle tone)
Interactivity/mental status
Consolability
Look or gaze
Speech or cry

WORK OF BREATHING
Body position
Visible movement (chest/abdomen)
Ventilatory rate
Ventilatory effort
Audible airway sounds

Appearance reflects the adequacy of oxygenation, ventilation, brain perfusion, homeostasis, and central nervous system function

Breathing reflects the adequacy of airway, oxygenation, and ventilation

Appearance | Breathing
Circulation

CIRCULATION
Skin Color

Circulation reflects adequacy of cardiac output and perfusion of vital organs

Decision: Sick (unstable) or not sick (stable)?

Sick
• Proceed immediately with rapid assessment of airway, breathing, and circulation
• If a problem is identified, perform necessary interventions – "Treat as you find"

Not Sick
Proceed systematically:
• Primary survey (ABCDE survey)
• Secondary survey
  ○ Vital signs
  ○ Focused history
  ○ Physical examination
• Reassessment

Figure 2-10 The Pediatric Initial Assessment Algorithm.   *Continued*

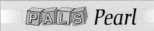

PALS Pearl

To determine the *minimum* systolic blood pressure for a child 1 to 10 years of age, the following formula may be used: 70 + (2 × age in years).

bladder completely encircling the extremity and the width covering one half to two thirds the length of the upper arm or upper leg. Use of a cuff that is too large will result in a falsely low reading. Use of a cuff that is too small will result in a falsely high reading.

• Pulse pressure

  • **Pulse pressure** is the difference between the systolic and diastolic blood pressures.

  • Indicator of **stroke volume** (the amount of blood ejected by either ventricle during one contraction).

  • Narrowed pulse pressure is an indicator of circulatory compromise.

PEDIATRIC INITIAL ASSESSMENT ALGORITHM
PRIMARY SURVEY (ABCDE)

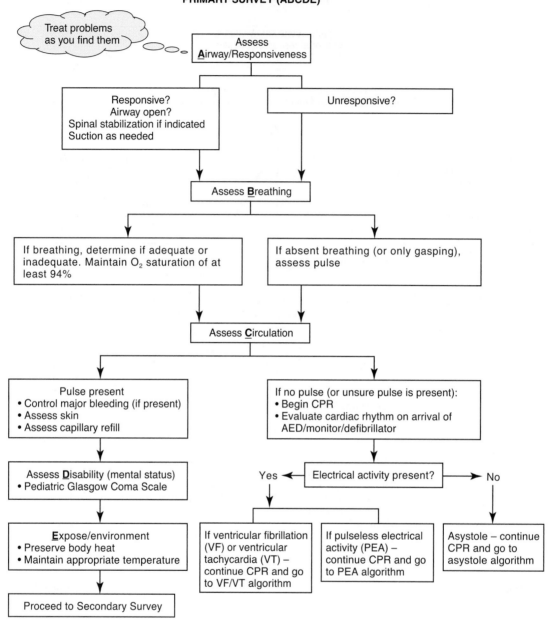

Figure 2-10, *cont'd.*

Continued

- Weight
  - Whenever possible, obtain a measured weight. If obtaining a measured weight is not possible, use a length-based measuring tape to estimate the child's weight if 35 kg or less, or ask the caregiver the child's last weight.
  - Pediatric weight formula
    - Weight in kg = 8 + (2 × age in years)
    - Use 3 kg for newborns
    - Use 7 kg for 6-month-olds

PEDIATRIC INITIAL ASSESSMENT ALGORITHM
SECONDARY SURVEY (ABCDEF)

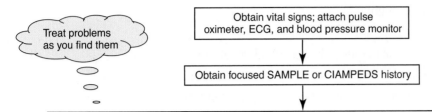

Treat problems as you find them

Obtain vital signs; attach pulse oximeter, ECG, and blood pressure monitor

↓

Obtain focused SAMPLE or CIAMPEDS history

↓

AIRWAY
• Reassess effectiveness of initial airway maneuvers and interventions
• Consider insertion of advanced airway if needed

BREATHING
• Reassess ventilation
• If applicable, confirm tracheal tube placement (or other airway device) by at least two methods
• Provide positive-pressure ventilation (if applicable) and evaluate effectiveness of ventilations

CIRCULATION
• Establish vascular access / administer medications, if appropriate

DETAILED (OR FOCUSED) EXAMINATION, DIFFERENTIAL DIAGNOSIS, DIAGNOSTIC PROCEDURES
• If unresponsive or significant mechanism of injury, perform detailed (head-to-toes) physical exam. If responsive or no significant mechanism of injury, perform focused exam.
• Search for, find, and treat reversible causes
• Glucose check
• Laboratory and radiographic studies

EVALUATE interventions, pain management
FACILITATE family presence for invasive and resuscitative procedures

↓

Reassessment

• Reassess airway patency, oxygen saturation
• Reassess breathing effectiveness with capnography
• Reassess pulse rate and quality, perfusion status, cardiac rhythm
• Reassess capillary refill (if younger than 6 years)
• Reassess mental status and activity level
• Reassess and document vital signs
• Reevaluate emergency care interventions

Figure 2-10, *cont'd.*

TABLE 2-8 *Lower Limit of Normal Systolic Blood Pressure by Age*

Age	Lower Limit of Normal Systolic Blood Pressure
Term neonate (0 to 28 days)	More than 60 mm Hg or strong central pulse
Infant (1 to 12 months)	More than 70 mm Hg or strong central pulse
Child 1 to 10 years	More than 70 + (2 × age in years)
Child 10 years or older	More than 90 mm Hg

- Weight conversion
  - Weight (lb) $\times$ 0.45 = Weight (kg)
  - Weight (kg) $\times$ 2.2 = Weight (lb)

Focused History

The history is often obtained simultaneously during the physical examination and while therapeutic interventions are performed. While performing the physical examination, ask the patient, family, bystanders, or others questions regarding the patient's history. SAMPLE is a mnemonic used to organize the information obtained when taking a patient history.

- **S**igns/symptoms: assessment findings and history as they relate to the chief complaint.
  - When did it start/occur (time, sudden, gradual)? What was the child doing when it started/occurred?
  - How long did it last? Does it come and go? Is it still present?
  - Where is the problem? Describe character and severity if painful (use pain scale).
  - Radiation? Aggravating or alleviating factors?
  - Previous history of same? If yes, what was the diagnosis?
- **A**llergies: to medications, food, environmental causes (e.g., pollen), and products (e.g., latex).
- **M**edications
  - Prescription and over-the-counter medications the child is currently taking.
  - Determine name of medication, dose, route, frequency, and indication for the medication.
- **P**ast medical history
  - Is the child currently under a physician's care?
  - Serious childhood illnesses: age, complications
  - Hospitalizations: age, reason for admission, length of stay
  - Surgical procedures: age, reason for procedure, complications
  - Trauma/injuries and fractures/ingestions, burns: age, circumstances surrounding event, treatment, complications
  - Immunization status with regard to diphtheria, tetanus, pertussis, varicella, poliomyelitis, *Haemophilus influenza* type B, hepatitis B, rubeola, rubella, mumps, and so forth.
  - For infants and toddlers, obtain a birth history.
    - Maternal age, gestational duration, prematurity, birth weight
    - Complications during pregnancy or delivery (e.g., cesarean delivery, forceps delivery)
    - Congenital anomalies
    - "Did the baby go home with you?"

- *L*ast oral intake
  - Time of last meal and fluid intake.
  - Changes in eating pattern or fluid intake.
  - For infants, determine if breast fed or bottle fed; if formula is used, which type; feeding difficulties.
- *E*vents leading to the illness or injury
  - Onset, duration, and precipitating factors
  - Associated factors such as toxic inhalants, drugs, alcohol
  - Injury scenario and mechanism of injury
  - Treatment given by caregiver

The Emergency Nurses Association (ENA) recommends use of the CIAMPEDS mnemonic:

- *C*hief complaint
  - Reason for the child's visit to the emergency department (ED)
  - Duration of complaint
- *I*mmunizations/isolation
  - Evaluate scheduled immunizations for the child's age.
  - Evaluate the child's exposure to communicable diseases (e.g., chickenpox, meningitis).
- *A*llergies: to medications, food, environmental causes (e.g., pollen), products (e.g., latex), and environment
- *M*edications
  - Prescription and over-the-counter medications the child is currently taking.
    - Include herbal and dietary supplements
  - Determine name of medication, dose, route, frequency, and indication for the medication.
- *P*ast medical history
  - Child's health status including prior illnesses, injuries, hospitalizations, surgeries, and chronic physical and psychiatric illnesses.
  - Use of alcohol, tobacco, drugs, or other substances of abuse.
  - The neonate's history should include the prenatal and birth history including maternal complications during pregnancy or delivery, infant's gestational age and birth weight, and number of days infant remained hospitalized after delivery.
  - Date and description of last menstrual period.
  - The history for sexually active patients should include type of birth control used, barrier protection, prior treatment for sexually transmitted diseases, pregnancies (gravida) and births, miscarriages, abortions, living children (para).
- *P*arent's/caregiver's impression of the child's condition
  - Identify the patient's primary caregiver.

OPQRST is an acronym that may be used when evaluating pain.

- *O*nset: What were you doing when the pain started?
- *P*rovocation: What makes the pain better or worse? Coughing/deep breathing, anxiety/fear, treatment/procedure, movement/positioning, parent/caregiver not present
- *Q*uality: What does the pain feel like (dull, sharp, pressure, burning, squeezing, stabbing, gnawing, shooting, throbbing)?
- *R*egion/radiation: Where is the pain? Is the pain in one area or does it move?
- *S*everity: On a scale of 0 to 10, with 0 being the least and 10 being the worst, what number would you assign your pain or discomfort?
- *T*ime: How long ago did the problem/discomfort begin? Have you ever had this pain before? When? How long did it last?

- Consider cultural differences that may affect the caregiver's impressions.
  - Evaluate the caregiver's concerns and observations of the child's condition.
- **E**vents surrounding illness/injury
  - Illness: duration, including date of onset and sequence of symptoms; treatment provided before arrival at ED
  - Injury: date/time of injury, mechanism of injury including use of restraints/protective devices, suspected injuries, prehospital vital signs and treatment, circumstances leading to the injury, witnessed or unwitnessed
- **D**iet/diapers
  - Time of last meal and fluid intake, changes in eating pattern or fluid intake.
  - For infants, determine if breast fed or bottle fed; if formula is used which type; feeding difficulties.
  - Special diet or dietary restrictions.
  - Evaluation of child's urine and stool output.
- (Associated) **S**ymptoms
  - Symptom identification and progression since onset of illness or injury

Physical Examination

The purpose of the physical examination in the Secondary Survey is to detect **non–life-threatening** conditions and provide care for those conditions/injuries. A detailed physical examination is presented here for completeness. A focused physical examination may be more appropriate, based on the patient's presentation and chief complaint.

- Inspect and palpate each of the major body areas for DCAP-BLS-TIC (**D**eformities, **C**ontusions, **A**brasions, **P**enetrations/punctures, **B**urns, **L**acerations, **S**welling/edema, **T**enderness, **I**nstability, **C**repitus).
- Auscultate breath and heart sounds.
  Head/Face
- Scalp and skull
  - Inspect for DCAP-BLS.
  - Palpate for DCAP-BLS-TIC, depressions, and protrusions.
  - In a child younger than 14 months, gently palpate the anterior and posterior fontanelles on the top of the head with the child in a sitting position (if no trauma is suspected).
    - The posterior fontanelle normally closes by 2 months of age. In most infants, the anterior fontanelle closes between 7 and 14 months of age (Figure 2-11).

The assessment procedure outlined here appears as a head-to-toes sequence; however, the sequence should be reversed (toes-to-head) in infants and young children. Infants and young children find it particularly threatening when strangers want to touch their faces. By beginning with the extremities and proceeding backward, you reduce the likelihood of frightening the child. Try to gain the child's trust as you proceed by being calm, friendly, and reassuring.

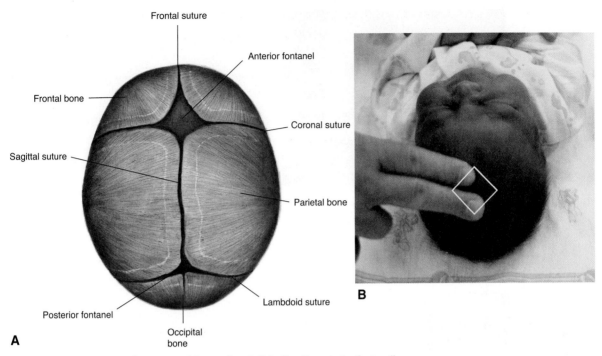

Frontal suture

Anterior fontanel

Frontal bone

Coronal suture

Sagittal suture

Parietal bone

Lambdoid suture

Posterior fontanel

Occipital bone

A

B

Figure 2-11   A, Location of sutures and fontanelles. **B,** Palpating the anterior fontanelle.

- A bulging anterior fontanelle may be due to crying, coughing, vomiting, or increased intracranial pressure (ICP) due to a head injury, meningitis, or hydrocephalus. A depressed anterior fontanelle is seen in dehydrated or malnourished infants.

To quickly assess the cranial nerves in a child who can follow commands, ask children to close their eyes, open their eyes wide, follow a finger with their eyes, open their mouth, and stick out their tongue.

- Ears
  - Inspect for DCAP-BLS, postauricular ecchymosis (Battle's sign), blood, or clear fluid.
  - Palpate for tenderness or pain.
- Face
  - Inspect for DCAP-BLS, singed facial hair, and symmetry of facial expression.
  - Palpate the orbital rims, zygoma, maxilla, and mandible for DCAP-BLS-TIC, neurovascular impairment, muscle spasm, false motion, or motor impairment.
- Eyes
  - Inspect for DCAP-BLS, foreign body, blood in the anterior chamber of the eye (hyphema) (Figure 2-12), presence of eyeglasses or contact lenses, periorbital ecchymosis (raccoon eyes) (Figure 2-13), color of sclera and conjunctiva, periorbital edema, pupils (size, shape, equality, reactivity to light), and eye movement (dysconjugate gaze, ocular muscle function).
  - Determine Pediatric Coma Scale score or GCS score.

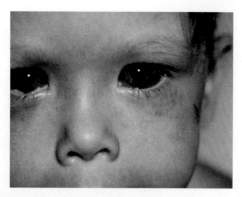

Figure 2-12 Blood in the anterior chamber of the eye (hyphema).

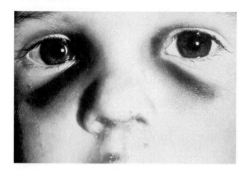

Figure 2-13 Raccoon eyes (periorbital ecchymosis).

- Nose
  - Inspect for DCAP-BLS, blood or fluid from the nose, singed nasal hairs, nares for flaring.
  - Palpate nasal bones.
- Mouth/throat/pharynx
  - Inspect for DCAP-BLS, blood, absent or broken teeth, gastric contents, foreign objects (e.g., loose teeth, gum, small toys); injured or swollen tongue; color of the mucous membranes of the mouth; note presence and character of fluids; vomitus; note sputum color, amount, and consistency.
  - Listen for hoarseness, inability to talk.
  - Note unusual odors (e.g., alcohol, feces, acetone, almonds).
  Neck
- Inspect for DCAP-BLS, neck veins (flat or distended), use of accessory muscles, presence of a stoma, and presence of a medical identification device. It is difficult to assess distended neck veins in infants and young children.

- Palpate for DCAP-BLS-TIC, subcutaneous emphysema, and tracheal position.

Chest

- Inspect: work of breathing (Figure 2-14), symmetry of movement, use of accessory muscles, retractions, note abnormal breathing patterns, DCAP-BLS, vascular access devices.
- Auscultate
  - Equality of breath sounds
  - Adventitious breath sounds (e.g., crackles, wheezes)
  - Heart sounds for rate, rhythm, murmurs, bruits, gallops, friction rub, muffled heart tones
- Palpate for DCAP-BLS-TIC, chest wall tenderness, symmetry of chest wall expansion, subcutaneous emphysema.

Abdomen

- Inspect for DCAP-BLS, distention, scars from healed surgical incisions or penetrating wounds, feeding tubes, use of abdominal muscles during respiration, signs of injury, discoloration.
- Auscultate to determine presence or absence of bowel sounds in all quadrants.
- Palpate all four quadrants for DCAP-BLS, guarding or distention, rigidity, masses.

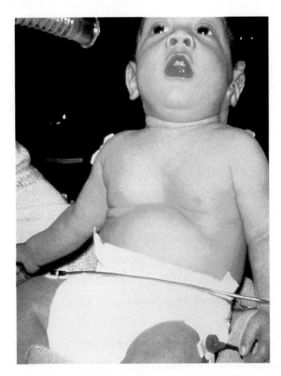

Figure 2-14 Inspect the chest and assess work of breathing, symmetry of movement, use of accessory muscles, and the presence of retractions.

Pelvis and Genitalia

- Inspect for DCAP-BLS
    - Discharge or drainage from the meatus
    - Priapism (spinal cord injury, sickle cell disease)
    - Scrotal bleeding or edema
- Palpate for DCAP-BLS-TIC
    - To assess the integrity of the pelvis:
        - First, gently palpate for point tenderness.
        - Next, place your hands on each iliac crest and press gently inward. If pain, crepitation, or instability is elicited, suspect a fracture of the pelvic ring. No further assessment is necessary if this assessment reveals positive findings.
        - If this assessment is negative, simultaneously push down on both iliac crests. Then place one hand on the pubic bone (over the symphysis pubis) and apply gentle pressure.
    - Assess strength and quality of femoral pulses.
    - In the hospital, assess anal sphincter tone.

Extremities

In an alert child, begin your assessment of the extremities by evaluating the lower extremities first. In an injured extremity, be sure to assess distal pulses and neurovascular integrity distal to the injury. Compare an injured extremity to an uninjured extremity and document your findings.

- Inspect for DCAP-BLS, vascular access devices, **purpura**, **petechiae** (Figures 2-15 and 2-16), presence of congenital anomalies (e.g., finger clubbing, club foot), abnormal extremity position, and medical identification bracelet.
- Palpate for DCAP-BLS-TIC
    - Assess skin temperature, moisture, and capillary refill in each extremity.
    - Assess the strength and quality of pulses, motor function, and sensory function (PMS) in each extremity.
        - If the child is alert, assess sensation by lightly touching the extremity and asking, "Do you feel me brushing your skin? Where?"
        - Assess motor function in an upper extremity in an alert patient by instructing the child to "Squeeze my fingers in your hand." To assess motor function in a lower extremity, instruct the child to "Push down on my fingers with your toes."

Posterior Body

- Inspect for DCAP-BLS, purpura, petechiae, rashes, and edema.
- Auscultate the posterior thorax.
- Palpate the posterior trunk for DCAP-BLS.

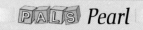 *Pearl*

If present, the following signs may help identify the nature and location of internal injuries:

- **Kehr's sign**: Left upper quadrant pain with radiation to the left shoulder; suggests injury to the spleen or liver (pain occurs because of blood or bile irritating the diaphragm)
- **Cullen's sign**: A bluish discoloration around the umbilicus that may indicate intraabdominal or retroperitoneal hemorrhage
- **Grey-Turner's sign**: Bruising of the flanks that may indicate intraabdominal hemorrhage, often splenic in origin

If trauma is suspected, ensure manual in-line stabilization of the head and spine is maintained during the exam.

Purpura—red-purple nonblanch-able discoloration greater than 0.5cm diameter. Cause: Intravascular defects, infection

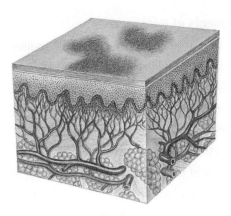

Figure 2-15 Purpura are reddish-purple nonblanchable discolorations in the skin greater than 0.5 cm in diameter. Purpura are produced by small bleeding vessels near the skin's surface.

Petechiae—red-purple nonblanch-able discoloration less than 0.5 cm diameter Cause: Intravascular defects, infection

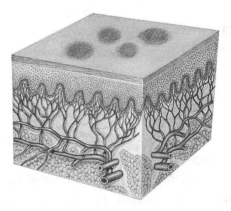

Figure 2-16 Petechiae are reddish-purple nonblanchable discolorations in the skin smaller than 0.5 cm in diameter.

Reassessment

Purpose

- Reevaluate the patient's condition.
- Assess the effectiveness of emergency care interventions provided.
- Identify any missed injuries or conditions.
- Observe subtle changes or trends in the patient's condition.
- Alter emergency care interventions as needed.

Reassessment should be:

- Performed on EVERY patient.
- Performed after ensuring completion of critical interventions.
- Performed after the detailed physical examination, if one is performed. (In some situations, the patient's condition may preclude performance of the detailed physical examination.)
- Repeated and documented every 5 minutes for an unstable patient.
- Repeated and documented every 15 minutes for a stable patient.

Components of Reassessment

- Reassess airway patency, oxygen saturation.
- Reassess breathing effectiveness:
  - Rise and fall of the chest
  - Ventilatory rate
  - Depth/equality of breathing
  - Rhythm of breathing
  - Signs of increased work of breathing (ventilatory effort)
  - Breath sounds
- Reassess pulse rate and quality, perfusion status, cardiac rhythm:
  - Look for changes in color of skin and mucous membranes.
  - Feel for changes in skin temperature and moisture.
  - Reassess capillary refill in infants and children younger than 6 years of age.
- Reassess mental status and activity level.
- Reassess and document vital signs.
- Reevaluate emergency care interventions:
  - Ensure suction is readily available
  - If an OPA or NPA has been placed, ensure it is properly positioned
  - If the patient is being ventilated with a bag-mask device:
    - Ensure the device is connected to oxygen at 10 to 15 L/min.
    - Reassess effectiveness of ventilation:
      - Ensure adequate rise and fall of the chest.
      - Ensure adequate face-to-mask seal.
      - Evaluate lung compliance (resistance to ventilation):
        - Increasing resistance suggests airway obstruction.
  - If oxygen is being delivered by nonrebreather mask:
    - Ensure the mask is connected to oxygen at 10 to 15 L/min.
    - Ensure the reservoir bag is not pinched off and remains inflated.
    - Ensure the inhalation valve is not obstructed.
  - If oxygen is being delivered by nasal cannula:
    - Ensure the oxygen flow rate is set at no more than 6 L/min.
    - Ensure the prongs are properly placed in the patient's nose.
    - Ensure open chest wounds have been properly sealed with an occlusive dressing.
    - Ensure bleeding is controlled. Assess and document the type and amount of drainage through dressings.
    - If intravenous (IV) fluids are administered, assess the IV site for patency. Document the type and amount of fluid administered.
    - If cardiopulmonary resuscitation (CPR) is performed, ensure pulses are produced with chest compressions.

- Ensure the trauma patient's cervical spine is adequately immobilized.
- Ensure injured extremities are effectively immobilized.
- Ensure open wounds are properly dressed and bandaged.

Pediatric Triage in the Emergency Department

Goals of Triage

- Rapidly identify patients with life-threatening conditions.
- Determine the most appropriate treatment area for patients presenting to the ED.
- Optimize use of resources.
- Decrease congestion in emergency treatment areas.
- Provide ongoing assessment of patients.
- Provide information to patients and families regarding services, expected care, and waiting times.

Triage Guidelines

The triage interview is performed to gather enough information to make a clinical judgment regarding the patient's priority of care. Effective triage requires the use of sight, hearing, smell, and touch.

The ability to triage patients effectively and accurately is based on the following:

- The PAT
- Physical assessment findings
- The patient's pertinent medical history
- Appropriate use of guidelines and triage protocols
- Practical knowledge gained through experience and training

A five-level triage classification system based on patient presentation and expected resource utilization has demonstrated reliability and is reviewed here.

Resuscitation (Critical)

A resuscitation condition is one that requires immediate medical attention and maximum use of resources. The patient presents with unstable vital functions with a high probability of mortality if immediate intervention is not begun to prevent further airway, respiratory, hemodynamic, and/or neurologic instability; a time delay would be harmful to the patient. Highest priority is given to conditions including the following:

- Apnea or severe respiratory distress
- Pale, diaphoretic, and lightheaded or weak
- Central cyanosis
- Unresponsive
- Pulseless
- Active seizure

An emergent condition is one that requires medical attention within 10 minutes and high resource utilization. The patient presents with threatened vital functions with a potential threat to life or limb. Highest priority is given to conditions including the following:

- Altered mental status
- Unstable vital signs
- Vomiting with head injury
- Severe pain or distress
- Fever with signs of severe dehydration
- Moderate to severe respiratory distress
- Extremity injury with neurovascular compromise
- Fever with excessive drooling or difficulty swallowing
- Fever in an infant younger than 6 months of age

Emergent (High Risk)

An urgent condition is one that requires prompt treatment within 30 to 60 minutes. The patient presents with stable vital functions that are not likely to threaten life and require medium resource utilization. The patient should be periodically reassessed (usually every 20 to 30 minutes) to ensure there is no deterioration in his or her condition.

- Infant fall more than 2 feet
- Foreign object ingested larger than a nickel
- Mild to moderate dehydration
- Mild to moderate respiratory distress
- Nonspecific chest pain
- Allergic reaction with hives over more than 50% of body
- Abdominal pain with suspected abuse
- Moderate pain
- Nonpenetrating eye injury

Urgent (Moderate Risk)

A semi-urgent condition is one that may safely wait 1 to 2 hours to be evaluated without risk of morbidity or mortality. The patient presents with stable vital functions and has a low need for resource utilization. The patient's illness or injury has a low probability of progression to more serious disease or development of complications. The patient with a semi-urgent condition should be periodically reassessed (usually every 30 to 60 minutes) to ensure there is no deterioration in his or her condition.

- Simple laceration
- History of seizure (now awake and alert)
- Fever in a child 3 months to 3 years old
- Head trauma without symptoms

Semi-Urgent (Low Risk)

Non-Urgent (Low Risk) — A non-urgent condition is one that may safely wait 2 hours or more to be evaluated without risk of morbidity or mortality; the patient presents with stable vital functions and does not require resource utilization. The patient's illness or injury has a low probability of progression to more serious disease or development of complications. The patient with a non-urgent condition should be periodically reassessed (usually every 60 to 120 minutes) to ensure there is no deterioration in his or her condition.

- Upper respiratory infection (URI)
- Fever in a child older than 36 months
- Impetigo
- Conjunctivitis
- Isolated soft-tissue injury
- Diaper rash
- Cold or flu
- Ear discomfort
- Sore throat
- Mild gastroenteritis
- Thrush

Case Study Resolution

Based on the information provided, this child is "not sick" (i.e., stable). Proceed systematically. Perform an initial assessment (i.e., primary survey), secondary survey (including vital signs, focused history, and detailed physical examination), and a reassessment.

If the child appeared "sick" (unstable), you would proceed immediately with rapid assessment of airway, breathing, and circulation. If a problem were identified, you would perform necessary interventions ("Treat as you find").

References

1. Walsh C, MacMillan HL, Jamieson E. The relationship between parental substance abuse and child maltreatment: findings from the Ontario Health Supplement. *Child Abuse Negl* 2003;27:1409–1425.

Chapter Quiz

1. The Pediatric Assessment Triangle (PAT):
   A) Is used to quickly determine if a child is "sick" or "not sick."
   B) Is a hands-on assessment of an infant or child.
   C) Is performed systematically from head-to-toes and requires the use of a stethoscope and blood pressure cuff.
   D) Should be repeated every fifteen to thirty minutes if the child appears very sick.

2. List the components of the Pediatric Assessment Triangle.

3. TICLS is a mnemonic used to recall the areas to be assessed related to a child's appearance. Explain the meaning of each of the letters of this mnemonic.
   T =
   I =
   C =
   L =
   S =

Questions 4–8 refer to the following patient situation:

A 2-year-old presents with shortness of breath. Mom states her son has had a three day history of a productive cough and runny nose. The child is holding a blanket and intently watching your movements while being held in his mother's arms. His respiratory rate appears to be within normal limits for his age with no evidence of increased work of breathing. Chest expansion appears equal and his skin is pink.

4. From the information provided, complete the following documentation regarding the Pediatric Assessment Triangle:
   Appearance:
   Breathing:
   Circulation:

5. Based on the information provided, is this child "sick" or "not sick?" How should you proceed?

6. To gain the child's cooperation you should:
   A) Introduce yourself and try to hold him.
   B) Sit down and listen attentively while speaking with the child's mother.
   C) Remove the child's clothing and inspect his airway with a pen light.
   D) Separate the mother and child and perform an initial assessment.

7. List the components of the Primary Survey.

8. A normal ventilatory rate for a child of this age is _____ . A normal heart rate for a child of this age is _____ .

9. True or False: Ventilations in a child younger than 8 years are primarily abdominal.

10. Select the *incorrect* statement regarding assessment of blood pressure:
    A) Use of a blood pressure cuff that is too large will result in a falsely low reading.
    B) Blood pressure is one of the least sensitive indicators of adequate circulation in children.
    C) Blood pressure should be measured only after assessing pulse and respiration.
    D) To ensure an accurate patient assessment, it is essential to obtain serial blood pressure measurements in children younger than 3 years.

11. A 7-month-old infant has a two day history of poor feeding. Which of the following should be used to assess a central pulse in this infant?
    A) Carotid pulse
    B) Femoral pulse
    C) Radial pulse
    D) Brachial pulse

12. The formula used to approximate the lower limit of systolic blood pressure in children 1 to 10 years of age is:
    A) $70 + (2 \times \text{age in years})$
    B) Age in years $\times 2.2$
    C) $16 + \text{age in years}/4$
    D) $2 \times 90/\text{age in years}$

Chapter Quiz Answers

1. A. The PAT is used to 1) establish the severity of the child's illness or injury (sick or not sick), 2) identify the general category of physiologic abnormality (e.g., cardiopulmonary, neurologic, etc.), and 3) determine the urgency of further assessment and intervention. Because approaching an ill or injured child can increase agitation, possibly worsening the child's condition, the PAT is an "across the room" assessment that is performed before approaching or touching the child and can usually be completed in 60 seconds or less. No equipment is required.

2. The components of the Pediatric Assessment Triangle are:
   1) Appearance
   2) Breathing
   3) Circulation.

3. TICLS is a mnemonic used to recall the areas to be assessed related to the child's appearance. TICLS stands for:

   Tone (muscle tone)

   Interactivity/mental status (e.g., level of responsiveness, interaction with parents/guardian, and response to you or other healthcare professionals)

   Consolability

   Look or gaze

   Speech or cry

4. Pediatric Assessment Triangle (first impression) findings:

   Appearance: Awake and alert, intently observing healthcare provider

   Breathing: Ventilatory rate within normal limits for age, no evidence of increased breathing effort, symmetrical chest expansion

   Circulation: Skin is pink

5. Based on the information provided, this patient is "not sick" (i.e., stable). Proceed systematically. Perform an initial assessment (i.e., primary survey), secondary survey (including vital signs, focused history, and detailed physical examination), and reassessment. If the child appeared "sick" (unstable), you would proceed immediately with rapid assessment of airway, breathing, and circulation. If a problem were identified, you would perform necessary interventions ("Treat as you find").

6. B. To gain the child's cooperation, sit down and listen attentively while speaking with the child's mother. Toddlers distrust strangers, are likely to resist examination and treatment, and do not like having their clothing removed. They fear pain, separation from their caregiver, and separation from transitional objects (e.g., blanket, toy). Approach the child slowly and talk to him at eye level using simple words and phrases and a reassuring tone of voice. The child will understand your tone, even if he does not understand your words.

7. The primary survey is performed to determine if life-threatening conditions exists and consists of **ABCDE**:

   Airway, level of responsiveness, and cervical spine protection

   Breathing

   Circulation

   Disability (mini-neurologic exam)

   and **E**xpose/environment

8. A normal ventilatory rate for a toddler (1 to 3 years of age) is 24 to 40 breaths/min. A normal heart rate for a child of this age is 90 to 150 beats/min.

9. True. Ventilations in infants and children younger than 6 or 7 years are primarily abdominal (diaphragmatic) because the intercostal muscles of the chest wall are not well developed and fatigue easily from the work of breathing. The transition from abdominal breathing to intercostal breathing begins between 2 and 4 years of age and is complete by 7 to 8 years of age.

10. D. Use of a blood pressure cuff that is too large will result in a falsely low reading. Blood pressure is one of the least sensitive indicators of adequate circulation in children. Blood pressure should be measured only after assessing a pulse and breathing. Children often become agitated during this procedure, which increases their pulse and ventilatory rate. Measure blood pressure in children older than 3 years. In children younger than 3 years, a strong central pulse is considered an acceptable sign of adequate blood pressure.

11. D. The location for assessment of a central pulse varies according to the age of the child. In the newly born, assess the strength and quality of a central pulse by palpating the base of the umbilical cord between your thumb and index finger or auscultating the apical pulse. In an infant, assess the brachial pulse. Assess the carotid or femoral pulse in any child over one year.

12. A. The formula used to approximate the lower limit of systolic blood pressure in children 1 to 10 years of age is $70 + (2 \times \text{age in years})$.

3 Respiratory Distress and Respiratory Failure

Case Study

A 2-year-old boy is having difficulty breathing. His parents tell you the child has had a cold for the past 2 days. According to mom, she picked the child up from daycare an hour ago because he was having difficulty breathing and noticed "a whistling sound when he breathes out." She recalls the child has had four or five similar breathing episodes during the past year, but none as severe as this one. Mom is unsure if the child has had a fever and says there is a family history of asthma. Both parents are smokers. The child has no allergies. The child's older brother had a cough and cold about 5 days ago, but he is fine now.

Using the Pediatric Assessment Triangle (PAT), your general impression reveals the child is awake and aware of your presence. His ventilatory rate is faster than normal for his age. You observe moderate subcostal and supraclavicular retractions and hear expiratory wheezing. His skin color is pink.

Based on the information provided, is this child sick or not sick? What should you do next?

Objectives

1. Identify key anatomic and physiologic characteristics of infants and children and their implications in the patient with respiratory distress or respiratory failure.
2. Define respiratory distress, respiratory failure, and respiratory arrest.
3. Describe the physiologic progression of respiratory distress, failure, and arrest.
4. Discuss the assessment findings associated with respiratory distress and respiratory failure in infants and children.
5. Differentiate between upper airway obstruction and lower airway disease.
6. Describe the general approach to the treatment of children with upper airway obstruction or lower airway disease.

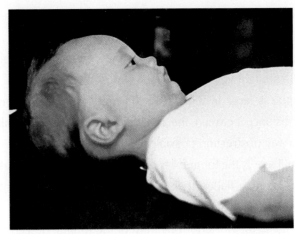

Figure 3-1   Because of the large occiput, the airway may be flexed when a child younger than 3 years is placed in a supine position. Placing a thin layer of padding under the child's shoulders helps obtain a neutral position.

Respiratory System: Anatomic and Physiologic Considerations

Head

The sniffing position allows for maximal airway patency. Sniffing position is a midposition of the head with slight extension.

- The head is large in proportion to the body with a larger occipital region.
  - Because of the large occiput, the airway may be flexed when the patient is in a supine position (Figure 3-1).
  - Different airway positioning techniques:
    ○ Place a thin layer of padding under the *shoulders* of a child younger than 3 years to obtain a neutral position (Figure 3-1).
    ○ Place a folded sheet under the *occiput* of a child older than 3 years to obtain a sniffing position (if no trauma is suspected).
  - Muscles that support the head are weak. Head bobbing often occurs when the child experiences respiratory distress.

Nose and Pharynx

Nasal flaring is an early sign of respiratory distress.

- Nasal passages are soft, narrow, distensible, have little supporting cartilage, and have more mucosa and lymphoid tissue than an adult's nasal passages.
- Infants younger than 6 months are obligate nose breathers.
  - Keep the nares clear. Any degree of obstruction (e.g., swelling of the nasal mucosa, accumulation of mucus, use of nasogastric tubes) can result in respiratory difficulty and problems with feeding.
- Tonsils and adenoids are large and may force the child to become a mouth breather.
  - In children of preschool age, the tonsils and adenoids occupy a larger proportion of the airway than in any other age group. Visual-

ization of the vocal cords during tracheal intubation may be impeded.

- Passageway through the turbinates to the posterior nasopharynx is more of a straight line.
- The tongue is large in relation to the mouth. The large tongue and shorter distance between the tongue and hard palate makes rapid upper airway obstruction possible.
  - Up until age 2, the tongue lies entirely in the oral cavity. Babies lying supine tend to flatten their tongue against the soft palate during inspiration.
  - After age 2, the posterior one third of the tongue descends into the neck and forms the anterior wall of the pharynx.

- The larynx connects the pharynx and trachea at the level of the cervical vertebrae and is a tubular structure composed of cartilage, muscles, and ligaments. The walls of the trachea are supported and held open by a series of C-shaped rings of cartilage that are open (incomplete) on the posterior surface. These rings are open to permit the esophagus, which lies behind the trachea, to bulge forward as food moves from the esophagus to the stomach. The three largest cartilages of the larynx are the thyroid cartilage, the epiglottis, and the cricoid cartilage.
  - The thyroid cartilage is the largest and most superior cartilage. In an adult, the glottic opening (the space between the true vocal cords) is located behind the thyroid cartilage and is the narrowest part of the adult larynx. A tracheal tube passing through an adult's glottic opening will pass through the cricoid cartilage.
  - The cricoid cartilage is the most inferior of the laryngeal cartilages and the first tracheal ring. It is the only completely cartilaginous ring in the larynx and helps protect the airway from compression. The cricothyroid membrane is a fibrous membrane located between the cricoid and thyroid cartilages.
  - The epiglottis is a small, leaf-shaped cartilage located at the top of the larynx. The adult epiglottis is broad and flexible. In infants and toddlers, the epiglottis is large, long, and U-shaped. It extends vertically beyond the opening of the cords, making a clear complete view of the airway difficult.
- In an adult, the larynx is located opposite the fourth to seventh cervical vertebrae (C4–C7).
  - The larynx of the pediatric airway is more anterior and superior in the neck.
  - In a newborn, the larynx is located between C1 and C4. The epiglottis can pass behind the soft palate and lock into the

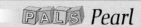
PALS Pearl

Any child with an altered mental status is at risk of an upper airway obstruction secondary to a loss of muscle tone affecting the tongue.

The tongue is a common cause of airway obstruction in children. Proper head/airway positioning is essential.

Larynx and Trachea

The tracheal rings are soft and susceptible to compression with improper positioning of the neck.

The narrowest part of the upper airway is at the level of the vocal cords in the older child and adult.

nasopharynx. This creates two separate channels—one for air and one for food (i.e., the infant can breathe and eat at the same time). The connection between the epiglottis and soft palate is constant except during crying and disease. Oral breathing begins at 5 to 6 months.

- At age 7, the larynx level is between C3 and C5. At this point, the epiglottis no longer connects with the soft palate (i.e., the child does not have two separate channels for food and air).
- The larynx of the newborn and young child resembles a funnel with the narrowest portion being at the cricoid ring. This area creates a natural seal (a physiologic cuff) around a tracheal tube.

The narrowest portion of the upper airway of an infant and young child is at the level of the cricoid ring.

- The trachea is smaller and shorter than that of an adult.
  - Movement of a tracheal tube may occur during changes in head position. The small, short trachea may result in intubation of the right primary bronchus or inadvertent extubation. Securing a tracheal tube before movement of an intubated infant or child is important to prevent tube displacement.
  - A small change in airway size results in a significant increase in resistance to air flow when edema or a foreign body is present. A marked increase in airway resistance can result in partial or complete airway obstruction.

Chest and Lungs

Use of the diaphragm leads to a characteristic "seesaw" or abdominal breathing pattern.

- The diaphragm is the primary muscle of inspiration.
  - The diaphragm must generate significant negative intrathoracic pressure to expand the child's underdeveloped lungs.
  - The diaphragm is horizontal in infants and results in decreased contraction efficiency. (The diaphragm is oblique in adults.) Efficiency of the diaphragm increases with age. Because this is the main way for pediatric patients to breathe, any compromise is serious.
- The intercostal muscles are immature and fatigue easily from the work of breathing.
  - The intercostal muscles act more as rib stabilizers and not as efficient rib elevators.
  - Accessory muscles of breathing are quiet during normal breathing, but may be activated during periods of respiratory distress.
- Effective ventilation may be jeopardized when diaphragmatic movement is compromised because the chest wall cannot compensate.
  - Restraint for immobilization may impair chest wall movement.
  - Consider insertion of an orogastric or nasogastric tube if gastric distention is present and impairs ventilation.
- The chest wall of the infant and young child is pliable because it is composed of more cartilage than bone and the ribs are more horizontal.

- Offers less protection to underlying organs.
- Significant internal injury can be present without external signs.
- Because of the flexibility of the ribs, children are more resistant than adults to rib fractures, although the force of the injury is readily transmitted to the delicate tissues of the lung and may result in a pulmonary contusion, hemothorax, or pneumothorax.
- Due to their pliability, the ribs may fail to support the lungs, leading to paradoxic movement during active inspiration, rather than lung expansion.
- The thin chest wall allows for easily transmitted breath sounds. It is easy to miss a pneumothorax or misplaced tracheal tube because of transmitted breath sounds.
- Thoracic volume is small.
  - Children have fewer and smaller alveoli. Thus, the potential area for gas exchange is less. Lung volume increases to 200 mL by age 8.
  - Fluids or air can more easily enter the interstitium (i.e., pneumothorax, pulmonary edema).
  - The oxygen requirements of infants and children are approximately twice those of adolescents and adults (6 to 8 mL/kg/min in a child; 3 to 4 mL/kg/min in an adult).
  - Children have a proportionately smaller functional residual capacity, and therefore proportionally smaller oxygen reserves. Hypoxia develops rapidly because of increased oxygen requirements and decreased oxygen reserves.
    - "Grunting" can help maintain functional residual capacity because it breaks the expiratory flow.
    - Grunting is not effective if there is reduced lung compliance (e.g., pneumonia, shock lung), impaired neurologic control (trauma, meningitis, drug effects), or an intubated trachea. Therefore, the volume left in the lungs may not be enough to keep the alveoli open.

The compliant chest wall of an infant or young child should expand easily during positive-pressure ventilation. If the chest wall does not expand equally during positive-pressure ventilation, ventilation is inadequate or the airway may be obstructed.

Respiratory Distress, Failure, and Arrest

Definitions

- **Respiratory distress** is increased work of breathing (ventilatory effort).
- **Respiratory failure** is a clinical condition in which there is inadequate blood oxygenation and/or ventilation to meet the metabolic demands of body tissues.
- **Respiratory arrest** is the absence of breathing.

Respiratory Distress

Respiratory distress is characterized by the presence of increased ventilatory effort, rate, and work of breathing.

Causes of Respiratory Distress in Children

Respiratory distress may result from a problem in the tracheobronchial tree, lungs, pleura, or chest wall (Figure 3-2).

- Asthma/reactive airway disease (RAD).
- Aspiration.
- Foreign body.
- Congenital heart disease.
- Infection (e.g., pneumonia, croup, epiglottitis, bronchiolitis).
- Medication or toxin exposure.
- Trauma.

Signs of Respiratory Distress

- Alert, irritable, anxious, restless
- Stridor
- Grunting
- Gurgling
- Audible wheezing
- Ventilatory rate faster than normal for age (tachypnea)
- Increased depth of breathing (hyperpnea)
- Intercostal retractions
- Head bobbing
- Seesaw ventilations (abdominal breathing)
- Nasal flaring
- Neck muscle use
- Central cyanosis that resolves with oxygen administration
- Mild tachycardia

Respiratory Failure

- Respiratory failure is the most common cause of cardiopulmonary arrest in children. It is often preceded by respiratory distress in which the child's work of breathing is increased in an attempt to compensate for hypoxia.

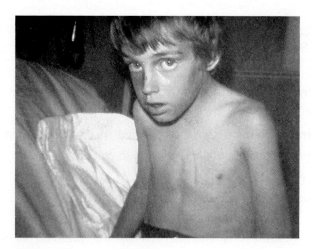

Figure 3-2   A child exhibiting signs of respiratory distress.

- *Potential* respiratory failure is based on clinical observation of signs of respiratory distress.
- Failure to improve (or deterioration) after treatment for respiratory distress indicates respiratory failure.

Causes of Respiratory Failure in Children

- Infection (e.g., croup, epiglottitis, bronchiolitis, pneumonia).
- Foreign body.
- Asthma/reactive airway disease.
- Smoke inhalation.
- Submersion syndrome.
- Pneumothorax, hemothorax.
- Congenital abnormalities.
- Neuromuscular disease.
- Medication or toxin exposure.
- Trauma.
- Heart failure.
- Metabolic disease with acidosis.

Signs of Respiratory Failure

- Sleepy, intermittently combative, or agitated (Figure 3-3)
- Decreased muscle tone
- Decreased level of responsiveness or response to pain
- Inadequate ventilatory rate, effort, or chest excursion
- Tachypnea with periods of bradypnea; slowing to bradypnea/agonal breathing

Signs of Respiratory Arrest

- Mottling; peripheral and central cyanosis
- Unresponsive to voice or touch
- Absent chest wall motion

Respiratory Arrest

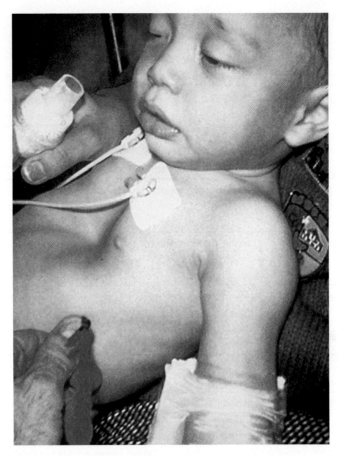

Figure 3-3   An infant exhibiting signs of respiratory failure.

- Absent breathing
- Weak to absent pulses
- Bradycardia or asystole
- Limp muscle tone

Respiratory Assessment

Scene Safety

On arrival, ensure the scene is safe before proceeding with your assessment of the patient.

Initial Assessment

Remember, the PAT is your general impression of the patient. From a distance, evaluate the child's appearance, work of breathing, and circulation to determine the severity of the child's illness or injury (Table 3-1) and assist you in determining the urgency for care (Table 3-2).

If the child appears sick (unstable), proceed immediately with the primary survey and treat problems as you find them. If the child appears "not sick" (stable), complete the initial assessment. Perform a focused or detailed physical examination, based on the patient's presentation and chief complaint. Remember: Your patient's condition can change at any time. A patient that initially appears "not sick" may rapidly deteriorate and appear "sick." Reassess frequently.

TABLE 3-1 *General Impression of Respiratory Emergencies*

Assessment	Respiratory Distress	Respiratory Failure	Respiratory Arrest
Mental status	Alert, irritable, anxious, restless	Decreased level of responsiveness or response to pain	Unresponsive to voice or touch
Muscle tone	Able to maintain sitting position (children older than 4 mo)	Normal or decreased	Limp
Body position	May assume tripod position	May assume tripod position May need support to maintain sitting position as he/she tires	Unable to maintain sitting position (infant older than 7 to 9 mo)
Ventilatory rate	Faster than normal for age	Tachypnea with periods of bradypnea; slowing to bradypnea/agonal breathing	Absent
Ventilatory effort	Intercostal retractions Nasal flaring Neck muscle use Seesaw breathing	Inadequate ventilatory effort or chest excursion	Absent
Audible airway sounds	Stridor, wheezing, gurgling	Stridor, wheezing, grunting, gasping	Absent
Skin color	Pink or pale; central cyanosis resolves with oxygen administration	Central cyanosis despite oxygen administration; mottling	Mottling; peripheral and central cyanosis

TABLE 3-2 *Immediate Interventions for Respiratory Emergencies Based on the General Impression*

	Interventions
Respiratory distress	Approach promptly, but work at a moderate pace Permit the child to assume a position of comfort Correct hypoxia by giving oxygen without causing agitation Provide further interventions based on assessment findings
Respiratory failure	Move quickly Open the airway and suction if necessary Correct hypoxia by giving supplemental oxygen Begin assisted ventilation if the patient does not improve Provide further interventions based on assessment findings
Respiratory arrest	Move quickly Check pulse; if no pulse, begin chest compressions If pulse present, immediately open the airway, suction if necessary, and begin assisted ventilation with supplemental oxygen Reassess for return of spontaneous ventilation Provide further interventions based on assessment findings

Modified from Foltin GL, Tunik MG, Cooper A, et al. *Teaching resource for instructors in prehospital pediatrics for paramedics.* New York: Center for Pediatric Emergency Medicine, 2002.

Focused History and Physical Examination

Focused History

In addition to the SAMPLE or CIAMPEDS history, consider the following questions when obtaining a focused history for a condition affecting the respiratory system. This list will require modification on the basis of the patient's age and chief complaint.

- Is the child having any trouble breathing?
- When did it start/occur (time, sudden, gradual)? What was the child doing when it started/occurred?
- How long did it last? Does it come and go? Is it still present?
- Does the child have a cough? If yes, what does the cough sound like? When does it occur? Does he or she bring up any sputum when he coughs? What does the sputum look like?
- History of a similar episode? If yes, what was the diagnosis?
- Does anything make the symptoms better or worse? (e.g., cool air, tripod position, use of inhaler)
- Allergies to medications, foods, pets, dust, perfume, pollen, or cigarette smoke? If yes, how does the child's allergy affect his or her breathing?
- History of asthma/RAD? Ever hospitalized or intubated for this condition?
- Medications: What are they (prescription, over-the-counter, recreational)? Last dose?
- Recent cold, flu, earache, pneumonia, other infection?
- Recent injuries/accidents (e.g., chest trauma, near-drowning)?
- Possibility of foreign body aspiration?
- History of trauma?
- Will the child drink? Has he been drooling?
- Has the child had a fever? For how long?
- Has the child's voice changed?
- Are siblings sick?
- Treatment given by caregiver?

Focused Physical Examination

A child presenting with a sudden onset of respiratory distress accompanied by fever, drooling, hoarseness, stridor, and tripod positioning may have a partial airway obstruction. Because agitation tends to worsen respiratory distress, keep the child as calm and as comfortable as possible, usually in the arms of the caregiver. Administer supplemental oxygen as discreetly as possible, usually via blow-by oxygen while the child is sitting on the caregiver's lap. Allow the child to assume a position of comfort and disturb the child as little as possible. Avoid procedures that may agitate the child until after the airway has been secured.

A quiet child is a sick child; a strong cry is a good cry.

- Determine if the airway is patent, maintainable, or unmaintainable:
  - Patent: able to be maintained independently.
  - Maintainable with positioning, suctioning.
  - Unmaintainable: requires assistance (e.g., tracheal intubation, crico-thyrotomy, foreign body removal).
- Assess for signs of airway obstruction. Signs include absent breath sounds, tachypnea, intercostal retractions, stridor or drooling, choking, bradycardia, and/or cyanosis.
- Assess oxygen saturation.
- Adequate breathing requires a patent airway, an adequate tidal volume, and an acceptable ventilatory rate (the rate is age dependent).
- Observe the chest wall for equal bilateral movement and time spent on inspiration and expiration (Table 3-3).
- Tachycardia is commonly seen in the child with respiratory distress. Bradycardia is seen with severe hypoxemia and acidosis due to respiratory failure. Bradycardia in a child with respiratory failure is a warning of imminent cardiopulmonary arrest (Figure 3-4).
- Agitation and irritability may indicate hypoxemia. Lethargy and decreased responsiveness may signal severe hypoxemia and/or carbon dioxide retention.
- Expose the child as needed to complete your examination.

For tachypnea without a distressed-looking patient, consider cardiac causes.

TABLE 3-3 *Signs of Increased Work of Breathing*

Visible Signs (Look)	Audible Signs (Listen)
Anxious appearance, concentration on breathing	Stridor
Ventilatory rate faster than normal for age	Wheezing
Use of accessory muscles	Crackles
Leaning forward to inhale	Grunting
Inspiratory retractions	Gurgling
Nasal flaring	Gasping
Head bobbing	
Seesaw (chest/abdominal) movement	

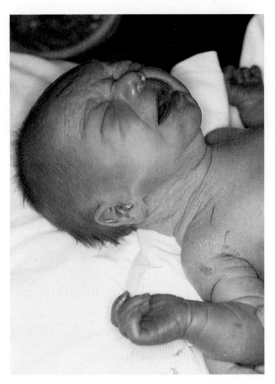

Figure 3-4   This ill infant exhibits cyanosis and poor skin perfusion.

Common Pediatric Upper Airway Emergencies

Croup

Description

Croup (laryngotracheobronchitis) is a respiratory infection that affects the upper respiratory tract. The area below the glottis is most commonly affected, resulting in swollen, inflamed mucosa with associated hoarseness, inspiratory stridor, and a barklike cough. The diagnosis is usually based on history and physical examination (Figure 3-5).

Etiology

Croup is caused by a respiratory virus. Parainfluenza types 1, 2, and 3 are the most common cause in up to 80% of cases[1], but it may also result from adenovirus, respiratory syncytial virus (RSV) (most common in patients younger than 5 years), varicella, herpes simplex virus measles, enteroviruses, *Mycoplasma pnemoniae*, and influenza viruses A and B.

Epidemiology and Demographics

- Primarily affects children ages 6 months to 3 years; peaks at age 2 years.
- The three parainfluenza viruses are observed most frequently in the

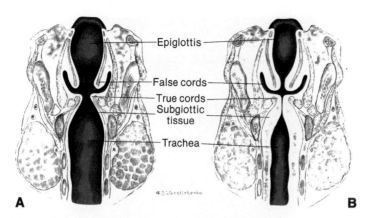

Figure 3-5   **A,** Normal larynx. **B,** Obstruction and narrowing resulting from edema of croup.

fall. RSV has a midwinter peak and can be found in increasing numbers in the spring.

- Spread via person-to-person contact or by large droplets and contaminated nasopharyngeal secretions.
- Incubation period: 2 to 4 days.

History

- Typical history of symptoms of upper respiratory infection (URI) for 1 to 2 days, but may be spasmodic (usually wakes from a nap or sleep). Croup is usually worse at night or when the child is agitated.
- Obtain a thorough history to narrow diagnosis:
  - Trauma
  - Cough or choking after playing with small toys

Physical Examination

- Vital signs: increased ventilatory rate, increased heart rate, low grade fever (usually below 102.2° F [39° C]).
- Loud stridor with hoarse voice and barky (seal-like) cough. Stridor becomes less as muscles fatigue.
- Nasal flaring.
- Retractions.

Croup Severity

- Mild croup: Normal color, normal mental status, air entry with stridor audible only with stethoscope, no retractions.
- Moderate croup: Normal color, audible stridor, mild to moderate retractions, slightly diminished air entry in an anxious child (Figure 3-6).
- Severe croup: Cyanosis, loud stridor, significant decrease in air entry, marked retractions in a highly anxious child.

The Westley croup score (Table 3-4) is a tool that may be used to characterize the severity of respiratory distress in children who have croup. The croup score is based on a child's color, level of alertness,

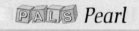
PALS *Pearl*

A radiograph of the neck may be a useful aid in diagnosing croup, but should be reserved for the child in whom epiglottitis is *not* suspected. The radiograph may reveal laryngeal narrowing 5 to 10 mm below the vocal cords. This finding is referred to as the typical "steeple sign" associated with viral croup (see Figure 3-7). However, the steeple sign may be absent in patients with croup, may be present in patients without croup as a normal variant, and may be present in patients with epiglottitis.[2]

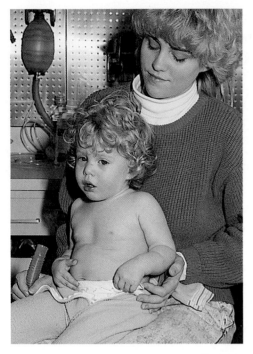

Figure 3-6   Croup. This toddler with moderate upper airway obstruction caused by croup had suprasternal and subcostal retractions. Her anxious expression was the result of mild hypoxia confirmed by pulse oximetry.

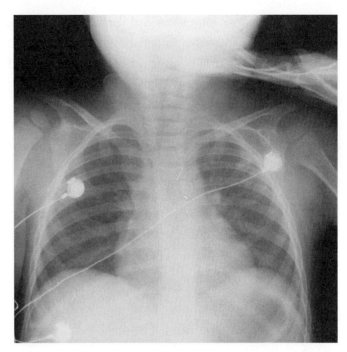

Figure 3-7   Croup. Radiograph of the airway of a patient with croup, showing typical subglottic narrowing ("steeple sign").

Patients who are younger than 6 months when they first present with croup, those who have an unusually long duration of symptoms (longer than 1 week), those who have unusually severe symptoms, and those who have recurrent croup should be evaluated for congenital or acquired airway narrowing.[1]

TABLE 3-4 *Westley Croup Score*

Criteria		Points
Retractions	None	0
	Mild	1
	Moderate	2
	Severe	3
Air entry	Normal	0
	Decreased but easily audible	1
	Severely decreased	2
Stridor	None	0
	Only with agitation/excitement	1
	At rest, with stethoscope	2
	At rest, without stethoscope	3
Cyanosis	None	0
	With agitation	4
	At rest	5
Alertness /level of responsiveness	Alert	0
	Restless, anxious	2
	Altered mental status	5

Croup score less than 3, mild croup; croup score 3 to 6, moderate croup; croup score 7 or higher, severe croup degree of stridor, air movement, and degree of retractions. Zero points are given if these findings are normal or not present. Up to 5 points are given for more severe symptoms. In general, a score of 3 necessitates hospitalization if unresponsive to therapy.

Acceptable Interventions

- Use personal protective equipment.
- Perform an initial assessment and obtain a focused history.
- Assist the child into a position of comfort, usually sitting up on the caregiver's lap.
- Maintaining an airway takes precedence over any other procedures.
- Avoid agitating the child. Keep the child as calm and as comfortable as possible, usually in the arms of the caregiver.
- Assess for foreign body airway obstruction (FBAO) (by history). Do not examine the oropharynx (may agitate the child and worsen respiratory distress).
- Initiate pulse oximetry. Maintain an oxygen saturation of 94% or higher. Note: The use of pulse oximetry in croup can be inaccurate. This is because a large degree of upper airway obstruction is required to produce hypoxia in an otherwise previously healthy child.[3]
- If ventilation is adequate and the patient exhibits signs of respiratory distress, give supplemental oxygen in a manner that does not agitate the child. If signs of respiratory failure or respiratory arrest are present, assist ventilation using a bag-mask device with supplemental oxygen.
- If the patient shows signs of respiratory failure or respiratory arrest, establish vascular access and administer normal saline at a rate sufficient to keep the vein open. In the field, do not delay transport to establish vascular access.
- In the child with mild croup, nebulized saline with no medication added may be used to provide a water vapor to help reduce inflammation and swelling.
- Moderate to severe croup:
  - Epinephrine has been used since the early 1970s to treat croup. The alpha-adrenergic effect of epinephrine is beneficial by reducing mucosal edema. Smooth muscle relaxation due to beta-adrenergic effects may benefit those children with croup who are also wheezing.[3] After nebulized therapy (using racemic or levo-epinephrine), these effects are generally noted within 10 to 30 minutes and last for about 1 hour. Epinephrine use is typically reserved for patients who have moderate to severe respiratory distress because of the potential for adverse effects, including tachycardia and hypertension. Observe for *at least* 3 to 4 hours after treatment to monitor for "rebound" symptoms. Rebound

A pulse oximeter provides information about oxygenation. It does not reflect the adequacy of ventilation. Capnography provides information about ventilation but does not reflect the adequacy of oxygenation.

For many years the use of cool, humidified air was thought to improve airflow through the edematous subglottis by decreasing the viscosity of secretions. However, studies have failed to demonstrate the benefit of cool mist in the outcome of moderate to severe croup.[4, 5]

symptoms refer to an improvement in the child's condition for a short period after treatment, with a subsequent return to the pretreatment level of obstruction or deterioration to a more severe state a few hours later.

- ◦ Administer with supplemental oxygen.
- ◦ Cardiac monitoring is **required** due to the tachycardic effect and potential for dysrhythmias.

- Systemic steroids (such as dexamethasone 0.6 mg/kg, maximum dose 8 mg) are often used for mild to severe croup because of their anti-inflammatory effects and can be administered by way of nebulization and oral and intravenous routes.
- Heliox (a non-toxic gas that combines helium with oxygen) is an alternative therapy that may improve airflow through the respiratory tract in patients with a compromised airway. Although one small study has reported benefits from the use of heliox similar to those of racemic epinephrine[6], there is a lack of evidence to establish the effect of heliox inhalation in the treatment of croup in children.[7]
- The child with severe croup may progress to respiratory failure. If tracheal intubation is required, use a tracheal tube 0.5 to 1.0 mm smaller than that calculated for age because of the swelling and inflammation of the trachea at the subglottic level.

Unacceptable Interventions

- Failure to use personal protective equipment.
- Failure to recognize signs of respiratory distress and the need for interventions.
- Failure to allow the child to assume a position of comfort.
- Failure to measure oxygen saturation and give supplemental oxygen, if indicated.
- Agitating the child with the placement of an intravenous (IV) line, a facemask, blood pressure assessment, or medication administration unless the treatment is immediately lifesaving.
- Failure to assist ventilation with a bag-mask device and supplemental oxygen if signs of respiratory failure or respiratory arrest are present.
- Performing tracheal intubation in a child who responds to less invasive interventions.
- Failure to recognize signs of deterioration to respiratory failure or arrest and the need for more aggressive interventions.
- If tracheal intubation is required, failure to confirm tracheal tube position using assessment and mechanical methods.
- Failure to administer nebulized epinephrine (racemic or levo-epinephrine) to a child with moderate to severe croup.

- Failure to monitor the cardiac rhythm if signs of respiratory failure or respiratory arrest are present, or if epinephrine is administered.
- Medication errors.
- Ordering a dangerous or inappropriate intervention.
- Performing any technique resulting in potential harm to the patient.

Description

Epiglottitis is a bacterial infection of the upper airway that may progress to complete airway obstruction and death within hours unless adequate treatment is provided (Figure 3-8). Diagnosis is often based on history and observation of the child from a distance.

Epiglottitis is more accurately called acute supraglottitis, because inflammation of the supraglottic structures can cause the symptoms of epiglottitis, without actually involving the epiglottis.

Etiology

In the past, *Haemophilus influenzae* type b (HiB) was the most commonly identified cause of acute epiglottitis. Due to the widespread use of the HiB vaccine in the United States, the incidence of epiglottitis due to HiB in pediatric patients has been significantly reduced. *Streptococcus pyogenes*, *Streptococcus pneumoniae*, and *Staphylococcus aureus* now represent a larger proportion of pediatric cases of epiglottitis.

Epiglottitis

The "three Ds" (drooling, dysphagia, and distress) are considered the classical clinical findings of acute epiglottitis.

Drug Pearl
Epinephrine

- Epinephrine relaxes the smooth muscle of the bronchioles and reduces tissue swelling of related structures.
- Inhaled epinephrine may be used for children with stridor at rest, associated reduced air entry, and/or retractions.
- In anaphylaxis, epinephrine is administered by subcutaneous or intramuscular injection.
- Adverse reactions include transient, moderate anxiety, apprehensiveness, restlessness, tremor, weakness, dizziness, sweating, palpitations, pallor, nausea and vomiting, and headache.

PALS *Pearl*

- Generally, sedatives should not be used in the child with croup because (a) they can depress the respiratory drive and (b) restlessness is used as one means of evaluating the severity of airway obstruction and the need for intubation. Opiates should not be used because they may depress breathing and dry secretions.

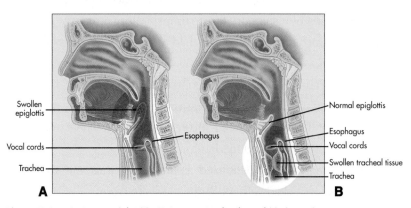

Figure 3-8   **A**, Acute epiglottitis. **B**, Laryngotracheobronchitis (croup).

Epidemiology and Demographics

- Can occur at any age; typically affects children 2 to 7 years of age.
- Decreased incidence in children because of widespread use of *H. influenzae* vaccine; increasing prevalence in adolescents and adults.
- No seasonal preference.

History

- Absence of a cough is an important diagnostic clue.
- Sudden onset of high fever.
- Typically, no other family members are ill with an acute upper respiratory illness.

Physical Examination

- Vital signs: increased ventilatory rate, increased heart rate, elevated temperature, usually 102° F to 104° F (38.89° C to 40° C).
- Difficulty swallowing, sore throat, drooling.
- Muffled voice.
- Shallow breathing.
- Prefers to sit up and lean forward (tripod position), with the mouth open (Figure 3-9).
- Stridor is a late finding and suggests near-complete airway obstruction.
- Child appears acutely ill ("toxic").

Acceptable Interventions

Because an aggressive physical examination, attempt to visualize the epiglottis, laboratory tests, or IV placement can precipitate complete airway obstruction, these procedures should be deferred until the diagnosis of epiglottitis is confirmed and the airway is secured. Close observation and frequent reassessment are essential.

- Use personal protective equipment.
- Perform an initial assessment and obtain a focused history.
- Assist the child into a position of comfort, usually sitting up on the caregiver's lap.
- Avoid agitating the child. Keep the child as calm and as comfortable as possible, usually in the arms of the caregiver.
- Do not examine the oropharynx (may agitate the child and worsen respiratory distress).
- Initiate pulse oximetry.
- If ventilation is adequate and the patient exhibits signs of respiratory distress, give supplemental oxygen in a manner that does not agitate the child. If signs of respiratory failure or respiratory arrest are present, assist ventilation using a bag-mask device with supplemental oxygen. Maintain an oxygen saturation of 94% or higher.
- Do not administer anything by mouth.

The child's muffled voice may be referred to as "hot potato" voice because it sounds as if the child is talking with a hot potato in his or her mouth.

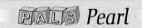 *Pearl*

Never force a child with respiratory distress to lie down. This may compromise the airway and cause immediate obstruction.

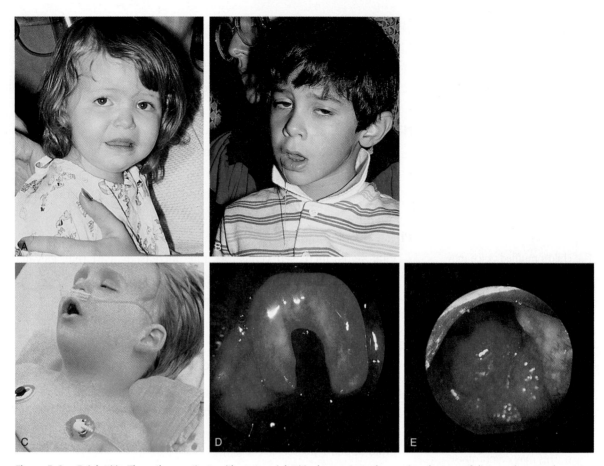

Figure 3-9   Epiglottitis. These three patients with acute epiglottitis demonstrate the varying degrees of distress that may be seen, depending on age and time of presentation. **A,** This 3-year-old seen a few hours after the onset of symptoms was anxious and still but had no positional preference or drooling. **B,** This 5-year-old, who had been symptomatic for several hours, holds his neck extended with the head held forward, is mouth breathing and drooling, and shows signs of tiring. **C,** This 2-year-old was in severe distress and was too exhausted to hold his head up. **D** and **E,** In the operating room, the epiglottis was visualized and appears intensely red and swollen. It may retain its omega shape or resemble a cherry.

- Management options:[8]
    - If the child is unstable (unresponsive, cyanotic, bradycardic), the clinician most skilled in pediatric intubation should emergently intubate. Tracheal intubation should be performed using a tracheal tube 0.5 to 1 mm smaller than that calculated for age.
    - If the child is stable with a high suspicion of epiglottitis, the patient should be escorted with an epiglottitis team (e.g., senior pediatrician, anesthesiologist, critical care intensivist, and otolaryngologist) for endoscopy and intubation under general anesthesia.
    - If the child is stable with a moderate or low suspicion of epiglottitis, and no evidence of obstruction exists, some clinicians prefer to obtain a radiograph of the nasopharynx and upper airway before direct visualization of the pharynx.

- ◦ A child with suspected epiglottitis should be accompanied by a clinician capable of intubating the patient and intubation equipment *at all times*, including the trip to and from the radiology department.
- ◦ The radiograph may show swelling of the epiglottis, also known as the "thumb" sign, because it resembles the size and shape of the human thumb (Figure 3-10); however, in many patients, the lateral neck film may not be diagnostic.[9]
- After the airway is secured, an IV should be established and fluid therapy begun. Blood cultures, cultures of the epiglottis and supraglottic surfaces, and other tests may be performed and antibiotic therapy started. The patient should be monitored in the intensive care unit (ICU).

Unacceptable Interventions

- Failure to use personal protective equipment.
- Failure to recognize signs of respiratory distress and the need for interventions.
- Failure to allow the child to assume a position of comfort.
- Failure to measure oxygen saturation and give supplemental oxygen, if indicated.
- Agitating the child with the placement of an IV line, a facemask, blood pressure assessment, or medication administration unless the treatment is immediately lifesaving.
- Failure to assist ventilation with a bag-mask device and supplemental oxygen if signs of respiratory failure or respiratory arrest are present.
- Failure to reassess respiratory status after initiating assisted ventilations.
- Performing tracheal intubation in a child who responds to less invasive interventions.

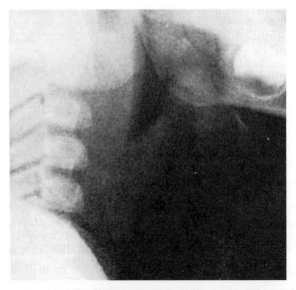

Figure 3-10 Epiglottitis. A lateral radiograph of the upper airway reveals a swollen epiglottis.

- Failure to recognize signs of deterioration to respiratory failure or arrest and the need for more aggressive interventions.
- Failure to monitor the cardiac rhythm if signs of respiratory failure or respiratory arrest are present.
- Failure to ensure a child with suspected epiglottitis is accompanied to and from the radiology department by a clinician capable of intubating the patient and with appropriate equipment.
- If tracheal intubation is required, failure to confirm tracheal tube position using assessment and mechanical methods.
- Attempting a needle or surgical cricothyrotomy before attempting assisted ventilations via bag-mask or tracheal tube and supplemental oxygen.
- Ordering a dangerous or inappropriate intervention.
- Performing any technique resulting in potential harm to the patient.

Bacterial Tracheitis

Description

Bacterial tracheitis (also called membranous tracheitis or pseudomembranous croup) is an acute bacterial infection of the subglottic area of the upper airway that can cause a life-threatening airway obstruction. The diagnosis is based on evidence of bacterial upper airway disease, high fever, purulent airway secretions, and an absence of the classic findings of epiglottitis.

Etiology

Bacterial tracheitis is most often caused by *Staphylococcus aureus* and *Streptococcus pyogenes.*[1]

Epidemiology and Demographics

- Bacterial tracheitis can occur at any age and in any season.[10]
- There are no clear gender differences in incidence or severity.
- Controversy exists as to whether bacterial tracheitis exists alone, or whether it is a bacterial complication of a preexistent viral respiratory infection (such as croup).
- This life-threatening illness is now more common than epiglottitis.[2]

History

- The patient with bacterial tracheitis frequently has a several-day history of viral upper respiratory symptoms, such as fever, cough, and stridor, similar to croup. This may be followed by a rapid onset of high fever, respiratory distress, and a toxic appearance. Drooling is usually absent.
- Patients frequently have concurrent sites of infection, with pneumonia being the most common.
- Bacterial tracheitis is associated with swelling of the mucosa at the level of the cricoid cartilage that is complicated by copious thick, purulent secretions. The child may decompensate quickly due to airway obstruction from a purulent membrane that has loosened.

Signs and symptoms are usually intermediate between epiglottitis and croup.

The usual treatments for croup are ineffective for bacterial tracheitis. Close observation and frequent reassessment are essential.

Physical Examination

- Inspiratory stridor with or without expiratory stridor.
- Barklike or brassy cough.
- Hoarseness.
- Variable degrees of respiratory distress: retractions, dyspnea, nasal flaring, and cyanosis.
- Sore throat (minimal).
- Dysphonia.
- Typically, no drooling.
- Worsening or abruptly occurring stridor or respiratory distress.

Acceptable Interventions

- Use personal protective equipment.
- Perform an initial assessment and obtain a focused history.
- Assist the child into a position of comfort.
- Avoid agitating the child. Keep the child as calm and as comfortable as possible, usually in the arms of the caregiver.
- Initiate pulse oximetry.
- If ventilation is adequate and the patient exhibits signs of respiratory distress, give supplemental oxygen in a manner that does not agitate the child. Maintain an oxygen saturation of 94% or higher. If signs of respiratory failure or respiratory arrest are present, assist ventilation using a bag-mask device with supplemental oxygen.
- If required, tracheal intubation should be performed using a tracheal tube 0.5 to 1 mm smaller than that calculated for age because of the swelling and inflammation of the trachea at the subglottic level. Frequent suctioning is often necessary to maintain the patency of the tube.
- After the airway is secured, establish IV access and begin antibiotic therapy.

Unacceptable Interventions

- Failure to use personal protective equipment.
- Failure to recognize signs of respiratory distress and the need for interventions.
- Failure to allow the child to assume a position of comfort.
- Failure to measure oxygen saturation and give supplemental oxygen, if indicated.
- Agitating the child with the placement of an IV line, a facemask, blood pressure assessment, or medication administration unless the treatment is immediately lifesaving.
- Failure to assist ventilation with a with a bag-mask and supplemental oxygen if signs of respiratory failure or respiratory arrest are present.
- Performing tracheal intubation in a child who responds to less invasive

interventions.

- Failure to recognize signs of deterioration to respiratory failure or arrest and the need for more aggressive interventions.
- Failure to monitor the cardiac rhythm if signs of respiratory failure or respiratory arrest are present.
- If tracheal intubation is required, failure to confirm tracheal tube position using assessment and mechanical methods.
- If suctioning is required, failure to limit suctioning to 10 seconds or less per attempt.
- Ordering a dangerous or inappropriate intervention.
- Performing any technique resulting in potential harm to the patient.

Description

Foreign Body Airway Obstruction

Foreign body airway obstruction (FBAO) may be seen at any age, but children younger than 5 years of age are especially vulnerable. One third of aspirated objects are nuts, particularly peanuts.[11] Laryngotracheal foreign bodies typically produce an acute obstruction. A foreign body in a bronchus may result in a more subtle presentation.

Etiology

- Common causes of foreign body aspiration in children include small foods such as nuts, raisins, sunflower seeds, watermelon seeds, popcorn, and improperly chewed pieces of meat, grapes, hot dogs, raw carrots, or sausages. Other items commonly found in the home that may cause FBAO include disc batteries, pins, rings, nails, buttons, coins, plastic or metal toy objects, and marbles (Figure 3-11).
  - Grapes, hot dogs, sausages, and balloons are more likely to cause tracheal obstruction and asphyxiation because they are round or smooth, or both.
  - Popular fruit-flavored gel snacks have been associated with an increased risk of aspiration in children.[12]
  - Hot dogs and bread are two of the most common causes of fatal aspiration.
- Because they absorb moisture, dried foods (such as beans and peas) may cause progressive airway obstruction.
- Peanut butter is particularly difficult to remove by coughing or with the use of instruments.

Epidemiology and Demographics

- Although an FBAO can occur in individuals of any age, it occurs most often in children younger than 5 years. Children younger than 3 years account for 73% of cases of FBAO.[11]
- Children are at risk of FBAO because of the following:
  - They are inherently curious.

Ages at highest risk of FBAO: 6 months to 5 years.

"A positive history must never be ignored. A negative history may be misleading."[12]
Suspect foreign body airway obstruction in any previously well, afebrile child with a sudden onset of respiratory distress and associated coughing, choking, stridor, or wheezing.

Children will eat, swallow, and place into any body cavity anything they can get hold of, even if it is "yucky" tasting or "yucky" appearing. Never doubt that they could or would!

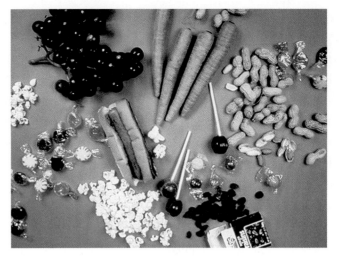

Figure 3-11 Common causes of foreign body aspiration in children include small foods such as nuts, raisins, sunflower seeds, popcorn, and improperly chewed pieces of meat, grapes, hot dogs, raw carrots, or sausages. Other items commonly found in the home that may cause foreign body airway obstruction include disc batteries, pins, rings, nails, buttons, coins, plastic or metal toy objects, and marbles.

- Infants and young children learn about their world by putting an object in their mouth.
- They lack molar teeth, decreasing their ability to sufficiently chew food.
- They tend to talk, laugh, and run while chewing.
- Parents may have unrealistic expectations regarding what their child should be able to eat or do at a given age.
- In adults, an FBAO most often occurs during eating. In infants and children, most episodes of choking occur during eating or play. Occasionally, poor supervision by adults or older siblings is a contributing factor.

History
- Fewer than 50% of children will have a history of witnessed or suspected foreign body aspiration or a choking spell.
- Frequently, the child presents after a sudden episode of coughing or choking while eating with subsequent wheezing, coughing, or stridor.

Physical Examination
- General signs and symptoms:
  - Sudden onset of respiratory distress; abnormal respiratory sounds including wheezing, inspiratory stridor, or decreased breath sounds; coughing or gagging, agitation, cyanosis, facial petechiae may be present because of increased intrathoracic pressure.
- Laryngeal foreign body:
  - Croupy, hoarse cough; dysphagia; stridor; pain; inability to speak

The symptoms, physical findings, and complications produced by a foreign body depend on the following:
- The size and composition of the material aspirated (e.g., inert, caustic, organic)
- The location of the foreign body (i.e., esophagus, larynx, trachea, bronchus)
- The degree and duration of obstruction

(with profound obstruction); hemoptysis; dyspnea with wheezing; cyanosis.

- Tracheal foreign body (diagnosis often requires bronchoscopy):
  - Stridor, cough, hoarseness, dyspnea, cyanosis.
  - Choking and aspiration occurs in 90% of patients with tracheal foreign bodies, stridor in 60%, and wheezing in 50%. Postero-anterior and lateral soft-tissue neck radiographs (airway films) show abnormal findings in 92% of children, whereas chest radiographs show abnormal findings in only 58%.[11]
- Bronchial foreign body:
  - Cough, wheezing, limited chest expansion, dull (i.e., atelectasis) or hyperresonant (i.e., overinflation) percussion note, diminished breath sounds distal to the foreign body.
- Esophageal foreign body:
  - Dysphagia, food refusal, weight loss, drooling, emesis/hematemesis, foreign body sensation, chest pain, sore throat, stridor, cough, unexplained fever, altered mental status.

Acceptable Interventions

- Use personal protective equipment.
- Perform an initial assessment and obtain a focused history.
- If an FBAO is present, position the child to facilitate drainage and suction the mouth. If solid material is visualized, remove it with a gloved finger covered in gauze.
- If a foreign body obstruction is suspected but not visualized, clear the obstruction by performing abdominal thrusts (if the patient is 1 year of age or older) or back slaps and chest thrusts (if the patient is younger than 1 year).
- Insert an airway adjunct as needed to maintain an open airway.
- If ventilation is adequate and the patient exhibits signs of respiratory distress, give supplemental oxygen in a manner that does not agitate the child. Maintain an oxygen saturation of 94% or higher. If signs of respiratory failure or respiratory arrest are present, assist ventilation using a with bag-mask device and supplemental oxygen.

Unacceptable Interventions

- Failure to use personal protective equipment.
- Failure to recognize signs of respiratory distress and the need for interventions.
- Failure to correctly perform FBAO maneuvers, if indicated.
- Failure to assist ventilation with a bag-mask device with supplemental oxygen if signs of respiratory failure or respiratory arrest are present.

Interventions depend on whether the patient is an infant or a child and conscious or unconscious. Procedures to relieve a FBAO are discussed in Chapter 4.

A comparison of upper-airway emergencies is shown in Table 3-5.

- Failure to recognize signs of deterioration to respiratory failure or arrest and the need for more aggressive interventions.
- Performing tracheal intubation in a child who responds to less invasive interventions.
- Ordering a dangerous or inappropriate intervention.
- Performing any technique resulting in potential harm to the patient.

TABLE 3-5 *Comparison of Upper Airway Emergencies*

	Croup	**Epiglottitis**	**Bacterial Tracheitis**	**Foreign Body**
Age	6 mo to 3 y	2 to 7 y	Any age	Younger than 5 y most common
Cause	Viral	Bacterial	Bacterial	Food, toys, coins
Incidence	80%	8%	2%	2%
Seasonal preference	Late fall, early winter	None	None	None
Onset	Gradual	Sudden	Gradual	Sudden
Fever	Low	High	High	No
Appearance	Nontoxic	Toxic	Toxic	Varies depending on location
Posture	No preference	Upright, leaning forward, drooling	Upright	Varies depending on location
Sore throat	No	Yes	Minimal	Varies depending on location
Cry	Bark, stridor	Muffled	Bark, stridor	Varies depending on location

Common Pediatric Lower Airway Emergencies

Asthma is a reversible obstructive airway disease characterized by chronic inflammation, hyperreactive airways, and episodes of bronchospasm.

Wheezing occurs commonly in young children and has been associated with certain viral infections. Due to emotional, financial, and other implications involved with a diagnosis of asthma, some physicians have been reluctant to call these children "asthmatics." Therefore, they sometimes call the clinical presentation, "reactive airway disease," or RAD.[13]

Etiology

- Allergens trigger the release of immunoglobulin E (IgE), causing mast cell release of histamine and other inflammatory mediators. The resulting edema of the bronchial mucosa, bronchospasm, cellular infiltration, and mucus plugging vary in severity depending on the age of the child, the size and anatomy of the airways, the type of irritant that precipitates the obstruction, and the duration and severity of the asthma attack.[14]

  - The increased work of breathing caused by use of accessory muscles and increased obstruction to airflow results in increased oxygen consumption and cardiac output.

  - This level of exertion is difficult for young children to maintain because of their small glycogen reserves and the likelihood that caloric intake is inadequate because of illness.

  - In most children, both larger and smaller airways are obstructed. The obstruction results from hypertrophy of smooth muscle, inflammatory exudate, and mucus plugs. Ineffective ventilation results in hypoxemia, which stimulates hyperventilation with hypocapnia and respiratory alkalosis.

    - As the obstruction becomes more severe, there is air trapping, inadequate ventilation, more severe hypoxemia, and hypercapnia (hypoventilation) with respiratory acidosis. Respiratory failure is imminent.

Epidemiology and Demographics

- Asthma is the most common pediatric chronic disease, affecting nearly 5 million children younger than 18 years in the United States.[15]
- Although allergens play an important role in asthma, 20% to 40% of children with asthma have no evidence of allergic disease.[16]
- The prevalence of asthma is greater in African Americans than in whites.

Asthma/Reactive Airway Disease

Upper airway obstruction typically produces *inspiratory* symptoms whereas lower airway obstruction produces more *expiratory* symptoms.

Risk factors for death from asthma include the following:
- History of sudden severe exacerbations
- Prior intubation for asthma
- Prior admission for asthma to an intensive care unit
- Two or more hospitalizations for asthma in the past year
- Three or more emergency care visits for asthma in the past year
- Hospitalization or emergency department visit for asthma in past month
- Use of more than two metered-dose inhaler (MDI) canisters of short-acting inhaled β_2-agonist per month
- Current use of oral corticosteroids or recent withdrawal from oral corticosteroids
- Serious psychiatric disease, including depression, or psychosocial problems
- Difficulty perceiving airflow obstruction or its severity

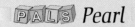 *Pearl*

Poor perception of the severity of asthma on the part of the patient and healthcare professional has been cited as a major factor causing delay in treatment and may contribute to increased severity and mortality from asthma exacerbations.[17]

Evaluate the asthma patient's ability to complete a sentence (age dependent), presence of a cough, breathlessness, and chest tightness. Assess pulse rate, ventilatory rate, breath sounds, use of accessory muscles, and presence of suprasternal retractions. Close monitoring is *essential*.

- Factors influencing asthma development and factors that trigger asthma symptoms (some do both) include the following:
  - Personal or family history of asthma or allergy.
  - Viral respiratory infections.
  - Indoor allergens (domestic mites, furred animals, cockroach allergen, fungi, molds, yeasts).
  - Outdoor allergens (pollens, fungi, molds, yeasts).
  - Occupational sensitizers.
  - Tobacco smoke.
  - Air pollution.
  - Diet.

History
- Recurrent respiratory symptoms (cough, wheeze, difficulty breathing, chest tightness) that are often worse at night.
- Wheezing, chest tightness, or cough after exposure to airborne allergens or pollutants.
- Symptoms occur or worsen in the presence of exercise, viral infections, animals with fur (dogs, cats, mice), house dust mites, molds, smoke (tobacco, wood), pollen, changes in weather, and strong emotional depression (Table 3-6).

Physical Examination
- Wheezing (most common finding).
- Dry cough.
- Chest tightness.
- Shortness of breath with exertion.
- Retractions.
- Tachypnea.
- Poor air entry.
- Prolonged expiratory phase.

Acceptable Interventions
Goals of treatment are to reverse bronchospasm, improve hypoxia, and correct dehydration.
- Use personal protective equipment.
- Perform an initial assessment and obtain a focused history.
- Assist the child into a position of comfort.
- Initiate pulse oximetry.
- If ventilation is adequate and the patient exhibits signs of respiratory distress, give supplemental oxygen in a manner that does not agitate the child. Maintain an oxygen saturation of 95% or higher. If signs of respiratory failure or respiratory arrest are present, assist ventilation using a bag-mask device with supplemental oxygen.

Continue monitoring oxygen saturation until a clear response to therapy has occurred.

An infant or young child can become quickly dehydrated because of an increased ventilatory rate and decreased oral intake. Be sure to assess fluid status and treat appropriately.

TABLE 3-6 *Severity of Asthma Exacerbations*[a]

	Mild	Moderate	Severe	Respiratory Arrest Imminent
Symptoms				
Breathless	Walking	Talking Infant—softer shorter cry; difficulty feeding Prefers sitting	At rest Infant stops feeding	
Talks in	Sentences	Phrases	Words	
Alertness	May be agitated	Usually agitated	Usually agitated	Drowsy or confused
Signs				
Ventilatory rate	Increased	Increased	Often more than 30 breaths/min	
Accessory muscles and suprasternal retractions	Usually not	Usually	Usually	Paradoxic thoracoabdominal movement
Wheeze	Moderate, often only end expiratory	Loud	Usually loud	Absence of wheeze
Pulse/min (bpm)	Slower than 100	100 to 120	Faster than 120	Bradycardia
Functional Assessment				
PEF after initial bronchodilator % predicted or % personal best	Over 80%	Approximately 60% to 80%	< 60% predicted or personal best or response lasts < 2 h	
Pao$_2$ (on air) and/or	Normal Test not usually necessary	> 60 mm Hg	< 60 mm Hg Possible cyanosis	
Paco$_2$	< 45 mm Hg	< 45 mm Hg	> 45 mm Hg: Possible respiratory failure	
Sao$_2$% (on air)	> 95%	91% to 95%	< 90%	
	Hypercapnia (hypoventilation) develops more readily in young children than in adults and adolescents.			

Adapted from *Global Initiative for Asthma*, Revised for 2009; http://ginasthma.org/Guidelineitem.asp??l1=2&l2=1&intID=1561, Accessed 8/19/2010.
bpm, beats per minute; PEF, peak expiratory flow; SaO$_2$, saturation oxygen.
[a]Note: The presence of several parameters, but not necessarily all, indicates the general classification of the exacerbation.

- Place the child on a cardiac monitor.
- Obtain vascular access if the patient shows signs of severe respiratory distress, respiratory failure, or respiratory arrest.
- If the patient shows signs of respiratory distress or respiratory failure with clinical evidence of bronchospasm or a history of asthma, give an inhaled rapid-acting β2-agonist continuously for 1 hour. Watch for tachycardia and vomiting.

PALS *Pearl*

- Wheezing is an unreliable sign when evaluating the degree of distress in an asthmatic patient. An absence of wheezing may represent severe obstruction. With improvement, wheezing may become more prominent.

- In infants, breathlessness sufficiently severe to prevent feeding is an important symptom of impending respiratory failure.

In children with asthma, PEF can be normal as airflow obstruction and gas trapping worsen. Therefore PEF can underestimate the degree of airflow obstruction.

- Evaluate the patient's response to the initial inhaled albuterol treatments.
  - Because peak expiratory flow (PEF) measurements require the child's cooperation in making a maximal expiratory effort (and coaching by a person trained in making these measurements), PEF measurements are used to assess the severity of an episode and the response to therapy in children older than 5 years.
  - The effort required to produce a PEF measurement is a full inspiration to total lung capacity followed by a short maximal exhalation in a standing position. PEF measurements should be compared with the patient's own previous best measurements.

Many asthma medications (e.g., glucocorticosteroids, β_2-agonists, theophylline) are metabolized faster in children than in adults, and young children tend to metabolize drugs faster than older children do.

- Administer systemic glucocorticosteroids if no immediate response, if the patient recently took an oral glucocorticosteroid, or if the episode is severe. The time to peak effect of systemic corticosteroids is at least 4 hours. The early use of steroids can shorten recovery time and reduce the need for hospitalization or shorten the hospital stay.
- Tracheal intubation may be necessary in the asthmatic patient with acute respiratory failure.

Drug Pearl
Albuterol (Proventil, Ventolin)

- Albuterol is a sympathomimetic bronchodilator that possesses a relatively selective specificity for β_2 (pulmonary) receptors and therefore is less likely to cause unwanted cardiovascular effects.
- Before administration, inquire about the medications the patient may have already taken. If the patient has been using an inhaler, ascertain the frequency and last application.
- The onset of action of inhaled bronchodilators is within

5 minutes. Their duration of action in severe asthma and may vary with the severity of the disease.
- Continuous cardiac monitoring is essential during bronchodilator administration because these medications may cause tachycardia and other dysrhythmias.
- After administration, reassess pulse and ventilatory rate, oxygen saturation, and peak expiratory flow rate. Any deterioration may require prompt intervention.

Drug Pearl
Methylxanthines

- Methylxanthines (e.g., theophylline, aminophylline) produce bronchodilation, increase pulmonary blood flow, and strengthen diaphragmatic contractions (reduce diaphragm fatigue). In higher doses, methylxanthines increase heart rate (chronotropy) and force of contraction (inotropy).
- Methylxanthines have an equivalent bronchodilator effect to inhaled β-2 agonists, but because of increased adverse effects, methylxanthines should only be considered as an alternative therapy.
- Before administration, obtain a theophylline level if the child is currently receiving a theophylline preparation.
- Assess the patient's ventilatory rate, tidal volume, breath sounds, heart rate, electrocardiogram (ECG) findings, and blood pressure before, during, and after administration. Continuous ECG monitoring is essential during administration of methylxanthines. Watch closely for signs of cardiac irritability, particularly premature ventricular complexes (PVCs) and tachycardia.
- Hypotension may occur following rapid administration.

- If the patient is experiencing a moderate episode (PEF 60% to 80% predicted/personal best, physical examination reveals moderate symptoms, accessory muscle use), give oxygen, an inhaled β2 agonist and inhaled anticholinergic every 60 minutes, and oral glucocorticosteroids; continue for 1 to 3 hours, provided there is improvement.

- If the patient is experiencing a severe episode (PEF less than 60% predicted/personal best, physical examination reveals severe symptoms at rest, chest retractions; history of high-risk patient; no improvement after initial treatment), give oxygen, an inhaled β2 agonist and inhaled anticholinergic, systemic glucocorticosteroids, and IV magnesium.

- Nonpharmacologic interventions:
  - Environmental control.
  - Irritant and allergen avoidance.

Unacceptable Interventions

- Failure to use personal protective equipment.
- Failure to recognize signs of respiratory distress and the need for interventions.
- Failure to allow the child to assume a position of comfort.
- Failure to measure oxygen saturation and give supplemental oxygen, if indicated.
- Failure to administer a bronchodilator for a child in respiratory distress with a history of asthma.

Drug Pearl
Ipratropium Bromide (Atrovent)

- Ipratropium bromide (Atrovent) blocks the contraction of bronchiolar smooth muscle and the increase in mucous secretion resulting from increased vagal (i.e., parasympathetic) activity.
- Anticholinergics produce preferential dilation of the larger central airways, in contrast to β-agonists, which affect the peripheral airways.
- Continuous cardiac monitoring is essential during bronchodilator administration because these medications may cause tachycardia and other dysrhythmias.
- After administration, reassess pulse and ventilatory rate, oxygen saturation, and peak expiratory flow rate.

Injectable β₂-agonists tend to produce more adverse effects (tachycardia, headache, tremor) than inhaled agents do.

PEDIATRIC ASTHMA ALGORITHM

Perform an initial assessment

• **Mild episode** = PEF >
80% predicted or personal
best

• **Moderate episode** = PEF
60 to 80%
predicted/personal best,
physical exam reveals
moderate symptoms,
accessory muscle use

• **Severe episode** = < 60%
predicted / personal best,
physical exam reveals
severe symptoms at rest,
chest retractions; history
of high-risk patient; no
improvement after initial
treatment

• Permit the child to assume a position of comfort
• Attach pulse oximeter and ECG monitor, assess peak expiratory flow (PEF) rate
• Administer oxygen; establish vascular access if the patient shows signs of severe
  respiratory distress, respiratory failure, or respiratory arrest

Initial Treatment*
• Give oxygen to achieve O_2 saturation of 95% or greater
• Inhaled rapid-acting β_2-agonist, continuously for 1 hour
• Systemic glucocorticosteroids if no immediate response, or if patient recently
  took oral glucocorticosteroid, or if episode is severe

• Assess clinical signs of respiratory distress including pulse and ventilatory rate,
  oxygen saturation, and peak expiratory flow (PEF) rate. Any deterioration may
  require prompt intervention.
• Treatment for moderate episode includes oxygen, inhaled β2 agonist and inhaled
  anticholinergic every 60 minutes, and oral glucocorticosteroids; continue for
  1 to 3 hours, provided there is improvement.
• Treatment for severe episode includes oxygen, inhaled β2 agonist and inhaled
  anticholinergic, systemic glucocorticosteroids, and IV magnesium.

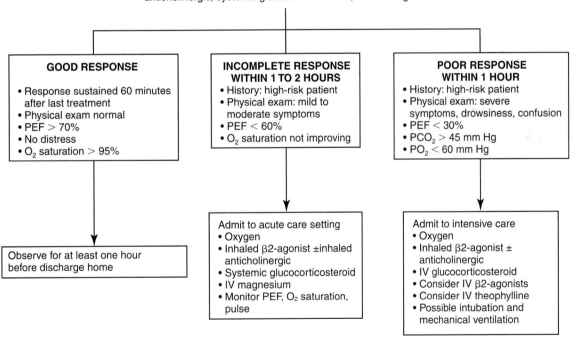

GOOD RESPONSE
• Response sustained 60 minutes
  after last treatment
• Physical exam normal
• PEF > 70%
• No distress
• O_2 saturation > 95%

INCOMPLETE RESPONSE WITHIN 1 TO 2 HOURS
• History: high-risk patient
• Physical exam: mild to
  moderate symptoms
• PEF < 60%
• O_2 saturation not improving

POOR RESPONSE WITHIN 1 HOUR
• History: high-risk patient
• Physical exam: severe
  symptoms, drowsiness, confusion
• PEF < 30%
• PCO_2 > 45 mm Hg
• PO_2 < 60 mm Hg

Observe for at least one hour
before discharge home

Admit to acute care setting
• Oxygen
• Inhaled β2-agonist ±inhaled
  anticholinergic
• Systemic glucocorticosteroid
• IV magnesium
• Monitor PEF, O_2 saturation,
  pulse

Admit to intensive care
• Oxygen
• Inhaled β2-agonist ±
  anticholinergic
• IV glucocorticosteroid
• Consider IV β2-agonists
• Consider IV theophylline
• Possible intubation and
  mechanical ventilation

Adapted from Global Initiative for Asthma, Revised 2009; http://ginasthma.org/Guidelineitem.asp??l1=2&l2=1&intId=1561,
Accessed 8/19/2010.

- Agitating the child with the placement of an IV line, a facemask, blood pressure assessment, or medication administration unless the treatment is immediately lifesaving.
- Failure to assist ventilation with a bag-mask device and supplemental oxygen if signs of respiratory failure or respiratory arrest are present.
- Performing tracheal intubation in a child who responds to less invasive interventions.
- Failure to recognize signs of deterioration to respiratory failure or arrest and the need for more aggressive interventions.
- Failure to monitor the cardiac rhythm if signs of respiratory failure or respiratory arrest are present, or if bronchodilators are administered.
- If tracheal intubation is required, failure to confirm tracheal tube position using assessment and mechanical methods.
- Failure to recognize signs of a tension pneumothorax.
- Medication errors.
- Ordering a dangerous or inappropriate intervention.
- Performing any technique resulting in potential harm to the patient.

Respiratory Syncytial Virus/Bronchiolitis

Bronchiolitis is an inflammation of the smaller bronchioles caused by a virus and characterized by thick mucus. It occurs primarily in late fall, winter, and early spring and is uncommon in children over 3 years of age. RSV is the primary cause of bronchiolitis and pneumonia in children younger than 1 year.

Etiology

- The cause of bronchiolitis is RSV in 45% to 75% of cases.
  - Parainfluenza viruses are the second most common cause.
  - Other agents that cause bronchiolitis include influenza virus, rhinovirus, adenovirus, and *Mycoplasma pneumoniae*.
- In bronchiolitis, airway obstruction is usually gradual and is caused by inflammation, secretions, and edema of varying degrees in the small bronchi and bronchioles. Areas of hyperinflation may exist with air trapping due to partial obstruction or areas of atelectasis or nonaeration resulting from total obstruction.
- RSV is highly contagious. The incubation period from exposure to first symptoms is about 4 days. The virus is shed in nasal secretions for varying periods, usually 5 to 12 days, although excretion of the virus for 3 weeks and longer has been documented.
  - RSV is spread from respiratory secretions through close contact with infected persons or contact with contaminated surfaces or objects. Infection can occur when infectious material contacts mucous membranes of the eyes, mouth, or nose, and possibly through the inhalation of droplets generated by a sneeze or cough.

Inflammation and edema make the small air passages in infants particularly vulnerable to obstruction.

- ◦ In the healthcare setting, RSV is often spread from child to child on the hands of caregivers.
- RSV in secretions can survive only a few hours on countertops, paper tissues, and cloth, and for 30 minutes on the skin. The virus is readily inactivated with soap and water and disinfectants.

Epidemiology and Demographics

- RSV occurs in yearly epidemics. In temperate climates, these epidemics occur each winter and last 4 to 5 months.
- RSV is most common in infants younger than 1 year.
- Fifty percent of all infants will be infected with RSV by the end of the first year of life. Infants 1 to 4 months old are at particular risk of severe infection and hospitalization.
- Almost all infants are infected by the virus by the end of their second winter, and half experience two infections during their first two winters.
- Risk factors for early-onset disease and subsequent hospitalization include low birth weight, prematurity, lower socioeconomic group, crowded living conditions, parental smoking, absence of breast feeding, chronic lung or cardiac conditions, and day care.

History

- URI with rhinorrhea and cough for several days.
  - Low-grade fever common.
  - Increasingly productive cough.
  - Increasing respiratory distress.
  - Caregiver often reports wheezing at home.
- Otitis media common.
- Contact with older siblings or children at day care who have viral respiratory symptoms.
- Hypoxemia in severe cases.
- Apnea may occur in former premature infants and infants younger than 4 months old.
- Family history of asthma or allergies.

Physical Examination

- RSV begins with signs and symptoms limited to an upper respiratory tract infection, such as rhinorrhea and pharyngitis.
  - Within 1 to 3 days, a cough usually appears and may be accompanied by sneezing and a low-grade (lower than 101° F) fever.
  - Wheezing develops soon after the cough appears and may be detectable without a stethoscope. Auscultation often reveals diffuse rhonchi, fine rales or crackles, and wheezes. A chest radiograph at this stage frequently has normal findings.
  - Mild cases of RSV may not progress beyond this stage.

Hand washing and the use of disposable gloves and gowns are important.

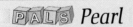 **PALS** *Pearl*

Because asthma and bronchiolitis present similarly, it may be difficult to distinguish between these conditions.

An RSV infection can affect any part of the respiratory tract.

- If RSV progresses, coughing and wheezing increase and air hunger follows. These signs and symptoms are accompanied by an increased respiratory rate, intercostal and subcostal retractions, hyperexpansion of the chest, restlessness, and peripheral cyanosis.
- Signs of dehydration (e.g., sunken eyes, dry mucous membranes, sunken fontanelle, and fatigue) may be present due to decreased fluid intake and increased fluid losses from fever and tachypnea.
- Tachypnea and tachycardia are often present.
- Signs of severe, life-threatening illness include central cyanosis, tachypnea of more than 70 breaths per minute, listlessness, and apnea spells.
  - At this stage, the chest may be greatly hyperexpanded and almost silent on auscultation because of poor air exchange.

Acceptable Interventions

- Use personal protective equipment.
- Perform an initial assessment and obtain a focused history.
- Assist the child into a position of comfort, usually sitting up on the caregiver's lap.
- Avoid agitating the child. Keep the child as calm and as comfortable as possible, usually in the arms of the caregiver.
- Initiate pulse oximetry.
- If ventilation is adequate and the patient exhibits signs of respiratory distress, give supplemental oxygen in a manner that does not agitate the child. Titrate oxygen therapy to maintain an oxygen saturation of 94% or higher. If signs of respiratory failure or respiratory arrest are present, assist ventilation using a bag-mask device with supplemental oxygen.
- Mild dehydration is often present. Fluid replacement is important; however, excessive fluid replacement may encourage interstitial edema formation. Close monitoring is essential.
- Severe episodes may require oxygen therapy, bronchodilators, and corticosteroids.

Oxygen administration and supportive care with fluid replacement are the mainstays of treatment.

Unacceptable Interventions

- Failure to use personal protective equipment.
- Failure to recognize signs of respiratory distress and the need for interventions.
- Failure to allow the child to assume a position of comfort.
- Failure to measure oxygen saturation and give supplemental oxygen, if indicated.
- Agitating the child with the placement of an IV line, a facemask, blood pressure assessment, or medication administration unless the treatment is immediately lifesaving.

- Failure to assist ventilation with a bag-mask device and supplemental oxygen if signs of respiratory failure or respiratory arrest are present.
- Failure to recognize signs of deterioration to respiratory failure or arrest and the need for more aggressive interventions.
- Performing tracheal intubation in a child who responds to less invasive interventions.
- Failure to monitor the cardiac rhythm if signs of respiratory failure or respiratory arrest are present, or if bronchodilators are administered.
- If tracheal intubation is required, failure to confirm tracheal tube position using assessment and mechanical methods.
- Medication errors.
- Ordering a dangerous or inappropriate intervention.
- Performing any technique resulting in potential harm to the patient.

Case Study Resolution

This child is sick. His presentation is consistent with acute bronchospasm. Move quickly. Use personal protective equipment. Perform an initial assessment and obtain a focused history. Assist the child into a position of comfort. Initiate pulse oximetry (initial SpO_2 on room air was 84%). Correct hypoxia by giving supplemental oxygen in a manner that does not agitate the child (blow-by oxygen was administered while the child was seated in mom's lap). Place the child on a cardiac monitor. Give nebulized albuterol and assess response. Begin assisted ventilation and establish vascular access if the child does not improve. Provide further interventions on the basis of assessment findings and the patient's response to therapy.

References

1. Sobol SE, Zapata S. Epiglottitis and Croup. Otolaryngol Clin North Am. 2008 Jun;41(3):551-66, ix. Review.
2. Roosevelt GE. Acute inflammatory upper airway obstruction. In: Behrman RE, Kliegman RM, Jenson HB, eds. *Nelson textbook of pediatrics,* 18th ed. Philadelphia: WB Saunders, 2007.
3. Wright RB, Pomerantz WJ, Joseph W. et al. New approaches to respiratory infections in children: bronchiolitis and croup. *Emerg Med Clin* North Am 2002;20:93–114.
4. Moore M, Little P. Humidified air inhalation for treating croup: a systematic review and meta-analysis. *Fam Pract* 2007;24(4):295–301.
5. Scolnik D, Coates AL, Stephens D, Da Silva Z, Lavine E, Schuh S. Controlled delivery of high vs low humidity vs. mist therapy for croup in emergency departments: a randomized controlled trial. *JAMA* 2006; 295:1274–80.

6. Weber JE, Chudnofsky CR, Younger JG. et al. A randomized comparison of helium-oxygen mixture (heliox) and racemic adrenaline for the treatment of moderate to severe croup. *Pediatrics* 2001;107:e96.

7. Vorwerk C, Coats T. Heliox for croup in children. Cochrane Database Syst Rev. 2010 Feb 17;2:CD006822.

8. Susil G. Respiratory emergencies. In: Custer JW, Rau RE, eds. *The Harriet Lane handbook: a manual for pediatric house officers,* 18th ed. Philadelphia: Mosby, 2009.

9. Barkin RM, Rosen P. Pulmonary disorders. In: Barkin RM, Rosen P, eds. *Emergency pediatrics: a guide to ambulatory care,* 5th ed. St. Louis: Mosby, 1999, pp. 786–788.

10. Schwartz RH. Infections related to the upper and middle airways. In: Long SS, ed. *Principles and practice of pediatric infectious diseases,* 3rd ed. Philadelphia: Churchill Livingstone, 2008.

11. Holinger LD. Foreign bodies of the airway. In: Behrman RE, Kliegman RM, Jenson HB, eds. *Nelson textbook of pediatrics,* 18th ed. Philadelphia: WB Saunders, 2007.

12. Oureshi S, Mink R. Aspiration of fruit gel snacks. *Pediatrics* 2003;111:687–689.

13. Hopp RJ. Recurrent wheezing in infants and young children: a perspective. *J Asthma* 1999;36:547–553.

14. Huether SE, McCance KL. Alterations of pulmonary function in children. In: Huether SE, McCance KL, eds. *Understanding pathophysiology,* 2nd ed. St. Louis: Mosby, 2000, pp. 775–788.

15. Lasley MV. Asthma. In: Kliegman RM, Marcdante KJ, Jenson HB, eds. *Nelson essentials of pediatrics,* 5th ed. Philadelphia: Elsevier, 2006.

16. Hueckel R, Wilson D. The child with respiratory dysfunction. In: Hockenberry MH, Wilson D, eds. *Wong's nursing care of infants and children,* 8th ed. Canada: Mosby, 2007.

17. Nowak RM, Pensler MI, Sarkar DD, et al. Comparison of peak expiratory flow and FEV1 admission criteria for acute bronchial asthma. *Ann Emerg Med* 1982;11:64–69.

Chapter Quiz

1. Which of the following should be suspected in any previously well, afebrile child with a sudden onset of respiratory distress and associated coughing, choking, stridor, or wheezing?
   A) Asthma.
   B) Epiglottitis.
   C) Foreign body airway obstruction.
   D) Croup.

2. Epiglottitis most commonly occurs in children _____ . Croup most commonly occurs in children _____ .
   A) 6 months to 3 years of age; 2 to 7 years of age.
   B) 3 months to 6 years of age; 6 to 12 years of age.
   C) 2 to 7 years of age; 6 months to 3 years of age.
   D) 6 to 12 years of age; 3 months to 6 years of age.

Questions 3–5 pertain to the following patient situation:

An 8-month-old infant presents with a cough, clear nasal discharge, and difficulty breathing. Mom states the infant has had a cold for the past 2 days. She is concerned because his breathing is "different" today and he has been feeding poorly. You note the infant appears tired and limp in his mother's arms and his color is dusky. His respiratory rate is rapid and shallow. Nasal flaring, and intercostal and subcostal retractions are visible.

3. From the information provided, complete the following documentation regarding the Pediatric Assessment Triangle:
   Appearance:
   Breathing:
   Circulation:

4. Your initial assessment reveals an open airway. The infant's ventilatory rate is 56/min. Auscultation of the chest reveals fine crackles and wheezes bilaterally. A brachial pulse is easily palpated at a rate of 148 beats/min. The skin is dusky and dry. Capillary refill is 2 to 3 seconds; temperature is 100.4°F. Based on the patient's age and clinical presentation, you suspect the patient has:
   A) Asthma
   B) Bronchiolitis
   C) Epiglottitis
   D) Pneumonia

5. Is this patient sick or not sick? Describe your approach to the initial management of this patient.

6. Which of the following is an *early* sign of impending respiratory difficulty?
   A) Delayed capillary refill.
   B) An increase in heart rate.
   C) An increase in ventilatory rate.
   D) A decrease in blood pressure.

7. The cough that accompanies croup is typically characterized as:
   A) A "whooping" sound.
   B) Barky (seal-like).
   C) Loose, productive.
   D) Brassy, dry.

8. Which of the following lists conditions that affect the upper airway?
    A) Bacterial tracheitis, epiglottitis, pneumonia.
    B) Bronchiolitis, croup, asthma.
    C) Asthma, bronchiolitis, pneumonia.
    D) Croup, epiglottitis, bacterial tracheitis.

Chapter Quiz Answers

1. C. Suspect a foreign body airway obstruction (FBAO) in any previously well, afebrile child with a sudden onset of respiratory distress and associated coughing, choking, stridor, or wheezing.

2. C. Epiglottitis most commonly occurs in children 2 to 7 years of age. Croup most commonly occurs in children 6 months to 3 years of age.

3. Pediatric Assessment Triangle (first impression) findings:
    Appearance: Awake but appears tired and limp
    Breathing: Respirations are rapid and shallow; increased work of breathing evident
    Circulation: Skin color is dusky; no evidence of bleeding

4. B. The patient's age and clinical presentation are consistent with bronchiolitis/respiratory syncytial virus (RSV). In bronchiolitis, airway obstruction is usually gradual and is caused by inflammation, secretions, and edema of varying degrees in the small bronchi and bronchioles. Inflammation and edema make the small air passages in infants particularly vulnerable to obstruction.

5. This infant is sick. Move quickly. Open the airway and suction if necessary. Correct hypoxia by giving supplemental oxygen. Begin assisted ventilation if the patient does not improve. Provide further interventions based on assessment findings.

6. C. An increase in the ventilatory rate (tachypnea) is an early sign of impending respiratory difficulty.

7. B. The cough that accompanies croup is typically described as barky or seal-like.

8. D. Croup, epiglottitis, and bacterial tracheitis are conditions that affect the upper airway. Pneumonia, asthma, and bronchiolitis are conditions that affect the lower airway.

Respiratory Interventions

4

Case Study

A 4-year-old girl has a fever and difficulty breathing. Mom states the child has had a cough and runny nose for the past 3 to 4 days, and the cough appears to be getting worse. Several family members have had symptoms of a cold recently. The child had a fever of 104° F yesterday that decreased to 101° F after she was given acetaminophen. Last night the child began breathing fast and her cough sounded "wet." The child's cough is productive for greenish-yellow sputum. Today she is "not acting right" and is having more difficulty breathing.

Using the Pediatric Assessment Triangle (PAT), your general impression reveals the child is awake, but is unconcerned about your presence. Her ventilatory rate is faster than normal for her age and shallow, and her skin is pale. The primary survey reveals the child is slow to respond to your questions. Her airway is patent. Her ventilatory rate is approximately 65 per minute, shallow and labored. Capillary refill is 5 seconds and the extremities are cool in a warm environment. Peripheral pulses are weak and rapid. The skin is pale and dry.

Based on the information provided, is this child sick or not sick? What should you do next?

Objectives

1. Describe the head tilt–chin lift and jaw-thrust without head tilt methods for opening the airway.
2. Describe the preferred method of opening the airway in cases of suspected cervical spine injury.
3. Describe the procedures used to relieve foreign body airway obstruction (FBAO) in infants and children.
4. Describe correct suctioning technique and complications associated with this procedure.
5. Discuss oxygen delivery systems used for infants and children.
6. Describe the oxygen liter flow per minute and estimated oxygen percentage delivered for a nasal cannula, simple face mask, partial non-rebreather mask, nonrebreather mask, and bag-mask device.
7. Describe the method of correct sizing, insertion technique, and possible complications associated with insertion of the oropharyngeal

airway (OPA) and nasopharyngeal airway (NPA).

8. Discuss appropriate ventilation devices for infants and children.

9. Discuss complications of improper use of ventilation devices with infants and children.

10. Discuss appropriate tracheal intubation equipment for infants and children.

11. Describe methods to confirm correct placement of an advanced airway.

Airway Maneuvers

In the unresponsive patient, a partial airway obstruction may occur if

- The tongue falls back against the back of the throat due to a loss of muscle control.
- The epiglottis acts as a flap to obstruct the airway at the level of the larynx.

If the patient is breathing, snoring respirations are a characteristic sign of airway obstruction due to displacement of the tongue. In the apneic patient, airway obstruction due to the tongue may go undetected until ventilation is attempted.

Ventilating an apneic patient with an airway obstruction is difficult. If the airway obstruction is caused by the tongue, repositioning of the patient's head and jaw may be all that is needed to open the airway.

Overview

The head tilt–chin lift is the preferred technique for opening the airway of an unresponsive patient without suspected cervical spine injury.

- Indications.
  - Unresponsive patient who does not have a mechanism for cervical spine injury.
  - Unresponsive patient who is unable to protect his or her own airway.
- Contraindications.
  - Awake patient.
  - Known or suspected cervical spine injury.
- Procedure.
  - Place the patient in a supine position.
  - Place the hand closest to the child's head on the forehead. Apply firm downward pressure with your palm to tilt the patient's head gently back into a neutral or slightly extended position (Figure 4-1).
  - Place the tips of the fingers of your other hand under the *bony* part of the patient's chin and gently lift the jaw upward and outward to open the airway.

Head Tilt–Chin Lift

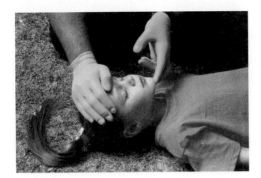

Figure 4-1   Head tilt–chin lift.

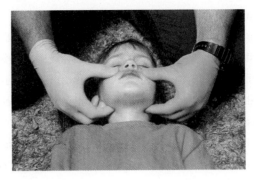

Figure 4-2   Jaw thrust without head tilt maneuver.

Studies have shown that this maneuver does cause some movement of the cervical spine. If an assistant is available, ask him or her to maintain manual in-line stabilization of the cervical spine to minimize movement of the head and neck when performing this maneuver.

The jaw thrust without head tilt maneuver is the preferred method of opening the airway when cervical spine injury is suspected.
- Indications.
  - Unresponsive patient with possible cervical spine injury.
  - Unable to protect own airway.
- Contraindications: Awake patient.
- Technique.
  - Place the patient in a supine position.
  - While stabilizing the patient's head in a neutral position, grasp the angles of the patient's lower jaw with both hands, one on each side, and displace the mandible forward (Figure 4-2).

Rescue Breathing

Assessment

- Assess the patient's level of responsiveness and quickly determine if the child is breathing. If the child is unresponsive and not breathing (or only gasping), check for a pulse. If no pulse is present, you are unsure if there is a pulse, or a pulse is present but the rate is slower than 60 beats per minute and there are signs of poor perfusion (i.e. pallor, mottling, cyanosis) despite support of oxygenation and ventilation, begin chest compressions.

Rescue Breathing

- If the child is responsive or unresponsive but has a pulse, determine if breathing is adequate or inadequate. Look for rise and fall of the chest and abdomen, and listen and feel for exhaled air. Rescue breathing should be performed if the patient has a pulse of 60 beats per minute or more but breathing is inadequate and should continue until adequate spontaneous breathing resumes.

- If ventilatory efforts are inadequate, the patient's breathing may be assisted by forcing air into the lungs (i.e., delivering positive pressure ventilations). Mouth-to-mouth, mouth-to-mask, and bag-mask ventilation (BMV) are methods that may be used to deliver positive pressure ventilation.

- Mouth-to-mouth ventilation is a basic method for providing positive pressure ventilation to apneic patients and requires no special equipment to perform. Mouth-to-mouth ventilation is capable of delivering excellent tidal volumes. Because expired air from your lungs contains approximately 16% oxygen, it will also deliver an adequate level of oxygen to the patient. To provide mouth-to-mouth ventilation, open the victim's airway, pinch the victim's nose, place your mouth over the victim's mouth, and create an airtight seal. Give two breaths, each breath given over 1 second, and give enough air to make the chest visibly rise. Take a regular breath before ventilating the victim. Taking deep breaths is unnecessary and may cause hyperventilation. If you experience difficulty in ventilating the victim (e.g., his chest does not rise with the first rescue breath), reposition his head and lift the chin, because an improperly opened airway is the most common cause of an inability to ventilate.

- A barrier device is a thin film of material, usually plastic or silicone, that is placed on the patient's face and used to prevent direct contact with the patient's mouth during positive pressure ventilation. One common type of barrier device is a face shield. A one-way valve or filter is present in the center of most face shields that diverts the patient's exhaled air away from you when you lift your mouth off the shield between breaths, reducing the risk of infection.

- The device used for mouth-to-mouth ventilation is commonly called a pocket mask, pocket face mask, ventilation face mask, or resuscitation mask. Mouth-to-mouth mask and bag-mask ventilation are discussed later in this chapter.

Although it has been said that the risk of disease transmission with mouth-to-mouth ventilation is very low[1], in this day of heightened awareness of communicable diseases, an issue of concern with this ventilation method is direct contact with oral secretions, possibly including blood. The U.S. Occupational Safety and Health Administration (OSHA) requires that healthcare professionals use standard precautions (such as a barrier device, pocket face mask, or bag-mask device) in the workplace, including during CPR.

Relief of Foreign Body Airway Obstruction

FBAO should be suspected in infants and children with a *sudden* onset of respiratory distress associated with coughing, gagging, stridor, or wheezing.

A "mild" airway obstruction is one in which the victim can cough or make some sounds.

- If the infant or child is conscious and maintaining his or her own airway *without* respiratory distress, do not interfere.
  - Allow the child to continue his or her efforts to attempt to clear the foreign body.
  - Allow the child to assume a position of comfort and administer supplemental oxygen if indicated.
  - Encourage the child to cough and provide emotional support.
  - Removal of the foreign body by bronchoscopy or laryngoscopy should be attempted in a controlled environment.
- If the infant or child is conscious and maintaining his or her own airway but respiratory distress is present, do not interfere.
  - Allow the child to continue his or her efforts to attempt to clear the foreign body.
  - Allow the child to assume a position of comfort and administer supplemental oxygen if indicated.
  - Encourage the child to cough and provide emotional support.
  - If the cough becomes ineffective and/or there is increasing respiratory difficulty accompanied by stridor, attempt to relieve the obstruction.

Performance Guidelines for a Conscious Choking Child

A "severe" airway obstruction is one in which the victim cannot cough or make any sound.

- Assess the infant. If the infant can cough or cry, watch him or her closely to ensure the object is expelled. If the infant is unable to cough or cry, provide care.
- Back slaps
  - While supporting the infant's head and neck, place the infant face down over one arm (Figure 4-3).
  - Position the infant's head slightly lower than the rest of the body.
  - Using the heel of one hand, deliver five back slaps forcefully between the infant's shoulder blades.
  - If the foreign body is not expelled, deliver chest thrusts.
- Chest thrusts
  - Support the infant's head and neck.
  - Position the infant between your hands and arms and turn the infant onto his or her back (Figure 4-4).
  - Imagine a line between the nipples. Place the flat part of your middle and ring fingers about one finger-width below this imaginary line. Deliver five quick downward chest thrusts.

Do not sweep the mouth unless the foreign body is visible. Blind sweeps may push the foreign body into the glottic opening, resulting in complete obstruction.

  - Check the patient's mouth. If the foreign body is seen, remove it. *Do NOT perform a blind finger sweep!*
- Open the airway and attempt rescue breathing.
  - If rescue breathing does not cause the infant's chest to rise, reposition the head and reattempt rescue breathing.

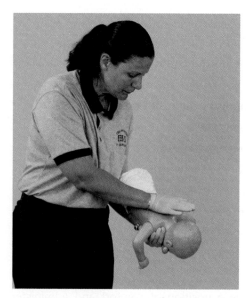

Figure 4-3   Back slaps and chest thrusts are used to dislodge an foreign body from a conscious infant's (under 1 year of age) airway. The infant is positioned prone on the rescuer's forearm with the head tilted slightly lower than the infant's torso. Support the infant's head at the chin. Avoid compressing the soft tissues under the chin because it can occlude the airway. With the heel of your other hand, deliver five forceful slaps to the middle of the back between the shoulder blades.

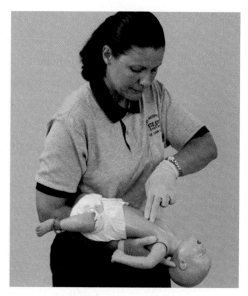

Figure 4-4   Next, while supporting the infant's head, transfer the infant to the other arm in the supine position. With the fingers of the rescuer's free hand, deliver five chest thrusts on the lower third of the infant's sternum. Repeat this sequence of maneuvers until the object is dislodged or the infant becomes unresponsive.

- If the chest does not rise (the airway remains obstructed), continue the sequence of five back slaps, five chest thrusts, and breathing attempts until the object is dislodged (and expelled) and rescue breathing is successful, or the victim becomes unconscious.

Performance Guidelines for an Unconscious Choking Infant or Child

- If the victim becomes unresponsive, begin CPR starting with chest compressions. Do not take the time to check for a pulse. After 30 chest compressions, open the airway. Look into the mouth and remove the foreign body, if visualized. Continue with cycles of chest compressions and ventilations until the object is expelled. Activate the emergency response system after 2 minutes if no one has already done so.
- If the obstruction is removed:
  - Assess breathing. Suction fluids and particulate matter if necessary. If the patient is breathing (and breathing is effective), turn the child to the side (recovery position) if trauma is not suspected (Figure 4-5). Many recovery positions have been used in the management of pediatric patients. The ideal position should enable maintenance of an open airway, maintenance of cervical spine stability, minimize the risk of aspiration, limit pressure on bony prominences and peripheral nerves, allow visualization of the child's ventilatory effort

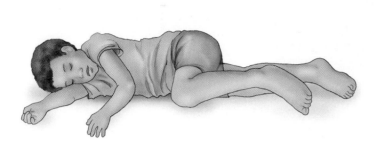

Figure 4-5 If the patient is breathing (and breathing is effective), turn the child to the side (recovery position) if trauma is not suspected.

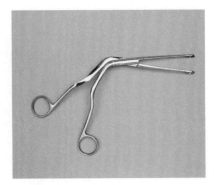

Figure 4-6 Magill forceps can be used to remove a visible foreign body.

and appearance, and permit access to the patient for procedures. Reassess frequently. If the patient is not breathing, give two breaths.

- Assess circulation.
  ○ If there is no pulse or other signs of circulation, or if the heart rate is less than 60 beats per minute with signs of poor perfusion, begin chest compressions.
  ○ If breathing is absent but a pulse is present, deliver one breath every 3 to 5 seconds (12 to 20 breaths per minute) and monitor the patient's pulse. Use the higher rate of ventilations for the younger child.
- Assess mental status.
- Expose as necessary to perform further assessments while maintaining the patient's body temperature.
- Perform a focused history and physical examination only if they will not interfere with lifesaving interventions.
- If basic airway maneuvers are not successful in clearing an obstructed airway:
  - Perform direct laryngoscopy (if you have been trained to do so) and attempt to locate the obstruction. Remove the foreign body using pediatric Magill forceps if it is clearly visible (Figure 4-6). If removal is successful, reassess breathing and resume bag–mask ventilation.
  - If unsuccessful, attempt tracheal intubation and ventilate the patient.
  - If child cannot be intubated, attempt bag–mask ventilation.
  - Needle crithyrotomy may be considered if complete airway obstruction exists and bag–mask ventilation is unsuccessful (check local protocol).
  - Removal of the foreign body by bronchoscopy should be attempted in a controlled environment.

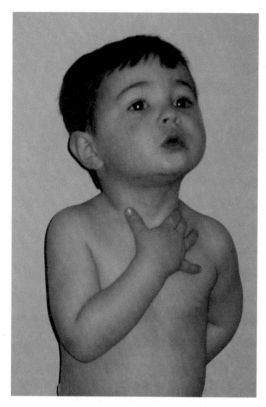

Figure 4-7   This child is demonstrating the universal distress signal for a choking emergency.

- The choking child may hold his neck or motion toward his throat with the thumb and fingers. This sign is the universal distress signal for a choking emergency (Figure 4-7). Assess the child's ability to speak or cough. Ask, "Are you choking?"
- If the child can cough or speak, watch him or her closely to ensure the object is expelled.
- If the child cannot cough or speak, perform abdominal thrusts (also called subdiaphragmatic thrusts or the Heimlich maneuver).
  - Stand or kneel behind the child and wrap your arms around the child's waist.
  - Abdominal thrusts should be delivered two finger's width above the naval. Make a fist with one hand. Place the fist thumb-side-in on the thrust site (Figure 4-8). Place your other hand on top of the fist (Figure 4-9). Perform a quick inward and upward thrust. Continue performing abdominal thrusts until the foreign body is expelled or the child becomes unresponsive.

Performance Guidelines for a Conscious Choking Child

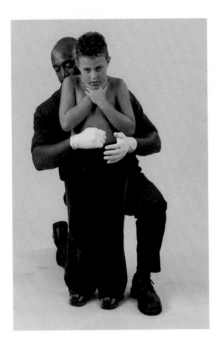

Figure 4-8   Stand or kneel directly behind the child. Place the flat, thumb side of one fist against the child's abdomen in the midline, slightly above the navel and well below the tip of the xiphoid process.

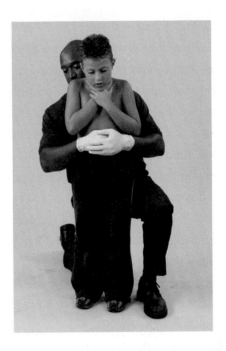

Figure 4-9   Grasp the fist with the other hand and deliver quick, inward and upward thrusts. Deliver each thrust as a separate, distinct movement with enough force to expel the obstruction. Continue until the object is expelled or the child becomes unresponsive.

Suctioning

Purpose of Suctioning

Before suctioning, note the child's heart rate, oxygen saturation, and color. Monitor the child's heart rate and clinical appearance during suctioning. Bradycardia may result from stimulation of the posterior pharynx, larynx, or trachea. If bradycardia occurs or the child's clinical appearance deteriorates, interrupt suctioning and ventilate with suppplemental oxygen until the child's heart rate returns to normal.

Suction Devices

- Remove vomitus, saliva, blood, meconium (in newly born infants), and other secretions from the patient's airway.
- Improve gas exchange.
- Prevent atelectasis.
- Obtain secretions for diagnosis.

- Bulb syringe (nasal aspirator).
  - A bulb syringe is most often used to remove secretions from the nose and mouth of newborns and infants up to approximately 4 months of age, but can also be used to clear the airway of a child.
- Soft suction catheters.
  - Also called "whistle-tip" or "French" catheters.
  - Long, narrow, flexible piece of plastic used to clear thin secretions from the mouth, trachea, nasopharynx, or tracheal tube.
  - A side opening is present at the proximal end of most catheters that is covered with the thumb to produce suction. (In some cases, suctioning is initiated when a button is pushed on the suction device itself.)
  - Can be inserted into the nares or mouth through an oropharyngeal or NPA or through a tracheal tube or tracheostomy tube.
- Rigid suction catheters.
  - Also called "hard," "tonsil tip," or "Yankauer" suction catheters.
  - The rigid suction catheter is made of hard plastic and is angled to aid in the removal of thick secretions and particulate matter from the mouth and oropharynx.
  - A rigid suction catheter typically has one large and several small holes at the distal end through which particles may be suctioned.
  - Because of its size, the rigid suction catheter is not used to suction the nares, except externally.

Suctioning Technique

- Using PPE, preoxygenate the patient for at least 30 seconds before suctioning when possible.
- Bulb syringe.
  - Depress the rounded end of the bulb to remove air from the syringe (Figure 4-10).

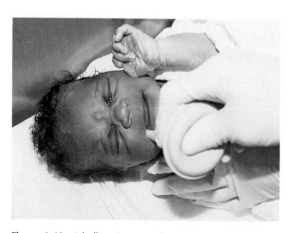

Figure 4-10 A bulb syringe may be used to suction the nose and mouth of newborns and infants.

- Place the tip of the syringe snugly into one side of the nose (or mouth).
- Release the bulb slowly; the bulb will operate as a vacuum to remove the secretions from the nose or mouth.
- When the bulb is reinflated, remove the syringe and empty the contents.
- Soft suction catheter (Figure 4-11).
  - Ensure the suction device is powered on and mechanical suction is present.
  - When preparing to suction the mouth, measure the proper distance the catheter should be inserted by holding the catheter next to the child's face and measuring from the tip of the nose to the ear lobe. To estimate the correct catheter depth for tracheobronchial suctioning, measure from the nose (or mouth) to the ear and add the distance from the ear to the sternal notch.
  - Gently insert the catheter up to the measured distance **without** applying suction. Apply intermittent suction while withdrawing the catheter.
  - Before repeating the procedure, ventilate the patient with supplmental oxygen for at least 2 minutes and rinse the suction catheter in sterile saline or water.
- Rigid suction catheter.
  - Ensure the suction device is powered on and mechanical suction is present. When using a rigid suction catheter, measure a length equal to the distance from the tip of the patient's nose to the earlobe (Figure 4-12).

PALS *Pearl*

Insertion of a suction catheter and suctioning should take no longer than 10 seconds per attempt. When suctioning to remove material that completely obstructs the airway, more time may be necessary.

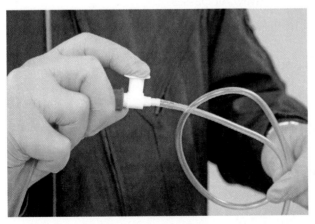

Figure 4-11 A soft suction catheter may be used to clear thin secretions from the mouth, trachea, nasopharynx, or tracheal tube. Before suctioning, turn on the power to the suction unit. Test for adequate suction by sealing the side port on the catheter with one finger. After confirming adequate suction is present, remove the finger from the port.

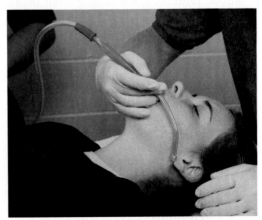

Figure 4-12 When using a rigid suction cathether, measure a length equal from the tip of the patient's nose to the earlobe.

- **Without** applying suction, gently place the tip of the catheter in the child's mouth along one side of the mouth until it reaches the posterior pharynx.
- Slowly withdraw the catheter, applying intermittent suction while sweeping from side to side to clear the airway.
- Before repeating the procedure, ventilate the patient with supplemental oxygen for at least 2 minutes and rinse the suction catheter in sterile saline or water.

Possible complications of suctioning include hypoxia, arrhythmias, increased intracranial pressure, local swelling, hemorrhage, tracheal ulceration, tracheal infection, bronchospasm, bradycardia and hypotension because of vagal stimulation, tachycardia because of sympathetic stimulation, and hypertension.

Suctioning: Possible Complications

Airway Adjuncts

Description and Function
- An OPA is a J-shaped plastic device designed for use in an unresponsive patient without a gag reflex.
- When correctly positioned, the OPA extends from the patient's lips to the pharynx. The flange of the device rests on the patient's lips or teeth. The distal tip lies between the base of the tongue and the back of the throat, preventing the tongue from occluding the airway. Air passes around and through the device.

Oropharyngeal Airway (OPA, Oral Airway)

An OPA does not protect the lower airway from aspiration.

Indications
- To aid in maintaining an open airway in an unresponsive patient who is not intubated.
- To aid in maintaining an open airway in an unresponsive patient with no gag reflex who is being ventilated with a bag-mask or other positive-pressure device.
- May be used as a bite block after insertion of a tracheal tube or orogastric tube.

Contraindications
- Patient with an intact gag reflex.

Sizing
- The size of the airway is based on the distance, in millimeters, from the flange to the distal tip.
- Available in many sizes varying in length and internal diameters (IDs).

An OPA should only be inserted by persons properly trained in their use.

- Proper airway size is determined by holding the device against the side of the patient's face and selecting an airway that extends from the corner of the mouth to the tip of the earlobe and the angle of the jaw (Figure 4-13).

Insertion

- Before inserting an OPA, use PPE, open the airway, and ensure the mouth and pharynx are clear of secretions, blood, and vomitus.
- After selecting an OPA of proper size, open the patient's mouth by applying thumb pressure on the chin.
- Depress the tongue with a tongue blade and gently insert the OPA with the curve downward. Place the airway over the tongue down into the mouth until the flange of the airway rests against the patient's lips (Figure 4-14).

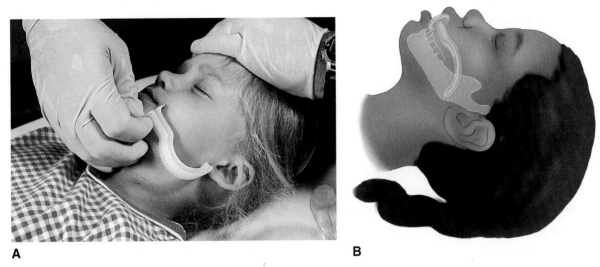

A   **B**

Figure 4-13   Proper airway size is determined by (**A**) holding the device against the side of the patient's face and selecting an airway that (**B**) extends from the corner of the mouth to the tip of the earlobe or angle of jaw .

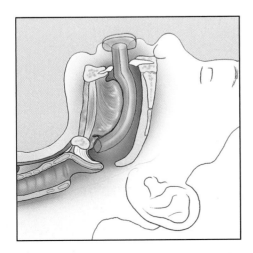

Figure 4-14   Place the oral airway over the tongue down into the mouth until the flange of the airway rests against the patient's lips. When correctly positioned, the distal tip of the oral airway lies between the base of the tongue and the back of the throat, preventing the tongue from occluding the airway.

Special Considerations

- The OPA should only be used in an unresponsive patient. Use in responsive or semiresponsive patients may stimulate the gag reflex when the back of the tongue or posterior pharynx is touched, resulting in retching, vomiting, and/or laryngospasm.
- Use of an OPA does not eliminate the need for maintaining proper head position.
- An improperly positioned OPA may compromise the airway.
    - If the airway is too long, it may press the epiglottis against the entrance of the larynx resulting in complete airway obstruction.
    - If the airway is too short, the tongue may be pushed back into the pharynx resulting in an airway obstruction, or the airway may advance out of the mouth.

Nasopharyngeal Airway (Nasal Trumpet, Nasal Airway)

Description and Function

- Soft, uncuffed rubber or plastic tube designed to keep the tongue away from the posterior pharynx.
- The device is placed in one nostril and advanced until the distal tip lies in the posterior pharynx just below the base of the tongue, while the proximal tip rests on the external nares.
- Available in many sizes varying in length and ID.

Indications

- To aid in maintaining an airway when use of an OPA is contraindicated or impossible (e.g., trismus, seizing patient, biting, clenched jaws or teeth).
- May be useful in patients requiring frequent suctioning (decreases tissue trauma, bleeding).
- Dental or oral trauma.

Contraindications

- Patient intolerance.
- Nasal obstruction.
- Significant mid-face trauma.
- Presence of cerebrospinal fluid drainage from the nose.
- Moderate to severe head trauma.
- Known or suspected basilar skull fracture.

Sizing

- Proper airway size is determined by holding the device against the side of the patient's face and selecting an airway that extends from the tip of the nose to the angle of the jaw or the tip of the ear (Figure 4-15).
    - If the NPA is equipped with an adjustable flange, adjust the flange up or down as necessary to obtain the appropriate length.

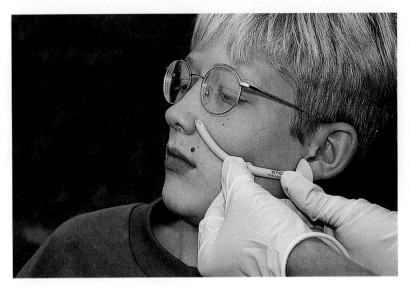

Figure 4-15 Sizing a nasal airway.

- An NPA that is too long may stimulate the gag reflex or enter the esophagus, causing gastric distention and hypoventilation. One that is too short may not be inserted far enough to keep the tongue away from the posterior pharynx.

Insertion

A NPA should only be inserted by persons properly trained in their use.

- Before inserting an NPA, use PPE and open the airway.
- Lubricate the distal tip of the device liberally with a water-soluble lubricant to minimize resistance and decrease irritation to the nasal passage.
- After selecting an NPA of the proper size, hold the device at its flange end like a pencil and slowly insert it into the patient's nostril with the bevel pointing toward the nasal septum.

If blanching of the nostril is present after insertion of an NPA, the diameter of the device is too large. Remove the NPA, select a slightly smaller size, and reinsert.

- Advance the airway along the floor of the nostril, following the natural curvature of the nasal passage, until the flange rests against the outside of the nostril.
  - The nasal cavity is very vascular. During insertion, do not force the airway because it may cause abrasions or lacerations of the nasal mucosa and result in significant bleeding, increasing the risk of aspiration.
  - If resistance is encountered, a gentle back-and-forth rotation of the device between your fingers may ease insertion. If resistance continues, withdraw the NPA, reapply lubricant, and attempt insertion in the other nostril.

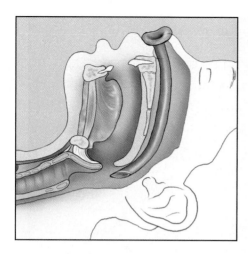

Figure 4-16 When correctly positioned, the nasal airway extends from the patient's nose to the pharynx. The flange of the device rests against the outside of the nostril. The distal tip lies between the base of the tongue and the back of the throat, preventing the tongue from occluding the airway.

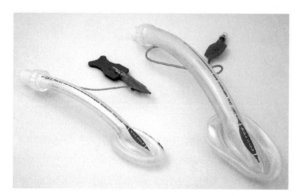

Figure 4-17   Laryngeal mask airways.

- When correctly positioned, the NPA extends from the patient's nose to the pharynx. The flange of the device rests against the outside of the nostril and the distal tip lies between the base of the tongue and the back of the throat, preventing the tongue from occluding the airway. Air passes around and through the device (Figure 4-16).

Special Considerations
- The NPA does not protect the lower airway from aspiration.
- Use of the NPA does not eliminate the need for maintaining proper head position.
- Small-diameter NPAs can become easily obstructed with blood, mucus, vomitus, or the soft tissues of the pharynx.
- Suctioning may be necessary to keep the NPA open; however, suctioning through an NPA is difficult.
- Although most responsive and semiresponsive patients can tolerate an NPA, the gag reflex may be stimulated in sensitive patients, precipitating coughing, laryngospasm, or vomiting.

Laryngeal Mask Airway

An LMA is a device that functions intermediately between an OPA and a tracheal tube and does not require direct visualization of the airway for insertion. The LMA is available in sizes for neonates, infants, young children, older children, and small, average, and large adults.

The LMA should only be inserted by persons properly trained in the use of the device.

Description and Function

The LMA consists of a tube fitted with an oval mask and an inflatable rim (Figure 4-17). The tube opens into the middle of the mask by means of vertical slits that prevent the tip of the epiglottis from falling back and blocking the lumen of the tube. The LMA is inserted through the mouth into the pharynx without visualization. The LMA is advanced until resistance is felt, using the right index finger to maintain firm pressure on the device against the hard palate. The rim of the mask is then inflated to seal the mask around the larynx and the base of the tongue, and the LMA is connected to a ventilation device.

The inflatable LMA mask does not ensure an airtight seal to protect the airway against gastric regurgitation. Leakage of the mask may allow aspiration of emesis and gastric distention may occur with misplacement.

Indications

- Patient in whom intubation has been unsuccessful and ventilation is difficult.
- Patient in whom airway management is necessary but healthcare provider is untrained in the technique of visualized orotracheal intubation
- Many elective surgical procedures.

Oxygen Delivery Systems

General Principles

The oxygen delivery systems described in this section may be used for the spontaneously breathing infant or child with effective ventilation (i.e., adequate chest movement and breath sounds). If spontaneous breathing is inadequate, assisted ventilation is required (discussed later in this chapter).

Administer supplemental oxygen to any seriously ill or injured child with signs or symptoms of respiratory compromise, shock, or trauma.

Indications for Oxygen Administration

- All cases of cardiopulmonary arrest.
- Suspected hypoxemia of any cause.
- Any condition of respiratory difficulty that may potentially lead to cardiopulmonary arrest.

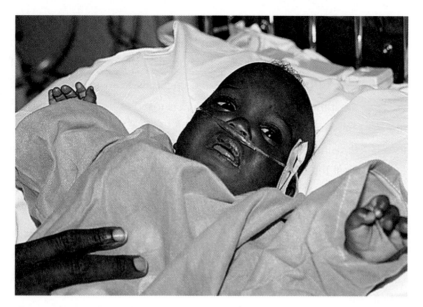

Figure 4-18 Nasal cannula.

Description and Function

- A nasal cannula is a piece of plastic tubing with two soft prongs that project from the tubing. The prongs are inserted into the patient's nares, and the tubing secured to the patient's face (Figure 4–18). Oxygen flows from the cannula into the patient's nasopharynx, which acts as an anatomic reservoir.
- Low-flow oxygen delivery device used for the infant or child who requires only low levels of supplemental oxygen.
    - Oxygen flow rate: 1 to 6 L/min.
    - Concentration delivered: up to 50%.
    - A high fraction of inspired oxygen (FIO_2) may result when the flow rate exceeds the patient's inspiratory flow and minute ventilation.

Advantages

- Easy to use.
- Allows the patient to eat and drink.
- Does not require humidification.
- No rebreathing of expired air.
- Does not interfere with patient assessment or impede patient communication with healthcare personnel.

Disadvantages

- Can only be used in the spontaneously breathing patient.
- Easily displaced.
- Nasal passages must be open.
- Drying of mucosa.
- May irritate nose.
- May cause sinus pain.

Nasal Cannula (Nasal Prongs)

Secure the nasal cannula in place and then slowly start the oxygen flow to avoid frightening the child.

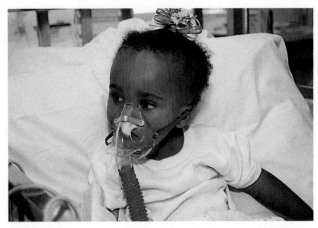

Figure 4-19   Child receiving oxygen via a face mask.

Simple Face Mask (Standard Mask)

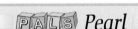

PALS *Pearl*

When using a simple face mask, the oxygen flow rate must be at least 6 L/min to flush the accumulation of the patient's exhaled carbon dioxide from the mask.

Description and Function

- A simple face mask is a plastic reservoir designed to fit over the patient's nose and mouth. Small holes on each side of the mask allow the passage of inspired and expired air. Supplemental oxygen is delivered through a small-diameter tube connected to the base of the mask (Figure 4-19). The mask is secured into position by means of an elastic strap around the back of the patient's head. The internal capacity of the mask produces a reservoir effect.
- Oxygen flow rate: 6 to 10 L/min.
- Concentration delivered: 35% to 60%.
- The patient's actual inspired oxygen concentration will vary because the amount of air that mixes with supplemental oxygen is dependent on the patient's inspiratory flow rate and breathing pattern.

Advantages

- Higher oxygen concentration delivered than by nasal cannula.
- Patient accessibility.

Disadvantages

- Can only be used with spontaneously breathing patients.
- Not tolerated well by severely dyspneic patients (feeling of suffocation).
- FIO_2 varies with inspiratory flow rate.
- Can be uncomfortable.
- Dangerous for the child with poor airway control and at risk for emesis.
- Difficult to hear the patient speaking when the device is in place.
- Must be removed at meals.
- Requires a tight face seal to prevent leakage of oxygen.

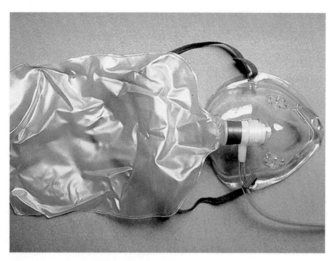

Figure 4-20 Partial rebreather mask.

Description and Function

- The partial rebreather mask is similar to a simple oxygen mask but has an attached oxygen-collecting device (reservoir) at the base of the mask that is filled before patient use (Figure 4-20).
- Depending on the patient's breathing pattern, mask fit, and the oxygen flowmeter setting, oxygen concentrations of 35% to 60% can be delivered when an oxygen flow rate (typically 6-10 L/min) is used that prevents the reservoir bag from completely collapsing on inspiration.
  - Fill the reservoir bag with oxygen *before* placing the mask on the patient.
  - After placing the mask on the patient, adjust the flow rate so the bag does not completely deflate when the patient inhales.

Advantages

- Higher oxygen concentration delivered than by nasal cannula.
- Patient accessibility.

Disadvantages

- Same as for simple mask.

Description and Function

- A nonrebreather mask is similar to a partial rebreather mask, but does not permit mixing of the patient's air with 100% oxygen. A one-way valve between the mask and reservoir bag and a flap over one of the exhalation ports on the side of the mask prevents inhalation of room air. When the patient breathes in, oxygen is drawn into the mask from the reservoir (bag) through the one-way valve that separates the bag from the mask. When the patient breathes out, the exhaled air exits through the open side port on the mask. The one-way valve prevents

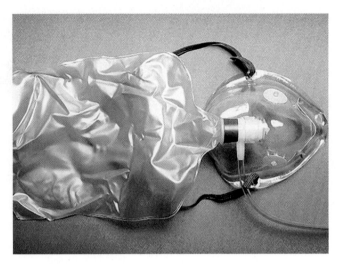

Figure 4-21   Nonrebreather mask.

When using a partial rebreather or nonrebreather mask, make sure that the bag does not collapse when the patient inhales. Should the bag collapse, increase the delivered oxygen by 2-liter increments until the bag remains inflated. The reservoir must remain at least 2/3 full so that sufficient supplemental oxygen is available for each breath.

the patient's exhaled air from returning to the reservoir bag (thus the name "nonrebreather"). This ensures a supply of 100% oxygen to the patient with minimal dilution from the entrainment of room air (Figure 4-21).

• Delivery device of choice when high concentrations of oxygen are needed in the spontaneously breathing patient because it can consistently deliver an inspired oxygen concentration of up to 95% at a flow rate of 10 to 15 L/min.

  • Fill the reservoir bag with oxygen *before* placing the mask on the patient.

  • After placing the mask on the patient, adjust the flow rate so the bag does not completely deflate when the patient inhales.

Advantages

• Higher oxygen concentration delivered than by nasal cannula, simple face mask, and partial rebreather mask.

Disadvantages

• Same as for simple mask.

Face Tent (Face Shield)

Description and Function

Large, soft plastic bucket that fits loosely around the child's face and lower jaw (Figure 4-22).

Advantages

• Permits access to the face and nose for suctioning.

• Can provide warmed or cooled humidified oxygen.

Disadvantages

• Oxygen concentrations in excess of 40% cannot be reliably provided, even with an oxygen flow rate of 10 to 15 L/min.

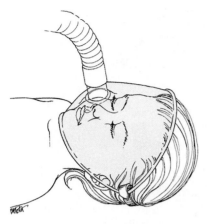

Figure 4-22 Face tent.

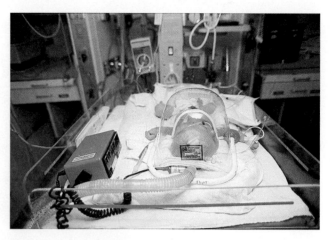

Figure 4-23 Oxygen administered to an infant by means of a plastic hood.

Description and Function

Oxygen Hood

- An oxygen hood is a clear plastic dome that encircles the child's head (Figure 4-23). The hood size should be adjusted to the patient's size.
- Used for neonates and infants weighing less than 10 kg who will not tolerate a face mask.
- Permits control of oxygen concentration, temperature, and humidity.
- At 10 to 15 L/min, can deliver an inspired oxygen concentration of approximately 80% to 90%.
- An oxygen flow rate of at least 10 L/min is required to flush accumulated carbon dioxide from inside the hood.

Advantages

- Oxygen concentration can be continuously monitored by means of a meter.
- Permits access to the chest, trunk, and extremities for continued care.

Disadvantages

- Generally not large enough to be used for children older than 1 year.
- "Raining out" on the walls of the hood may obscure the patient's head from observation.
- Noisy for the patient.

When an infant or child cannot tolerate supplemental oxygen delivery by means of a nasal cannula or face mask, blow-by oxygen may be used. The oxygen tubing or mask should be directed near the child's nose and mouth (Figure 4-24). Consider attaching the oxygen tubing to a toy and encourage the child to hold the toy near the face or try placing the tubing in a paper cup (Figure 4-25), then ask the child to "drink from the cup."

Blow-by Oxygen Delivery

When possible, allow the child's caregiver to administer blow-by oxygen.

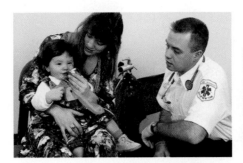

Figure 4-24 When an infant or child cannot tolerate supplemental oxygen delivery by means of a nasal cannula or face mask, blow-by oxygen may be used.

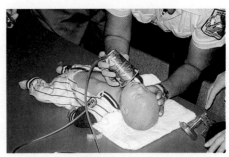

Figure 4-25 When administering blow-by oxygen, consider attaching the oxygen tubing to a toy and encourage the child to hold the toy near the face or try placing the tubing in a paper cup and then ask the child to "drink from the cup."

Ventilation Devices

If the patient's ventilatory efforts are inadequate, breathing may be assisted by forcing air into the lungs (i.e., delivering positive-pressure ventilation). Several methods may be used to deliver positive-pressure ventilation including mouth-to-mask ventilation and bag-mask ventilation. Regardless of the method used, effective positive-pressure ventilation requires the delivery of an adequate volume of air at an appropriate rate.

Cricoid Pressure (Sellick maneuver)

Purpose

Positive-pressure ventilation, especially if performed rapidly, may cause gastric distention. The cricoid cartilage is the most inferior of the laryngeal cartilages and is the only completely cartilaginous ring in the larynx. For many years, healthcare professionals have taught that by pressing down

TABLE 4-1 *Oxygen Percentage Delivery by Device*

Device	Approximate Inspired Oxygen Concentration	Liter Flow (L/min)
Nasal cannula	Up to 50%	1 to 6
Simple face mask	35% to 60%	6 to 10
Partial rebreather mask	35% to 60%	6 to 10
Nonrebreather mask	60% to 95%	10 to 15
Face tent	35% to 40%	10 to 15
Oxygen hood	80% to 90%	10 to 15
Blow-by (via face mask)	30% to 40%	10

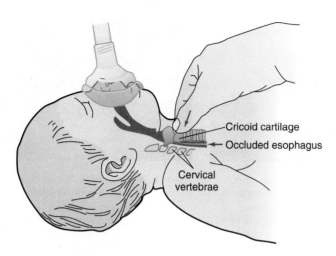

Figure 4-26 Compression of the cricoid cartilage pushes the trachea posteriorly, compressing the laryngopharynx.

on the cricoid cartilage, the esophagus is compressed between the cricoid cartilage and the cervical vertebrae, reducing inflation of the stomach during positive pressure ventilation and reducing the likelihood of vomiting and aspiration. Using magnetic resonance imaging, a 2009 study demonstrated that the laryngopharynx, not the esophagus, is what lies behind the cricoid ring and is compressed by cricoid pressure[2] (Figure 4-26). In this study, the mean anteroposterior diameter of the laryngopharynx was reduced by 35% with cricoid pressure and the lumen likely obliterated. Compression of the laryngopharynx may help minimize inflation of the stomach during ventilation, reducing the likelihood of vomiting and aspiration.

- Cricoid pressure (also called the Sellick maneuver) is used only in unresponsive patients and is usually applied by an assistant during positive-pressure ventilation. Pressure is applied on the cricoid cartilage with the thumb and index or middle finger, just lateral to the midline. In an infant or young child, cricoid pressure is applied using only one finger (Figure 4-27). Studies suggest that cricoid pressure is frequently applied incorrectly. In some studies, participants applied too little pressure, placing patients at risk of regurgitation, and in others excessive pressure was used.[3-8]

- Although some studies have not found cricoid pressure to cause a barrier to advanced airway insertion, most have shown that cricoid pressure impedes placement, impairs the rate of successful ventilation, and hinders ventilation. Aspiration can occur despite application of pressure.

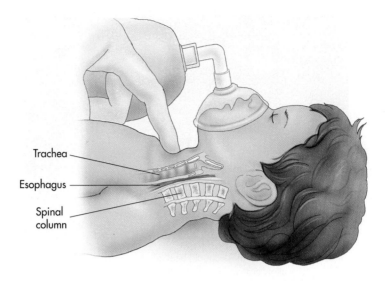

Trachea

Esophagus

Spinal
column

Figure 4-27 In an infant or young child, cricoid pressure is applied using only one finger.

- Current resuscitation guidelines state that cricoid pressure may be considered to minimized gastric inflation in the unresponsive patient but may require a third rescuer if cricoid pressure cannot be applied by the rescuer who is securing the mask (or bag-mask device) to the face.[9-10]
- If excessive pressure is applied, cricoid pressure can cause complete airway obstruction. If active regurgitation occurs while performing cricoid pressure, release cricoid pressure to avoid rupture of the stomach or esophagus.

Mouth-to-Mask Ventilation

Description and Function
- The device used for mouth-to-mask ventilation is commonly called a **pocket mask**, pocket face mask, ventilation face mask, or resuscitation mask. A ventilation face mask permits the rescuer to oxygenate and ventilate a patient. The device can be used with an NPA or OPA during spontaneous, assisted, or controlled ventilation.
- Some ventilation masks have an oxygen inlet on the mask, allowing delivery of supplemental oxygen; others do not.
- A ventilation mask should be made of transparent material to allow evaluation of the patient's lip color and detection of blood, vomitus, or secretions. It should be equipped with a one-way valve to divert the patient's exhaled air, reducing the risk of infection (Figure 4-28).

Advantages
- Aesthetically more acceptable than mouth-to-mouth ventilation.
- Easy to teach and learn.

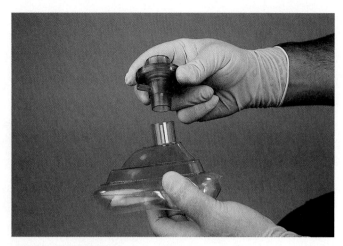

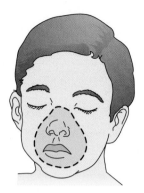

Figure 4-29 A proper fitting mask should extend from the bridge of the nose to the crease of the chin.

Figure 4-28 A pocket mask should be made of transparent material to allow evaluation of the patient's lip color and detection of blood, vomitus, or secretions and equipped with a one-way valve that diverts the patient's exhaled gas, reducing the risk of infection.

- Physical barrier between the rescuer and the patient's nose, mouth, and secretions.
- Reduces (but does not prevent) the risk of exposure to infectious disease.
- Use of a one-way valve at the ventilation port decreases exposure to patient's exhaled air.
- If the patient resumes spontaneous breathing, the mask can be used as a simple face mask by administering supplemental oxygen through the oxygen inlet on the mask (if so equipped).
- Can deliver greater tidal volume with mouth-to-mask ventilation than with a bag-mask device.
- With mouth-to-mask ventilation, the rescuer can feel the **compliance** of the patient's lungs. Compliance refers to the resistance of the patient's lung tissue to ventilation.

Disadvantages
- Rescuer fatigue.

Technique
- Using PPE, position yourself at the patient's head or side. If needed, clear the patient's airway of secretions or vomitus. Open the patient's airway with a head tilt–chin lift or, if trauma is suspected, perform the jaw thrust without head tilt maneuver. If the patient is unresponsive, insert an OPA.
- Select a mask of appropriate size and place it on the patient's face.
  - Ventilation masks are available in a variety of sizes. The mask should have limited dead space, have an inflatable rim, and provide a tight seal without pressure on the eyes. A mask of proper size should extend

from the bridge of the nose to the groove between the lower lip and chin (Figure 4-29).

- Apply the narrow portion (apex) of the mask over the bridge of the patient's nose and stabilize it in place with your thumbs.
- Lower the mask over the patient's face and mouth.
- Use your index fingers to stabilize the wide end (base) of the mask over the groove between the lower lip and chin. When in proper position, your thumb and index finger create a C. Use your remaining fingers to maintain proper head position. Your remaining fingers create an E.
- Ventilate the patient through the one-way valve on the top of the mask, and deliver each breath over 1 second. Stop ventilation when adequate chest rise is observed. Allow the patient to exhale between breaths.

Bag-Mask Ventilation

Description and Function

- The bag-mask device is the most common mechanical aid used to deliver positive-pressure ventilation in emergency care. A bag-mask device may also be referred to as a bag-valve-mask device or bag-mask resuscitator (when the mask is used), or a bag-valve device (when the mask is not used, i.e., when ventilating a patient with a tracheal tube in place).
- A bag-mask consists of a self-inflating bag; a nonrebreathing valve with an adapter that can be attached to a mask, tracheal tube, or other invasive airway device; and an oxygen inlet valve.
- A bag-mask used for resuscitation should have either no pop-off (pressure release) valve or a pop-off valve that can be disabled during resuscitation (Figure 4-30). Disabling the pop-off valve, or using a bag-mask with no pop-off valve, helps ensure delivery of adequate tidal volumes to the patient during resuscitation.
- Bag-mask devices are available in various sizes. It is important to select a device with sufficient volume for the patient's size:
  - At least 450 to 500 mL (pediatric bag) for full-term neonates, infants, and young children.
  - A 1000 mL or more (adult) bag for older children and adolescents.
  - A 250-mL (neonatal) bag may not provide sufficient volume or the longer respiratory times required by term neonates and infants. A child can be ventilated with a larger bag as long as proper technique is used: Squeeze the bag just until the chest begins to rise, then release the bag.

Oxygen Delivery

- A bag-mask used without supplemental oxygen will deliver 21% oxygen (room air) to the patient.

To disable a pop-off valve, depress the valve with a finger during ventilation or twist the pop-off valve into the closed position.

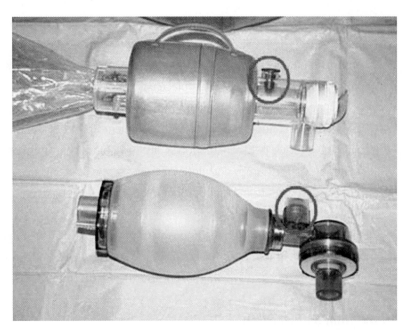

Figure 4-30 These bag-mask devices have pop-off valves. If used for resuscitation, the pop-off valve should be disabled. This can be done by depressing the valve with a finger during ventilation or twisting the pop-off valve into the closed position.

- A bag-mask should be connected to an oxygen source. Attach one end of a piece of oxygen-connecting tubing to the oxygen inlet on the bag-mask and the other end to an oxygen regulator.
    - A pediatric bag-mask used with supplemental oxygen set at a flow rate of 10 L/min will deliver approximately 30% to 80% oxygen to the patient.
    - An adult bag-mask used with supplemental oxygen set at a flow rate of 15 L/min will deliver approximately 40% to 60% oxygen to the patient.
- An oxygen-collecting device (reservoir) should be attached to the bag-mask to consistently deliver high-concentration oxygen. The reservoir collects a volume of 100% oxygen equal to the capacity of the bag. After squeezing the bag, the bag reexpands, drawing in 100% oxygen from the reservoir into the bag.
    - A pediatric bag-mask used with supplemental oxygen (set at a flow rate of 10 to 15 L/min) and an attached reservoir will deliver approximately 60% to 95% oxygen to the patient.
    - An adult bag-mask used with supplemental oxygen (set at a flow rate of 15 L/min) and an attached reservoir will deliver approximately 90% to 100% oxygen to the patient.

Advantages

- Provides a means for delivery of an oxygen-enriched mixture to the patient.

- Conveys a sense of compliance of the patient's lungs to the bag-mask operator.
- Provides a means for immediate ventilatory support.
- Can be used with the spontaneously breathing patient and the apneic patient.

Disadvantages

- The most frequent problems with bag-mask ventilation are the inability to deliver adequate ventilatory volumes and gastric inflation. Delivery of an inadequate ventilatory volume may be due to difficulty in providing a leak proof seal to the face while simultaeneously maintaining an open airway and/or incomplete bag compression. Gastric inflation may result if excessive force and volume are used during ventilation.

Bag-mask Ventilation: Technique

- Using PPE, position yourself at the top of the supine patient's head.
- Select an appropriate bag for ventilation based on the patient's size.
  - The bag should have an oxygen reservoir.
  - Connect one end of the oxygen tubing to an oxygen source and the other end to an oxygen flow meter. Set the flow meter to the appropriate liter flow.
- Open the patient's airway using a head tilt–chin lift or, if trauma is suspected, perform the jaw thrust without head tilt maneuver. If needed, clear the patient's airway of secretions or vomitus.
- If the patient is unresponsive, insert an oral airway.
- Select a mask of appropriate size and place it on the patient's face. Apply the narrow portion (apex) of the mask over the bridge of the patient's nose and the wide end (base) of the mask over the groove between the lower lip and chin. If the mask has a large, round cuff surrounding a ventilation port, center the port over the mouth.
- One-handed technique ("E-C clamp").
  - Stabilize the mask in place with your thumb and index finger, creating a "C" (Figure 4-31).
  - With gentle pressure, push down on the mask to establish an adequate seal.
  - Place your third, fourth, and fifth fingers along the patient's jaw, forming an "E." Use these fingers to lift the jaw along the bony portion of the mandible.
  - Connect the bag to the mask (if not already done) and ensure the bag is connected to oxygen.
  - Squeeze the bag with your other hand (or with one hand and your arm or chest if necessary).
  - If the infant or child has a perfusing rhythm but absent or

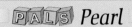
PALS *Pearl*

Gastric distention is a complication of positive-pressure ventilation that can lead to regurgitation and subsequent aspiration. Gastric distention also restricts movement of the diaphragm, impeding ventilation. Consider insertion of a gastric tube to alleviate gastric distention when the patient requires bag-mask ventilation.

Avoid compressing the soft tissues of the face and neck and ensure that the mask does not compress the eyes.

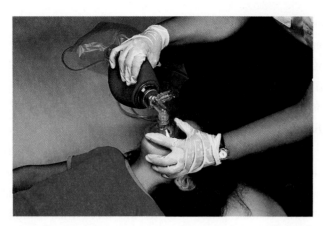

Figure 4-31 One-handed bag-mask ventilation using the "E-C clamp" technique.

inadequate ventilatory effort, give one breath every 3 to 5 seconds (12 to 20 breaths per minute), using the higher rate for the younger child. Allow 1 second per breath while watching for chest rise. As soon as chest rise is visible, release the bag.

- If the infant or child has no pulse and is not intubated, pause after 30 chest compressions (1 rescuer) or after 15 chest compressions (2 rescuers) to give two ventilations. If the infant or child is intubated, ventilate at the rate of about 1 breath every 6 to 8 seconds (8 to 10 times per minute) without interrupting chest compressions.
- Two-handed technique.
  - Bag-mask ventilation is optimally a two-rescuer operation—one to hold the mask to the face (ensuring a good mask to face seal) and maintain an open airway, the other to compress the bag with two hands.
  - Ask an assistant to squeeze the bag with two hands until the patient's chest begins to rise while you press the mask firmly against the patient's face with both hands and simultaneously maintain proper head position.
- Assess the effectiveness of ventilation.
  - Ensure the mask forms an airtight seal on the patient's face.
  - Evaluate lung compliance (resistance to ventilation).
  - Observe the rise and fall of the patient's chest with each ventilation.
  - Assess for an improvement in the color of the patient's skin or mucous membranes.
  - Assess for an improvement in the patient's mental status, heart rate, perfusion, and blood pressure.
  - Auscultate for bilateral breath sounds.

Increasing resistance during positive-pressure ventilation suggests airway obstruction.

Troubleshooting Bag-Mask Ventilation

- If the chest does not rise with bag-mask ventilation, ventilation is not effective: Either the airway is obstructed or more volume or pressure is needed to provide effective ventilation.
  - A common problem when ventilating with a bag-mask device is placing the mask tightly on the face without performing an adequate maneuver to open the patient's airway. This results in an airway obstruction because of improper airway positioning. Readjust the patient's head position, ensure the mouth is open, and reattempt to ventilate.
- Inadequate tidal volume delivery may be the result of gastric distention, an improper mask seal, or incomplete bag compression.
  - Gastric distention may cause regurgitation with a risk of subsequent aspiration. Gastric distention may also impair movement of the diaphragm, resulting in inadequate ventilation.
    - Considering insertion of an orogastric or nasogastric tube to decompress the stomach after placement of a tracheal tube. Insertion of a gastric tube before a tracheal tube can interfere with the gastroesophageal sphincter and result in vomiting.
  - An inadequate mask seal may result in hypoxia or hyperventilation. If air is escaping from under the mask, reposition your fingers and the mask. If the leak persists, ask for assistance with the patient's airway, consider using another mask, or use the two-handed technique.
  - Remember that in certain situations (e.g., severe asthma, cardio-pulmonary arrest), higher than normal inspiratory pressures may be required for adequate ventilation. Check to see if the bag-mask has a pop-off valve. If a pop-off valve is present, disable the valve and attempt to ventilate again.
- Reevaluate the effectiveness of bag compression.
  - Check for obstruction.
  - Lift the jaw.
  - Suction the airway as needed.
- If the chest still does not rise, suspect an airway obstruction.

Tracheal Intubation

Tracheal intubation is an advanced airway procedure in which a tube is placed directly into the trachea. This procedure requires special training and frequent refresher training to maintain skill proficiency.

Tracheal intubation may be performed for a variety of reasons including the delivery of anesthesia, assisting a patient's breathing with positive-pressure ventilation, and protection of the patient's airway from aspiration. Pulse oximetry and electrocardiogram (ECG) monitoring should be performed throughout this procedure. Special equipment and supplies required for this procedure include the following:

- Laryngoscope
  - A laryngoscope is an instrument that consists of a handle and blade used for examining the interior of the larynx, specifically visualization of the glottic opening (the space between the vocal cords).
- Laryngoscope blades
  - There are two primary types of laryngoscope blades: straight and curved.
    - During orotracheal intubation, the tip of the straight blade is positioned under the epiglottis. When the laryngoscope handle is lifted anteriorly, the blade directly lifts the epiglottis out of the way to expose the glottic opening.
    - The curved blade is inserted into the vallecula, the space (or "pocket") between the base of the tongue and the epiglottis. When the laryngoscope handle is lifted anteriorly, the blade elevates the tongue and indirectly lifts the epiglottis, allowing visualization of the glottic opening.
  - Select the appropriate blade size with the laryngoscope blade held next to the patient's face. A blade of proper size should reach between the patient's lips and larynx.
- Tracheal tube
  - A tracheal tube is a curved tube that is open at both ends. A standard 15-mm connector is located at the proximal end for attachment of a device for delivery of positive-pressure ventilation.
  - Tracheal tubes are measured in millimeters (mm) by their ID and external diameter (OD). Centimeter markings on the tracheal tube are used as reference points aiding in tube placement and assisting in detection of accidental tube displacement.
  - Some tracheal tubes have an inflatable balloon cuff that surrounds the distal tip of the tube. When the distal cuff is inflated,

Description and Function

For prehospital professionals with short transport times, oxygenation and ventilation of the patient using a bag-mask device is recommended instead of tracheal intubation because of the high incidence of misplaced and displaced tracheal tubes.

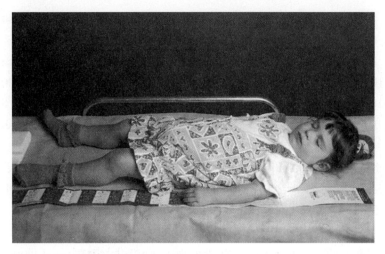

Figure 4-32 The Broselow resuscitation tape.

it contacts the wall of the trachea as it expands, sealing off the trachea from the remainder of the pharynx, reducing the risk of aspiration. The cuff is attached to a one-way valve through a side tube with a pilot balloon that is used to indicate if the cuff is inflated.

- Stylet
  - A stylet is a flexible plastic-coated wire inserted into a tracheal tube that is used for molding and maintaining the shape of the tube during intubation.
  - If a stylet is used, be sure the stylet is free of kinks to allow easy removal after successful intubation. Some advocate lubrication of the stylet with a water-soluble lubricant before placement in the tracheal tube. This aids removal once the tube has been placed, avoiding accidental extubation. A petroleum-based lubricant should never be used because it may damage the tracheal tube and cause tracheal inflammation.
  - When a stylet is used, the tip of the stylet must be recessed about 0.5 cm from the end of the tracheal tube to avoid trauma to the airway structures.

Tracheal Tube Sizing

Tracheal tube size can be estimated by using one of the following methods:

- Length-based resuscitation tape (e.g., Broselow tape) (Figure 4-32).
  - Useful and more accurate than age-based formula estimates for determining the correct tracheal tube size for children who weigh up to approximately 35 kg.
- If an uncuffed tracheal tube is used for intubation, use of a 3.5-mm ID tube for infants up to 1 year of age and a 4-mm ID tube for patients between 1 and 2 years of age is considered reasonable. After age 2, the

following formula can be used to estimate uncuffed tracheal tube size: Uncuffed tracheal tube ID (mm) = 4 + (age in years/4)[10]

- If a cuffed tracheal tube is used for intubation of an infant, use of a 3-mm ID tube is considered reasonable. Use of a 3.5-mm ID tube for children between 1 and 2 years of age is considered reasonable. After age 2, the following formula can be used to estimate cuffed tracheal tube size: Cuffed tracheal tube ID (mm) = 3.5 + (age in years/4)[10]

Because of the variation in patient sizes, it is important to have several sizes of tubes on hand. At a minimum, have available a tracheal tube that is 0.5 mm smaller and 0.5 mm larger than the estimated tube size.

Tracheal Tube Depth

- The pediatric trachea is shorter than the adult trachea. Failure to approximate the proper depth of tracheal tube insertion may result in hypoxia, perforation, or endobronchial intubation.
- The proper depth of tracheal tube insertion (in centimeters at the teeth or lips) is approximately three times the tracheal tube size. This formula assumes that the proper size tracheal tube is selected.
- Alternatively, the following formula may be used to determine proper depth of insertion (from the distal end of the tube to the alveolar ridge of the teeth) for children older than 2 years: (12 + age in years) ÷ 2.
- Some tracheal tubes have markings on them that can be used to visually determine the correct depth of tube insertion as the tube is passed through the vocal cords.

Tracheal Intubation: Indications

- Hypoxemia despite supplemental oxygen.
- Inadequate ventilation with less invasive methods.
- Actual or potential decrease in airway protective reflexes (e.g., drug overdose, head trauma).
- Respiratory failure or arrest, gasping or agonal breathing.
- Present or impending airway obstruction (e.g., stridor, significant increase in work of breathing, inhalation injury, epiglottitis, bleeding in the airway, asthma, severe pulmonary edema).
- Unstable chest wall, inadequate respiratory muscle function, or severe chest trauma (e.g., severe flail chest, pulmonary contusion, pneumothorax).
- When mechanical ventilatory support is anticipated (e.g., acute respiratory failure, chest trauma, increased work of breathing, shock, increased intracranial pressure).

Advantages

- Isolates the airway.
- Keeps the airway patent.
- Reduces the risk of aspiration of gastric contents.
- Ensures delivery of a high concentration of oxygen.

- Permits suctioning of the trachea.
- Provides a route for administration of some medications.
- Ensures delivery of a selected tidal volume to maintain lung inflation.

Disadvantages

- Considerable training and experience required.
- Special equipment needed.
- Bypasses physiologic function of upper airway (e.g., warming, filtering, humidifying of inhaled air).
- Requires direct visualization of vocal cords.

Technique

Using PPE (at a minimum, use gloves, protective eyewear, and a mask), open the patient's airway with a head tilt–chin lift (or jaw thrust without head tilt if trauma is suspected).

1. Oxygenate and ventilate the patient.
   - Ask an assistant to preoxygenate the patient while you auscultate bilateral lung sounds to establish a baseline. Preoxygenation is particularly important in children because they have less oxygen reserve in their lungs and their metabolic oxygen consumption is proportionately greater than that in adults.
   - Place the patient on a cardiac monitor and attach the pulse oximeter.
2. Prepare the equipment.
   - While your assistant continues to preoxygenate the patient, assemble and prepare the equipment needed for intubation, including suction equipment.

The *minimum* equipment prerequisites that must be present to ensure a safe intubation can be remembered by the mnemonic "SALTT": Suction, Airway (oral), Laryngoscope, Tube and Tape (or Tube holder).

   - Select the proper size blade and then assemble the laryngoscope. Attach the blade to the handle and check the blade for a "white, bright, light." After verifying the light is in working order, move the blade to its unlocked position to conserve battery life until the light is needed.
   - Select the proper size tracheal tube.
     ◦ If a cuffed tracheal tube is used, test the cuff for leaks. If there are no leaks, completely deflate the cuff. Refill the syringe with air and leave the syringe attached to the inflation valve on the tracheal tube.
     ◦ Be sure to have at least two additional tracheal tube sizes available (one 0.5 mm smaller and one 0.5 mm larger than the selected size).
   - If a stylet will be used, insert it into the tracheal tube making sure that the end of the stylet is recessed at least 0.5 cm from the tip of the tracheal tube.
3. Position the patient.

Do not place the patient's head in a sniffing position if trauma is suspected.

   - To achieve direct visualization of the laryngeal opening, the three axes of the pharynx-glottis, glottis-trachea, and mouth-pharynx must be aligned. Proper positioning of the patient's head and neck will vary depending on the patient's age and clinical situation.

- In the absence of trauma, use the sniffing position to align the axes of the airway. In the sniffing position, the child looks as if he is putting his head forward to sniff a flower.
- If trauma to the head, neck, or spine is suspected, do **not** place the patient in sniffing position. Instead, use an assistant to keep the head and neck in a neutral, in-line position throughout the procedure.

4. Provide suctioning and oxygenation.
   - If necessary, suction the patient's mouth and pharynx of secretions. After suctioning, ventilate the patient with supplemental oxygen for at least 2 minutes.
   - Stop ventilations and remove the ventilation face mask and OPA (if present). Do not exceed 30 seconds from ventilation to ventilation for each intubation attempt.

5. Open the patient's mouth.
   - Open the patient's mouth by applying thumb pressure on the chin.
   - Alternatively, an unresponsive patient's mouth may be opened using the crossed-finger method.
     ◦ Cross the fingers and thumb of your nondominant hand.
     ◦ Press your gloved thumb against the child's upper teeth and your fingers against the lower teeth and push them apart.

6. Control the patient's tongue.
   - The flange and tip of the laryngoscope blade are used to control the tongue and epiglottis.
   - Holding the laryngoscope in the left hand and with the tip of the blade pointing away from you, insert the blade into the right side of the patient's mouth, sweeping the tongue to the left.
   - Advance the laryngoscope blade slowly along the tongue until the distal end reaches the base of the tongue. Lift the laryngoscope to elevate the mandible without putting pressure on the front teeth and visualize the glottis. Do NOT use the patient's teeth or gums as a fulcrum. Do not allow the blade to touch the patient's teeth.

7. Control the patient's epiglottis.
   - After visualizing the epiglottis, place the blade in the proper position.
   - If you are using a straight blade, advance the tip under the epiglottis. If you are using a curved blade, advance the tip of the blade into the vallecula.

8. Locate landmarks for intubation (Figure 4-33).
   - When the straight blade is lifted anteriorly, the blade directly lifts the epiglottis out of the way to expose the glottic opening (Figure 4-34).
   - When the curved blade is lifted anteriorly, the blade indirectly lifts

The smaller the child, the greater the proportion between the size of the cranium and midface and the greater the propensity of the posterior pharyngeal area to "buckle" as the relatively large occiput forces passive flexion of the cervical spine.[11]

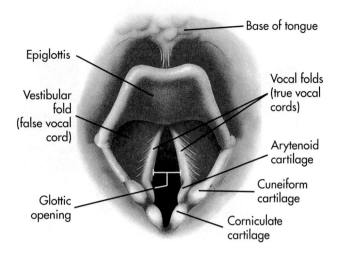

Figure 4-33 Landmarks for tracheal intubation.

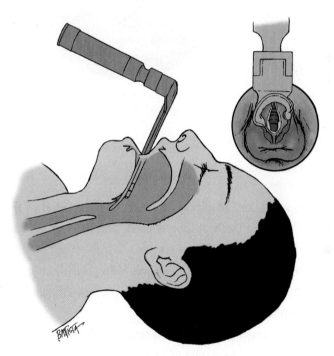

Figure 4-34 When the straight blade is lifted anteriorly, the blade directly lifts the epiglottis out of the way to expose the glottic opening.

the epiglottis to expose the glottic opening (Figure 4-35).

- Visualize the vocal cords.

9. Insert the tracheal tube.

- While holding the laryngoscope steady with your left hand, grasp the tracheal tube with your right hand and gently introduce it into the right corner of the patient's mouth.

- If the patient's vocal cords are open, advance the tube through the glottic opening. If they are closed, wait for them to open before advancing the tube.

- Visualize the distal tip of the tracheal tube and advance the tube

Do not attempt to pass the tracheal tube through the channel in the laryngoscope blade. Doing so will obstruct your view of the glottic opening.

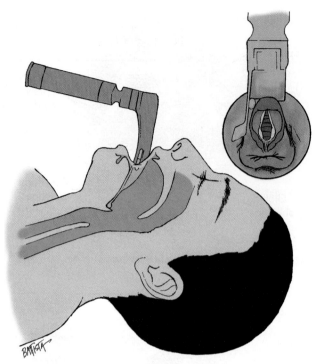

Figure 4-35 When the curved blade is lifted anteriorly, the blade indirectly lifts the epiglottis to expose the glottic opening.

until the vocal cord marker on the tube is at the level of the vocal cords. If a cuffed tracheal tube is used, advance the tube until the cuff lies just beyond the vocal cords.

- While holding the tracheal tube firmly with your thumb and index finger against the child's lip or upper gum, remove the laryngoscope blade from the patient's mouth.

- While continuing to hold the tracheal tube in place, remove the stylet from the tracheal tube (if used). If a cuffed tracheal tube was used, inflate the distal cuff with air; disconnect the syringe from the inflation valve. Check the pilot balloon on the tracheal tube to verify inflation.

- Detach the face mask from the bag-mask device. Attach the bag-mask device to the tracheal tube and ventilate the patient at an age-appropriate rate. If a cuffed tracheal tube was used, the distal cuff should be inflated just until the air leak heard during ventilation disappears.

10. Confirm correct placement.

    While holding the tube securely against the corner of the patient's mouth, use primary and secondary methods to confirm proper placement of a tracheal tube.

Fogging or vapor condensation on the inside of the tracheal tube is *not* a reliable indicator of proper tube position.

- **Primary** methods include clinical assessments.
  - Visualize the passage of the tracheal tube between the vocal cords.
  - Visualize symmetrical chest rise during positive-pressure ventilation.
  - Confirm the absence of sounds over the epigastrium during positive-pressure ventilation.
    - After intubation, the presence of bubbling or gurgling sounds during auscultation of the epigastrium suggests the tube is incorrectly positioned in the esophagus. To correct this problem, deflate the tracheal tube cuff (if a cuffed tube was used), remove the tube, and preoxygenate before reattempting intubation.
    - Breath sounds may be heard over the stomach in infants but should not be louder than midaxillary sounds.
  - Auscultate for bilateral breath sounds.
    - Auscultate for breath sounds in the second or third intercostal space in the anterior axillary line. Listen for two breaths on the right side of the chest, and then listen to the left side and compare.
    - If baseline breath sounds (i.e., breath sounds before intubation) were equal bilaterally, diminished breath sounds on the left side after intubation suggests that the tracheal tube has entered the right primary bronchus. To correct this problem, auscultate the left side of the chest while slowly withdrawing the tube until breath sounds are equal and chest expansion is symmetric.
    - If baseline breath sounds were equal bilaterally and are absent bilaterally after intubation, the tracheal tube is most likely in the esophagus. To correct this problem, deflate the tracheal tube cuff (if a cuffed tube was used), remove the tube, and preoxygenate before reattempting intubation.
  - Absence of vocal sounds after placement of the tracheal tube.
  - Assess the child's skin color and heart rate. If poor skin color and bradycardia persist after intubation, consider the following possible causes:
    - The tracheal tube is too small, allowing air leaks.
    - The tracheal tube cuff (if used) is underinflated.
    - The pop-off valve on the bag-mask device is not disabled.
    - The bag-mask device operator is not delivering an adequate volume for each breath.
    - A pneumothorax is present.
    - The tracheal tube is clogged or kinked.
    - Esophageal intubation.

- Primary bronchus intubation.
- There is a leak (or other malfunction) in the bag–mask device (mechanical failure).
- Disconnected oxygen source (mechanical failure).

- **Secondary** methods include the use of a mechanical device.
  - Use a capnometer to measure the concentration of CO_2 at the end of exhalation (discussed later in this chapter). Waveform capnography is preferred.
  - If the infant or child has a perfusing rhythm, oxygen saturation can be assessed using a pulse oximeter.
  - Verify tube placement with an esophageal detector device.
    - Esophageal detector devices (EDDs) are simple, inexpensive, and easy to use. An EDD is used as an aid in determining if a tracheal tube is in the trachea or esophagus.
    - These devices operate under the principle that the esophagus is a collapsible tube and the trachea a rigid one.
    - The syringe-type EDD is connected to a tracheal tube with the plunger fully inserted into the barrel of the syringe (Figure 4-36A). If the tracheal tube is in the trachea, the plunger can be easily withdrawn from the syringe barrel. If the tracheal tube is in the esophagus, resistance will be felt when the plunger is withdrawn because the walls of the esophagus will collapse when negative pressure is applied to the syringe.
    - The bulb-type EDD is compressed before it is connected to a tracheal tube (Figure 4-36B).
    - A vacuum is created as the pressure on the bulb is released. If the tracheal tube is in the trachea, the bulb will refill easily when pressure is released, indicating proper tube placement. If the tracheal tube is in the esophagus, the bulb will remain collapsed, indicating improper tube placement.
    - Special considerations.
      - Results may be misleading in cases of morbid obesity, late pregnancy, and status asthmaticus, and in the presence of copious tracheal secretions.
      - If an EDD is used to confirm placement of a cuffed tracheal tube, do NOT inflate the cuff before using the esophageal detector. Inflating the cuff moves the distal end of the tracheal tube away from the walls of the esophagus. If the tube was inadvertently inserted into the esophagus, this movement will cause the detector bulb to reexpand, falsely suggesting that the tube was in the trachea.

An EDD may be used in children with a perfusing rhythm who weigh more than 20 kilograms.

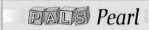
PALS Pearl

Movement of the head and neck of an intubated infant or child can affect the placement of the tube. Reassess and confirm the position of the tube:
- Immediately after tube insertion
- Whenever the patient is moved or repositioned
- Whenever a procedure is performed (e.g., suctioning, tracheal medication administration)
- When there is a change in the patient's clinical status
- During interhospital and intrahospital transport

- On chest radiography, the tip of the tracheal tube should be positioned midway between the vocal cords and the carina.

11. Secure the tube in place.
    - Secure the tracheal tube with a commercial tube holder or tape and provide ventilatory support with supplemental oxygen.
    - After securing the tube, reassess to ensure the tracheal tube is in proper position.
    - Record the tube depth at the patient's teeth.

12. Resume oxygenation and ventilation.

Troubleshooting inadequate ventilation or oxygenation (DOPE).

- **D**isplaced tube (e.g., right primary bronchus or esophageal intubation): reassess tube position.
- **O**bstructed tube (e.g., blood or secretions are obstructing air flow): suction.
- **P**neumothorax (tension): needle thoracostomy.
- **E**quipment problem/failure: check equipment and oxygen source.

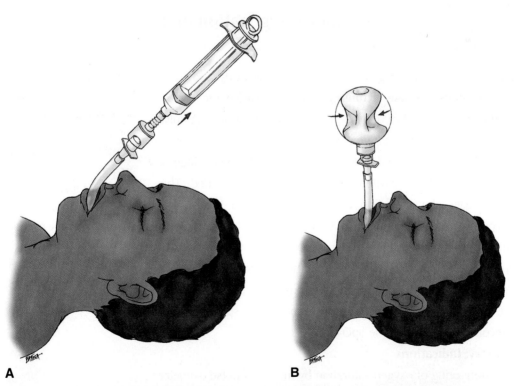

A   **B**

Figure 4-36 A) The syringe type esophageal detector device (EDD) is connected to a tracheal tube with the plunger fully inserted into the barrel of the syringe. If the tracheal tube is in the trachea, the plunger can be easily withdrawn from the syringe barrel. B) When using a bulb-type EDD, the bulb is compressed before it is connected to a tracheal tube. If the tracheal tube is in the trachea, the bulb will refill easily when pressure is released.

- Bleeding.
- Laryngospasm.
- Vocal cord damage.
- Mucosal necrosis.
- Barotrauma.
- Aspiration.
- Cuff leak.
- Esophageal intubation.
- Right primary bronchus intubation.
- Occlusion caused by patient biting the tube or secretions
- Laryngeal or tracheal edema.
- Tube occlusion.
- Hypoxia due to prolonged or unsuccessful intubation.
- Arrhythmias.
- Trauma to the lips, teeth, tongue or soft tissues of the oropharynx.
- Increased intracranial pressure.

Devices to Monitor Oxygenation and Ventilation

Oxygenation is the process of getting oxygen into the body and to its tissues for metabolism. **Pulse oximetry** is a noninvasive method of measuring the percentage of oxygen saturated peripheral tissues. A pulse oximeter (commonly called a *pulse ox*) is a small instrument with a light sensor. The oximeter quickly and accurately calculates the percentage of hemoglobin saturated with oxygen in a pulsating capillary bed. This calculation is called the saturation of peripheral oxygen (SpO_2). The sensor is typically applied to a finger, but the forehead, an earlobe, or a toe can be used with selection of a sensor appropriate for the chosen site. For example, an adhesive or clip-on sensor can be used for a finger, while a forehead is usually adhesive. Placement of a sensor in a central location, such as the earlobe, may reflect the most rapid oximeter response (within about 10 seconds) to a drop in the SpO_2).

Pulse Oximetry: Indications

Continuous monitoring of oxygen saturation by means of pulse oximetry is considered the standard of care in any circumstance in which detection of hypoxemia is important. However, in critical situations, do not delay lifesaving interventions to initiate pulse oximetry.

When using a pulse oximeter, check that the pulse rate according to the oximeter is consistent with that obtained by palpation to ensure an accurate measurement. Be aware that tissue injury may occur at the measuring site because of probe misuse (e.g., pressure sores from prolonged application.) Assess the site every 2 to 4 hours and replace the sensor every 24 hours.

Because pulsatile blood flow is necessary for a pulse oximeter to work, it may provide inaccurate results in a child with poor peripheral perfusion. Pulse oximetry may also be inaccurate in children with chronic hypoxemia (e.g., cyanotic heart disease, pulmonary hypertension).

Possible indications for continuous pulse oximetry include the following:

- The patient has a critical or unstable airway
- The patient requires oxygen therapy
- During the intrahospital and interhospital transfer of critically ill patients
- During hemodialysis
- The patient requires oxygenation monitoring during emergency airway management
- During ventilatior and oxygen therapy changes
- Evaluate of the adequacy of preoxygenation before tracheal intubation
- During the delivery and recovery from conscious sedation or surgery
- The patient has acute respiratory distress or a chronic respiratory condition
- The patient has a chest wall injury or chest pain
- The patient is morbidly obese
- The patient is receiving analgesics at a dose or by a route of administration that is likely to produce ventilatory depression.

A pulse oximeter is an adjunct to, not a replacement for, vigilant patient assessment. You must correlate your assessment findings with pulse oximeter readings to determine appropriate-treatment interventions for the patient.

After hypooxygenation, the oxyhemoglobin saturation detected by pulse oximetry may not decline for as long as 3 minutes—even when ventilation is ineffective.[10, 12, 13]

Exhaled or End-Tidal Carbon Dioxide Monitoring

An ETCO$_2$ detector can accurately confirm tracheal placement of a tracheal tube in children with spontaneous circulation who weigh more than 2 kg.

End-Tidal Carbon Dioxide Monitoring: Indications

Examples of situations in which exhaled CO$_2$ monitoring is commonly used include the following:

- Verification of tracheal tube placement (capnography should not be used as the only means of assessing tracheal tube assessment)
- Procedural sedation and analgesia
- Evaluation of mechanical ventilation and resuscitation efforts
- Continuous monitoring of tracheal tube position (including during patient transport)
- Monitoring of exhaled CO$_2$ levels in patients with suspected increased intracranial pressure
- Assessment of the adequacy of ventilation in patients with altered mental status, bronchospasm, asthma, anaphylaxis, heart failure, drug overdose, stroke, shock, or circulatory compromise

End-Tidal Carbon Dioxide Monitoring: Types of Devices

- Digital capnometers use infrared technology to analyze exhaled gas. These devices provide a quantitative measurement of the exhaled CO$_2$ in that they provide the exact amount of CO$_2$ exhaled. This is beneficial as trends in CO_2 levels can be monitored and the effectiveness of treatment can be determined.

- Capnography devices function through infrared technology. In addition to providing quantitative data as the digital capnometer does, they also provide information about air movement in and out of the lungs with a graphical waveform. The process of CO_2 elimination produces a characteristic waveform called a capnogram.

- A colorimetric capnometer functions through a pH change that occurs within the breath of a patient. The patient's breath causes a chemical reaction on pH-sensitive litmus paper housed in the detector. The capnometer is placed between a tracheal tube or advanced airway device, and a ventilation device. The presence of CO_2 (evidenced by the color change on the colorimetric device) suggests the placement of the tube in the trachea, however this type of capnometer is qualitative in that it simply shows the presence of CO_2. It has no ability to provide an actual CO_2 reading, indicate the presence of hypercarbia, and provides no opportunity for ongoing monitoring to ensure the tube remains in the trachea. A lack of CO_2 (no color change) suggests tube placement in the esophagus, particularly in clients with spontaneous circulation. Because CO_2 may inadvertently enter the stomach, ventilate the patient at least six times before evaluating tracheal tube placement using an exhaled CO_2 detector to quickly wash out any retained CO_2. If the tracheal tube is misplaced in the esophagus, six ventilations may lead to gastric distention, vomiting, and aspiration. In animals, false-positive results (CO_2 is detected despite tube placement in the esophagus) has been reported when large amounts of carbonated beverages were ingested before a cardiac arrest. False-negative results (lack of CO_2 detection despite tube placement in the trachea) may occur in cardiac arrest or in a patient who has a significant pulmonary embolus because of reduced CO_2 to the lungs. Colorimetric capnometers are susceptible to inaccurate results because of the age of the paper, exposure of the paper to the environment, patient secretions such as vomitus, or acidic drugs such as tracheally administered epinephrine.

Use a pediatric $ETCO_2$ detector for patients weighing 2 to 15 kg. Use an adult $ETCO_2$ detector if the patient weighs more than 15 kg.

Rapid Sequence Intubation

Rapid Sequence Intubation: Description

RSI is the use of medications to sedate and paralyze a patient to rapidly achieve tracheal intubation. In addition to sedatives and paralytics, other medications may be used to minimize or prevent the physiologic responses of intubation such as the cough reflex, gag reflex, cardiac dysrhythmias, increased intracranial pressure, pain, hypoxia, hypertension, and increased ocular pressure.

Rapid Sequence Intubation: Indications

- Excessive work of breathing, which may lead to fatigue and respiratory failure.
- Loss of protective airway reflexes (e.g., cough, gag).
- Combative patients requiring airway control.
- Uncontrolled seizure activity (to provide airway control).
- Functional or anatomic airway obstruction.
- Head trauma and Glasgow Coma Scale score less than 8.
- Severe asthma.
- Inadequate central nervous system control of ventilation.
- Need for high peak inspiratory pressure or positive-end expiratory pressure to maintain effective alveolar gas exchange.
- To permit sedation for diagnostic studies while ensuring airway protection and control of secretions.

Rapid Sequence Intubation: Procedure

Ensure all equipment is in working order.

The seven P's of rapid sequence intubation:
Preparation (0 –10 minutes)
Preoxygenate (0 –5 minutes)
Premedicate (0 –3 minutes)
Paralysis with sedation (0)
Protect the airway (0 + 15 seconds)
Pass the tube and proof of placement (zero + 45 seconds)
Postintubation management (zero + 60 seconds)

1. **Prepare** (zero minus 10 minutes).
   - Obtain a SAMPLE medical history and perform a focused physical examination.
   - Assemble age-appropriate equipment. Alternative airways should be readily available to assist in the management of a difficult airway such as LMAs, needle cricothyrotomy equipment, and surgical cricothyrotomy equipment.
   - Apply the cardiac monitor and pulse oximeter.
   - Assemble personnel.
     ○ If cervical spine injury is suspected, assign another assistant to manually stabilize the neck in a neutral position.
     ○ Assign another assistant to monitor the patient's heart rate, ECG rhythm, blood pressure, and pulse oximeter readings.
   - Establish an IV. Assemble and draw up all medications that will be used during the procedure.
2. **Preoxygenate** (0 minus 5 minutes) with 100% oxygen for 3 minutes.
3. **Premedicate** (0 minus 3 minutes).

- The initial medications administered during RSI are used to minimize the physiologic responses sometimes associated with intubation. These medications are referred to "adjunctive medications" or "adjunctive agents."
- Atropine.
  - Atropine is given to decrease airway secretions and minimize the bradycardia that may result from vagal stimulation during intubation.
    - Atropine administration should be standard for all children younger than 1 year, children who are bradycardic, children younger than 5 years who are to receive succinylcholine, and adolescents who receive a second dose of succinylcholine. Ketamine increases secretions. Atropine is suggested if ketamine is administered.
- Lidocaine.
  - Give lidocaine for head injury or increased intracranial pressure.
  - Lidocaine diminishes the cough and gag reflexes, and may diminish the rise in intracranial pressure (ICP) associated with intubation.
  - If indicated, administer 2 to 5 minutes before the RSI procedure.
  - Administration of a defasciculating dose (one tenth of the paralyzing dose) of a nondepolarizing paralytic agent (e.g., vecuronium, pancuronium) is recommended for children 5 years of age and older if succinylcholine is the paralytic agent selected for use.

4. **Paralyze and sedate** (0 minute).

- Agents used for sedation during RSI include barbiturates, benzodiazepines, opiates, nonbarbiturate sedatives, and dissociative agents. Select an appropriate sedative based on the patient's age,

> For maximum effect at the time of intubation, atropine should be given at least 1 to 2 minutes before the procedure.

PALS Pearl

"I SOAP ME" is a memory aid that can help you recall the equipment and medications required for rapid sequence intubation:

IV—Ensure a secure intravenous (IV) line is in place

Suction—Connect, power on, verify it is in working order.

Oxygen—Ensure patient is adequately ventilated and preoxygenated.

Airway equipment—Laryngoscope with various blade sizes, stylet, tracheal tube for body length and age plus tubes 0.5 mm larger and smaller, tape or a commercial tube holder, oropharyngeal and nasal airways, nasogastric tube, Magill forceps, alternative airways

Pharmacologic agents—Decide what medications will be used, calculate correct doses, and draw up.

Monitoring equipment—ECG monitor, pulse oximeter, capnometer, blood pressure.

Endotracheal versus esophageal detection method for confirmation of tube position.

clinical condition, and the effects of the medication being considered for administration. Select a sedative that lasts as long as or longer than the paralytic agent to be administered, or be prepared to administer additional sedation. Administer the sedative *before* the paralytic agent.

Fasciculations are muscle twitches. A defasciculation agent is a medication that is given to inhibit muscle twitching.

- Administer a paralytic agent. *Once a paralytic has been administered, you assume complete responsibility for maintaining an adequate airway and ventilation.*
  - Administration of a defasciculating dose (one tenth of the paralyzing dose) of a nondepolarizing paralytic agent (e.g., vecuronium, pancuronium) is recommended for children 5 years of age and older if succinylcholine is the paralytic agent selected for use.

Paralysis without sedation has been described as comparable to being buried alive. The patient should **never** be awake while paralyzed.

5. **Protect the airway** (0 + 15 seconds).
  - Position the patient for intubation. Ensure the patient is supine on a firm surface with the head in a midline and slightly extended position. Open the mouth with the right thumb and index finger. While maintaining direct visualization, insert the tracheal tube from the right corner of the mouth through the vocal cords.

6. **Pass the tube and proof of placement** (0 + 45 seconds).
  - Relaxation of the mandible and decreased resistance to manual ventilation indicates that the patient is ready to be intubated. Insert a tracheal tube of appropriate size to a depth of three times the tube diameter, remove the stylet (if used), and inflate the tracheal tube cuff (if so equipped).
  - If intubation is unsuccessful, maintain cricoid pressure and ventilate the patient with a bag-mask device. After the patient is reoxygenated, attempt another intubation or use an alternative airway technique.
  - Confirm tube placement.

7. **Postintubation management** (0 + 60 seconds).
  - Verify the tracheal tube is positioned at the correct depth (centimeters at the lips should be three times the tracheal tube diameter).
  - Secure the tube in place with tape or a commercial tracheal tube holder.
  - Begin mechanical ventilation.
  - Reassess the patient's vital signs, including pulse oximetry and waveform capnography.
  - Administer additional medications as necessary (e.g., sedatives, long-lasting muscle relaxants).
  - Obtain a chest radiograph to confirm correct tube placement.

Absolute Contraindications

- Patients in whom alternative airway control (i.e., cricothyrotomy) would be difficult or impossible due to anatomy or massive neck swelling.
- Patients who would be difficult or impossible to intubate after paralysis.
- Operator unfamiliarity with the medications used for the RSI procedure.

Relative Contraindications

The risk of complications must be weighed against the benefit of obtaining airway control.

- Severely increased intracranial pressure.
- Known hypersensitivity to the medications used for the procedure.
- Known unstable cervical spine injury or fracture.

- Prolonged apnea.
- Bradycardia.
- Fasciculations.
- Death due to anoxia in a patient who cannot be intubated or ventilated.
- Hypotension (secondary to sedative administration).
- Hyperkalemia (adverse effect associated with succinylcholine).
- Increased intragastric pressure.
- Malignant hyperthermia.

Rapid Sequence Intubation: Contraindications

Before initiating RSI, the individual performing the procedure must be trained, appropriately credentialed, and prepared to perform a cricothyrotomy in the event of a failed airway.

Rapid Sequence Intubation: Complications

Needle Cricothyrotomy

- Needle cricothyrotomy (also called percutaneous cricothyrotomy) is a method of providing ventilation by insertion of a large-bore, over-the-needle catheter into the cricothyroid membrane. This procedure may be indicated in cases of upper airway obstruction that *cannot be relieved by less invasive methods* such as head positioning, suctioning, foreign body airway maneuvers, bag-mask ventilation, and tracheal intubation.
- Needle cricothyrotomy may be extremely difficult to perform in infants and young children because of the mobility of the larynx and trachea and the softness of the laryngeal cartilage in these patients, making palpation of the landmarks for the procedure difficult and collapse of the upper airway with labored breathing more likely.[14] This procedure requires special training and frequent refresher training to maintain skill proficiency.

- Conditions in which intubation is difficult or impossible.
- Craniofacial abnormalities.
- Congenital laryngeal anomalies.
- Excessive oropharyngeal hemorrhage.

Description

Indications

- Massive traumatic or congenital deformities.
- Complete upper airway obstruction.
- Laryngeal fracture.
- Pharyngeal/laryngeal burns.
- Subglottic stenosis.
- Respiratory arrest or near arrest in patients who cannot be tracheally intubated.
- Cervical spine fracture with respiratory compromise in patients who cannot be tracheally intubated.

Contraindications

- Unavailable or inadequate equipment.

Advantages

- Allows rapid entrance to the airway for temporary oxygenation and ventilation.

Disadvantages

- Does not allow for efficient elimination of CO_2.
- Invasive procedure.
- Requires skilled rescuers to perform with frequent retraining.

Equipment Needed

- PPE.
- Oxygen source.
- Suction equipment.
- Antiseptic solution.
- Bag-mask device (size appropriate for patient).
- 14-gauge (or larger) over-the-needle catheter.
- 3-mL syringe.
- Adapter from the top of a 3-mm tracheal tube.
- Tape or commercial tube holder.

Procedure

- Place the patient in a supine position.
- Identify landmarks (Figure 4-35). Palpate the cricothyroid membrane between the thyroid and cricoid cartilages.
- Cleanse the site. Attach a 3-mL syringe to a 14-gauge (or larger) over-the-needle catheter.
- Stabilize the cricoid and thyroid cartilage between the thumb and finger of one hand. Using the over-the-needle catheter, carefully puncture the skin in the midline, directly over the cricothyroid membrane (Figure 4-36).
- Direct the needle and catheter toward the feet at a 45-degree angle. Carefully insert the needle and catheter through the cricothyroid membrane, maintaining negative pressure (pulling back) on the syringe as the needle is advanced. A return of air signifies entry into the tracheal lumen.

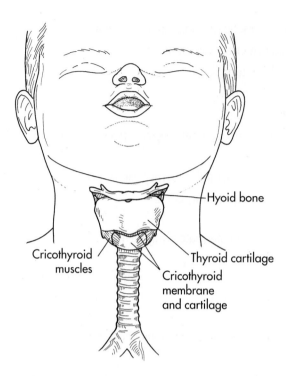

Figure 4-35 Anatomic landmarks for cricothyroidotomy.

- Advance the catheter over the needle, being careful to avoid the posterior tracheal wall, until the catheter hub is flush with the skin. Hold the catheter hub in place to prevent displacement.
- Withdraw the needle carefully, advancing the catheter downward into position in the trachea.
- Attach the hub of the IV catheter to a 3-mm pediatric tracheal tube adapter and ventilate with 100% oxygen using a bag-mask device. (Alternatively, attach the barrel of a 3-mL syringe to the IV catheter and an 8-mm tracheal tube adapter to the syringe barrel.)
- Monitor carefully for chest rise, and auscultate for adequate ventilation. Assess ETCO$_2$, pulse oximetry, ECG, and vital signs.
- Secure the catheter in place.

Complications

- Bleeding.
- Infection.
- Hematoma.
- Hypoxemia.
- Catheter dislodgement.
- Subcutaneous and/or mediastinal emphysema.
- Inadequate ventilation resulting in hypoxia and death.

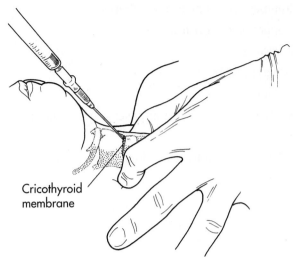

Cricothyroid
membrane

Figure 4-36 Stabilize the cricoid and thyroid cartilage between the thumb and finger of one hand. Using the over-the-needle catheter, carefully puncture the skin in the midline, directly over the cricothyroid membrane. Direct the needle and catheter toward the feet at a 45-degree angle.

Surgical Cricothyrotomy

Description

- A surgical cricothyrotomy is the creation of an opening into the cricothyroid membrane with a scalpel to allow rapid entrance to the airway for temporary oxygenation and ventilation. This procedure may be indicated in cases of upper airway obstruction that *cannot be relieved by less invasive methods* such as head positioning, suctioning, foreign body airway maneuvers, bag-mask ventilation, and tracheal intubation.
- Because surgical cricothyrotomy may be difficult to perform in infants and young children as a result of the difficulty in palpating and identifying the important landmarks of the neck, and because of the small diameter of the cricoid cartilage, the procedure is not recommended in children under the age of 10.[15] This procedure requires special training and frequent refresher training to maintain skill proficiency.

Indications

Surgical cricothyrotomy is rarely indicated for the infant or young child. If the procedure is necessary, it should be performed by the most experienced person available, preferably an experienced surgeon.

- Conditions in which intubation is difficult or impossible.
- Craniofacial abnormalities.
- Congenital laryngeal anomalies.
- Excessive oropharyngeal hemorrhage.

- Massive traumatic or congenital deformities.
- Complete upper airway obstruction.
- Laryngeal fracture.
- Pharyngeal/laryngeal burns.
- Subglottic stenosis.
- Respiratory arrest or near arrest in patients who cannot be tracheally intubated.
- Cervical spine fracture with respiratory compromise in patients who cannot be tracheally intubated.

- Children younger than 10 years.
- Adequate nonsurgical airway.
- Unavailable or inadequate equipment.
- Bleeding diatheses.

Contraindications

- Allows rapid entrance to the airway for temporary oxygenation and ventilation.

Advantages

- Invasive procedure.
- Requires skilled rescuers to perform with frequent retraining.

Disadvantages

- PPE.
- Oxygen source.
- Suction equipment.
- Antiseptic solution.
- Bag-mask device (size appropriate for patient).
- Scalpel.
- Tracheal tube or tracheostomy tube.
- Tape or commercial tube holder.

Equipment Needed

The most prominent structures in the anterior neck of the infant or child are the hyoid bone and the cricoid cartilage.

Procedure

- Place the patient in a supine position. If not contraindicated, extend the neck to expose landmarks.
- Identify landmarks (hyoid bone, thyroid cartilage, cricoid cartilage, cricothyroid membrane). Palpate the hyoid bone high in the neck. Next, locate the thyroid cartilage and then the cricoid cartilage. Identify the cricothyroid membrane between the thyroid and cricoid cartilages.
- Cleanse the site. Use a local anesthetic if the patient is conscious and if time permits.

In an older child, a horizontal incision may be made directly through the skin, muscle, and cricothyroid membrane if landmarks are obvious.

- Stabilize the larynx between the finger and thumb of one hand. Make a vertical incision over the thyroid and cricoid cartilages.
- Expose the cricothyroid membrane (Figure 4-37). Make a horizontal incision through the cricothyroid membrane into the airway and listen/feel for air flow.
- Insert a tracheostomy or tracheal tube of appropriate size through the cricothyroid membrane, directing the tube caudally into the lower trachea.
- Connect the tracheostomy (or tracheal) tube to a bag–mask device and ventilate the patient with 100% oxygen.
- Monitor carefully for chest rise and auscultate for adequate ventilation. Assess ETCO$_2$, pulse oximetry, ECG, and vital signs.
- Secure the tube to prevent dislodgement.

Complications

- Asphyxia.
- Aspiration (blood).
- Creation of a false passage into the tissues.
- Mediastinal emphysema.
- Hemorrhage or hematoma formation.

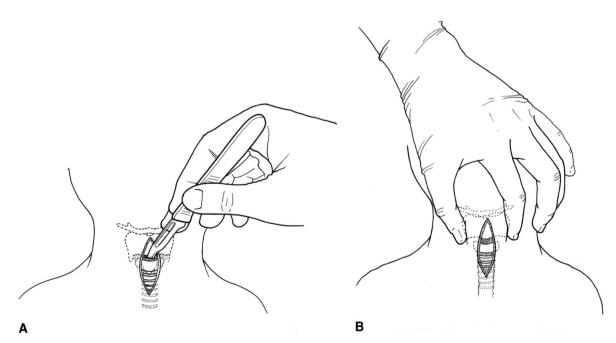

A   B

Figure 4-37 Identify the hyoid bone, thyroid cartilage, cricoid cartilage, and cricothyroid membrane. Stabilize the larynx between the finger and thumb of one hand. Make a vertical incision over the thyroid and cricoid cartilages. Expose the cricothyroid membrane. In an older child, a horizontal incision may be made directly through the skin, muscle, and cricothyroid membrane if landmarks are obvious.

- Vocal cord paralysis.
- Hoarseness.
- Laceration of the trachea/esophagus.
- Subglottic stenosis.
- Tube dislodgement.

Needle Thoracostomy

Description

Needle thoracostomy (also called needle decompression) is the insertion of an over-the-needle catheter into the chest to relieve a tension pneumothorax.

Indications

Suspected tension pneumothorax as evidenced by:
- Progressively worsening dyspnea.
- Tachypnea.
- Tachycardia.
- Poor ventilation despite an open airway.
- Restlessness and agitation.
- Increased airway resistance when ventilating patient (poor bag compliance).
- Hyperresonance to percussion on the affected side.
- Diminished or absent breath sounds on the affected side.
- Decreased level of responsiveness.
- Hypotension.
- Tracheal deviation away from side of injury (may or may not be present).
- Distended neck veins (may not be present if hypovolemia is present or hypotension is severe).
- Cyanosis.

Contraindications

There are no contraindications to this procedure if the patient's clinical presentation, history, and physical findings suggest the presence of a tension pneumothorax.

Equipment Needed

- PPE.
- Oxygen source.
- Antiseptic solution.
- 18-gauge over-the-needle catheter for children younger than 8 years.
- 14-gauge over-the-needle catheter for children 8 years of age and older.
- One-way valve (e.g., Heimlich valve).

Procedure

- Place the patient in a supine position and elevate the child's arm behind the head. Restrain as needed.
- Identify landmark—the second intercostal space at the midclavicular line.
- Cleanse the site. Use a local anesthetic if the patient is conscious and if time permits.
- Holding an over-the-needle catheter at a 90-degree angle to the chest wall, insert the needle through the skin.
  - Use an 18-gauge over-the-needle catheter for children younger than 8 years.
  - Use a 14-gauge over-the-needle catheter for children 8 years of age and older.
- Slowly advance the needle over the superior border of the rib until the pleural space is entered. Entry into the pleural space is evidenced by one or more of the following:
  - A "popping" sound or "giving way" sensation.
  - A sudden rush of air.
  - Ability to aspirate air into a syringe (if used).
- Remove the needle from the catheter, leaving the catheter in place.
- Connect the catheter to a one-way valve (e.g., Heimlich valve). (An improvised one-way valve may be constructed from the finger of a surgical glove.)
- Secure the catheter and valve to the patient's chest wall to prevent dislodgement.
- Assess the patient's response to the procedure by evaluating ventilatory status, breath sounds, jugular veins, tracheal position, and vital signs.

Definitive treatment of a tension pneumothorax requires insertion of a chest tube, after which the needle thoracostomy catheter may be removed.

Complications

- Pneumothorax.
- Pleural infection.
- Laceration of the lung.
- Laceration of the intercostal vessel(s) with resultant hemorrhage.

Case Study Resolution

This child is sick. The presence of a high fever, productive cough, and tachypnea suggests pneumonia with signs of respiratory failure. Move quickly. Use PPE. Initiate pulse oximetry (initial SpO_2 on room air was 83%). Correct hypoxia by giving supplemental oxygen in a manner that does not agitate the child (SpO_2 on a nonrebreather mask was 87%). Place the child on a cardiac monitor and establish vascular access. Provide further interventions based on assessment findings. (Note: This child had decreased breath sounds in the right middle and lower lobes. Lower lobe consolidation was observed on her chest radiograph. She was preoxygenated, RSI was performed, and IV antibiotics were started.)

References

1. Berg RA, Hemphill R, Abella BS, et al. Part 5: Adult basic life support: 2010 American Heart Association Guidelines for Cardiopulmonary Resuscitation and Emergency Cardiovascular Care. *Circulation.* 2010;122(suppl 3):S685–S705.

2. Rice MJ, Mancuso AA, Gibbs C, et al. Cricoid pressure results in compression of the postcricoid hypopharynx: the esophageal position is irrelevant. *Anesth Analg* 2009 Nov;109(5):1546-5152.

3. Howells TH, Chamney AR, Wraight WJ, Simons RS. The application of cricoid pressure: an assessment and a survey of its practice. *Anaesthesia* 1983;38(5):457-460.

4. Lawes EG. Cricoid pressure with or without the "cricoid yoke." Br J *Anaesth* 1986;58(12):1376-1379.

5. Flucker CJ, Hart E, Weisz M, et al. The 50-millilitre syringe as an inexpensive training aid in the application of cricoid pressure. *Eur J Anaesthesiol* 2000;17(7):443-447.

6. Koziol CA, Cuddeford JD, Moos DD. Assessing the force generated with application of cricoid pressure. *AORN J* 2000;72(6):1018-1028, 1030.

7. Kopka A, Crawford J. Cricoid pressure: a simple, yet effective biofeedback trainer. *Eur J Anaesthesiol* 2004;21(6):443-447.

8. Domuracki KJ, Moule CJ, Owen H, et al. Learning on a simulator does transfer to clinical practice. *Resuscitation* 2009;80(3):346-349.

9. Berg MD, Schexnayder SM, Chameides L, et al. Part 13: Pediatric basic life support: 2010 American Heart Association Guidelines for Cardiopulmonary Resuscitation and Emergency Cardiovascular Care. *Circulation* 2010;122(suppl 3):S862-S875.

10. Kleinman ME, Chameides L, Schexnayder SM, et al. Part 14: Pediatric advanced life support: 2010 American Heart Association Guidelines for Cardiopulmonary Resuscitation and Emergency Cardiovascular Care. *Circulation* 2010;122(suppl 3):S876 –S908.

11. McSwain NE, Frame S, Salomone JP, eds. *Special considerations in trauma of the child,* 5th ed. St. Louis: Mosby, 2003.

12. Poirier MP, Gonzalez Del-Rey JA, McAneney CM, DiGiulio GA. Utility of monitoring capnography, pulse oximetry, and vital signs in the detection of airway mishaps: a hyperoxemic animal model. *Am J Emerg Med* 1998;16:350–352.

13. Birmingham PK, Cheney FW, Ward RJ. Esophageal intubation: a review of detection techniques. *Anesth Analg* 1986;65:886–891.

14. Bower CM. The surgical airway. In: Dieckmann RA, Fiser DH, Selbst SM, eds. *Illustrated textbook of pediatric emergency and critical care procedures*, St. Louis: Mosby,1997.

15. Gerardi MG. Evaluation and management of the multiple trauma patient. In: Strange GR, Ahrens WR, Lelyveld S, et al, eds. *Pediatric emergency medicine: a comprehensive study guide*, 2nd ed. New York: McGraw-Hill, 2002.

Chapter Quiz

1. Which of the following is NOT a desirable feature of a bag-mask device used during cardiopulmonary resuscitation?
   A) A clear mask
   B) A compressible, self-refilling bag
   C) Availability in adult and pediatric sizes
   D) Pop-off (pressure release) valve

2. A 3-year-old child weighing 15 kilograms requires tracheal intubation.
   A) What size laryngoscope blade should be used?
   B) What size tracheal tube should be used?
   C) Should you use a cuffed or uncuffed tracheal tube for this child?
   D) When the tracheal tube has been inserted to the proper depth, what is the cm marking that should appear at the patient's lips?

3. A six-year-old child in cardiopulmonary arrest has been intubated. Which of the following would indicate inadvertent esophageal intubation?
   A) Subcutaneous emphysema
   B) External jugular vein distention
   C) Gurgling sounds heard over the epigastrium
   D) Breath sounds present on only one side of the chest

4. Select the correct statement regarding cricoid pressure.
   A) Health care professionals often apply cricoid pressure incorrectly.
   B) Cricoid pressure should be used in pediatric patients of all ages to aid insertion of an advanced airway.
   C) Cricoid pressure eliminates the risk of vomiting and aspiration during ventilation and advanced airway insertion.
   D) Cricoid pressure may be used in both responsive and unresponsive patients who require positive pressure ventilation.

5. Stridor is:
   A) A high-pitched "whistling" sound produced by air moving through narrowed airway passages
   B) A harsh, high-pitched sound heard on inspiration associated with upper airway obstruction
   C) Abnormally rapid breathing
   D) An abnormal respiratory sound associated with collection of liquid or semi-solid material in the patient's upper airway

6. Tracheal intubation:
   A) Is contraindicated in an unresponsive patient
   B) Eliminates the risk of aspiration of gastric contents
   C) Should be performed in less than 60 seconds
   D) Should be preceded by efforts to ventilate by another method

7. The maximum length of time for suctioning an infant or child is:
   A) 5 seconds
   B) 10 seconds
   C) 15 seconds
   D) 30 seconds

8. Under optimum conditions, a partial rebreather mask can deliver an oxygen concentration of at a flow rate of 6 to 10 L/min.
   A) Up to 50%
   B) 25 to 45%
   C) 35 to 60%
   D) 60 to 95%

9. List five potential complications of tracheal intubation.
   1. _____
   2. _____
   3. _____
   4. _____
   5. _____

10. When intubating a patient with a curved blade, the tip of the blade should be placed:
    A) In the vallecula
    B) In the glottic opening
    C) Under the epiglottis
    D) Under the thyroid cartilage

Questions 11–21 refer to the following patient situation.

A 7-year-old girl is having difficulty breathing. You find the child sitting upright and leaning forward, supported by her arms, with her mouth open. Although she is aware of your presence, she appears unconcerned. You note the child has nasal flaring, suprasternal retractions, and is using her intercostal muscles to breathe. You hear loud wheezes without the use of a stethoscope. Her skin color is pale. A family member states the child has a history of asthma. A neighbor visited their home about an hour ago and showed them a kitten she had acquired, not realizing that the patient is allergic to cats.

11. From the information provided, complete the following documentation regarding the Pediatric Assessment Triangle.
    Appearance:
    Breathing:
    Circulation:

12. Your initial assessment reveals labored breathing at a rate of 38/min. Auscultation reveals absent breath sounds bilaterally in the bases, and diminished breath sounds throughout the remaining lung fields. Her heart rate is 140 beats/min and blood pressure is 94/62. Her skin is pale, but warm and dry. Capillary refill is less than 2 seconds. Speech is limited to 2 to 3 words. Is this patient sick or not sick? Describe your approach to the initial management of this patient.

13. What is the normal ventilatory rate for a 7-year-old child?

14. What is the normal heart rate for a 7-year-old child?

15. This child's appearance and assessment findings are consistent with:
    A) Respiratory distress
    B) Respiratory failure
    C) Respiratory arrest
    D) Cardiopulmonary arrest

16. The patient is now unresponsive. You have two other advanced life support personnel to assist you. Emergency equipment is immediately available. How will you open the patient's airway?

17. The patient's airway is now open. How should you proceed?

18. The patient's airway is clear. How should you proceed?

19. The patient is apneic. How will you determine the proper size oropharyngeal airway (OPA) for this child?

20. An oropharyngeal airway has been inserted. The patient remains apneic. A pulse is present at 70 beats/min. A bag-mask is available to provide positive pressure ventilation.
    1. What size mask should be used for this child?
    2. What size resuscitation bag should be used to ventilate this child?
    3. At what rate/minute should ventilations be delivered?

21. Which of the following types of medications are often used in the treatment of asthma?
    A) Bronchodilators, diuretics
    B) Beta-blockers, methylxanthines
    C) Corticosteroids, bronchodilators
    D) Diuretics, beta-blockers

Chapter Quiz Answers

1. D. The bag-mask used for resuscitation should have either no pop-off (pressure-release) valve or a pop-off valve that can be disabled during resuscitation. Some resuscitation situations require higher than normal ventilatory pressure, such as drowning, CPR, pulmonary edema, asthma, partial upper airway obstruction, or initial resuscitation of the newly born. To effectively ventilate a patient in these situations, the ventilatory pressure needed may exceed the limits of the pop-off valve. Thus, a pop-off valve may prevent generation of sufficient tidal volume to overcome the increase in airway resistance.

2. Tracheal intubation of a 3-year-old, 15 kg child:
    A) A size 2 laryngoscope blade should be used.
    B) If an uncuffed tracheal tube is used, a 5-mm tube should be selected. Be sure to have a 4.5 mm and 5.5 mm immediately available. If a cuffed tracheal tube is used, select a 4-mm tube and be sure that a 3.5 mm and 4.5 mm tube are within arm's reach.
    C) Both cuffed and uncuffed endotracheal tubes are acceptable for intubating infants and children.
    D) When the tracheal tube has been inserted to the proper depth, the 14 to 15 cm marking should appear at the patient's lips.

3. C. After intubation, the presence of bubbling or gurgling sounds during auscultation of the epigastrium suggests the tube is incorrectly positioned in the esophagus. To correct this problem, deflate the tracheal tube cuff (if a cuffed tube was used), remove the tube, and preoxygenate before reattempting intubation.

4. A. Cricoid pressure may be considered to minimize gastric inflation in an unresponsive patient. Studies suggest that cricoid pressure is frequently applied incorrectly. In some studies, participants applied too little pressure, placing patients at a risk of regurgitation, and in others excessive pressure was used. Although some studies have not found cricoid pressure to cause a barrier to advanced airway insertion, most have shown that cricoid pressure impedes placement, impairs the rate of successful ventilation, and hinders ventilation. Aspiration can occur despite application of pressure.

5. B. Stridor is a harsh, high-pitched sound heard on inspiration associated with upper airway obstruction. Wheezes are high-pitched "whistling" sounds produced by air moving through narrowed airway passages. Tachypnea is abnormally rapid breathing. Gurgling is abnormal respiratory sound associated with collection of liquid or semi-solid material in the patient's upper airway.

6. D. Tracheal intubation should be preceded by attempts to ventilate by another method. Tracheal intubation reduces, but does not eliminate, the risk of aspiration of gastric contents. When attempted, tracheal intubation should be performed in less than 30 seconds.

7. B. Insertion of a suction catheter and suctioning should take no longer than 10 seconds per attempt. When suctioning to remove material that completely obstructs the airway, more time may be necessary.

8. C. A partial rebreather mask can deliver an oxygen concentration of 35 to 60% at a flow rate of 6 to 10 L/min.

9. Complications of tracheal intubation include bleeding, laryngospasm, vocal cord damage, mucosal necrosis, barotrauma, aspiration, cuff leak, esophageal intubation, right primary bronchus intubation, occlusion caused by patient biting the tube or secretions, laryngeal or tracheal edema, tube occlusion, hypoxia due to prolonged or unsuccessful intubation, arhythmias; trauma to the lips, teeth, tongue or soft tissues of the oropharynx; increased intracranial pressure

10. A. When intubating a patient with a curved blade, the tip of the blade should be placed in the vallecula.

11. Pediatric Assessment Triangle:
    Appearance: Awake, seated in tripod position; unconcerned about your presence
    Breathing: Spontaneous breathing; increased ventilatory effort evident
    Circulation: Pale skin color; no evidence of bleeding

12. This child is sick. Move quickly. Open the airway and suction if necessary. Correct hypoxia by giving supplemental oxygen. Begin assisted ventilation if the patient does not improve. Provide further interventions based on assessment findings.

13. The normal ventilatory rate for a 7-year-old is 18 to 30 breaths/min. This patient's ventilatory rate is elevated for her age.

14. The normal heart rate for a 7-year-old is 70 to 120 beats/min. This patient's heart rate is elevated for her age.

15. B. This child's appearance and assessment findings are consistent with respiratory failure.

16. Open the child's airway with a head tilt-chin lift.

17. Assess for sounds of airway compromise (snoring, gurgling, stridor) and look in the mouth for blood, gastric contents, foreign objects, etc.

18. Proper airway size is determined by holding the device against the side of the patient's face and selecting an airway that extends from the corner of the mouth to the angle of the jaw.

19. An adult mask should be used for this child. A child or adult resuscitation bag may be used. Deliver one ventilation every 3 to 5 seconds (12 to 20 breaths/minute).

20. C. Because beta-blockers impede bronchodilation, they are not routinely used in the management of asthma. Bronchodilators are used to improve airflow in the lungs. Corticosteroids are used to reduce airway swelling and inflammation. Methylxanthines (e.g., theophylline) may be used as an alternative therapy in some cases of severe asthma.

5 Cardiovascular Emergencies

Case Study

Your patient is a 4-year-old boy who presents with a swollen left foot, inspiratory stridor, and hives on his face, chest, back, and extremities. Mom says the boy had been outside playing with a friend and came in the house complaining that a bug bit him in the foot. Your general impression reveals an anxious child who is laboring to breathe. Inspiratory stridor is audible. The child has no allergies, but his older sister has an allergy to penicillin.

Is this child sick or not sick? What should you do next?

Objectives

1. Define the following terms: afterload, preload, cardiac output, stroke volume, and shock.
2. List assessment findings consistent with circulatory compromise.
3. Define shock (hypoperfusion).
4. Discuss the common causes of shock in infants and children.
5. Describe the clinical classifications of shock.
6. Describe the assessment findings that indicate shock in infants and children.
7. Differentiate between compensated and decompensated shock.
8. Describe the initial management of hypovolemic, cardiogenic, distributive (septic, anaphylactic, neurogenic), and obstructive shock in infants and children.
9. Describe assessment findings that indicate cardiopulmonary failure or arrest in children.
10. Discuss the primary etiologies of cardiopulmonary arrest in infants and children.
11. Identify the major classifications of pediatric cardiac dysrhythmias.
12. Identify four essential questions to ask in the initial emergency management of a pediatric patient with a dysrhythmia.
13. Recognize the following dysrhythmias: bradycardia, sinus tachycardia, supraventricular tachycardia (SVT), ventricular tachycardia (VT), ventricular fibrillation (VF), and asystole.

14. Differentiate sinus tachycardia from SVT and SVT from VT.

15. Recognize a "sick" (unstable) and "not sick" (stable) infant or child with a cardiac dysrhythmia.

16. Discuss the dysrhythmias associated with pediatric cardiopulmonary failure or arrest.

17. Discuss the management of cardiac dysrhythmias in infants and children.

18. Discuss the pharmacology of medications used during shock, symptomatic bradycardia, stable and unstable tachycardia, and cardiopulmonary arrest.

19. Given a patient situation, formulate a management plan (including assessment, airway management, cardiopulmonary resuscitation (CPR), pharmacologic, and electrical interventions where applicable) for a patient in shock, or presenting with symptomatic bradycardia, stable or unstable tachycardia, or cardiopulmonary arrest.

Cardiovascular System: Anatomic and Physiologic Considerations

Perfusion

- **Perfusion** is the circulation of blood through an organ or a part of the body. Perfusion delivers oxygen and other nutrients to the cells of all organ systems and removes waste products.
- **Hypoperfusion** (shock) is the inadequate circulation of blood through an organ or a part of the body.

Heart rate

- The heart is innervated by both the sympathetic and parasympathetic divisions of the autonomic nervous system (ANS).
- The sympathetic division mobilizes the body, allowing the body to function under stress ("fight or flight" response).
- The parasympathetic division is responsible for the conservation and restoration of body resources ("feed and breed" response).

Venous return

- The heart functions as a pump to propel blood through the systemic and pulmonary circulations. As the heart chambers fill with blood, the heart muscle is stretched.
- The most important factor determining the amount of blood pumped by the heart is the amount of blood flowing into it from the systemic circulation (**venous return**).

Cardiac output

- **Cardiac output** (CO) is the amount of blood pumped into the aorta

Review of the Cardiovascular System

Cardiac output = stroke volume × heart rate (CO = SV × HR).

each minute by the heart. It is calculated as the SV (amount of blood ejected from a ventricle with each heartbeat) times the HR and is expressed in liters per minute. Adequate cardiac output is necessary to maintain oxygenation and perfusion of body tissues.

- Normal cardiac output:
  - Neonates: 200 mL/kg/min.
  - Infants and children: 150 mL/kg/min.
  - Adolescents: 100 mL/kg/min.
- Changes in HR *OR* SV can affect cardiac output.
  - ↑ SV or HR → ↑ CO.
  - ↓ SV or HR → ↓ CO.
- Tachycardia is the initial compensatory response to the demand for increased CO.
  - Tachycardia shortens the length of time spent in diastole.
  - The coronary arteries are perfused during diastole. If the length of diastole is shortened (as in a prolonged tachycardias), there is less time for adequate ventricular filling and coronary artery perfusion.
  - This may result in decreased SV, decreased CO, and myocardial ischemia.
- **Blood pressure** is the force exerted by the blood on the inner walls of the blood vessels.
  - Systolic blood pressure is the pressure exerted against the walls of the large arteries at the peak of ventricular contraction.
  - Diastolic blood pressure is the pressure exerted against the walls of the large arteries during ventricular relaxation.
- **Vascular resistance** is the amount of opposition that the blood vessels give to the flow of blood.
  - Resistance is affected by the diameter and length of the blood vessel, blood viscosity, and the tone of the vessel. The most significant changes in resistance are caused by the arterioles (Figure 5-1).
  - Even at rest, vascular tone is maintained by constant input from the sympathetic division of the ANS. This results in partial vasoconstriction throughout the body to ensure continued circulation of blood.
- Blood pressure is equal to CO × peripheral vascular resistance.
  - Blood pressure is affected by any condition that increases peripheral resistance or CO.
  - Thus, an increase in either CO or peripheral resistance will result in an increase in blood pressure. Conversely, a decrease in either will result in a decrease in blood pressure.

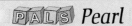 *Pearl*

Because of the immaturity of sympathetic innervation to the ventricles, infants and children have a relatively fixed stroke volume and are therefore dependent on an adequate heart rate to maintain adequate cardiac output.

An early sign of impending shock is a slight increase in diastolic pressure without a change in the systolic pressure (i.e., narrowed pulse pressure).

Tone is a term that may be used when referring to the normal state of balanced tension in body tissues.

PALS *Pearl*

Infants and children are capable of more effective vasoconstriction than adults are. As a result, a previously healthy infant or child is able to maintain a normal blood pressure and organ perfusion for a longer time in the presence of shock.

Effect of Resistance on Pressure

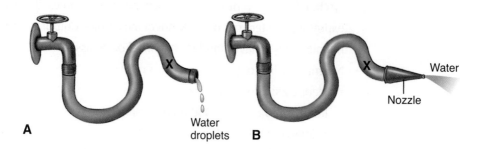

Effect of Resistance on Blood Pressure

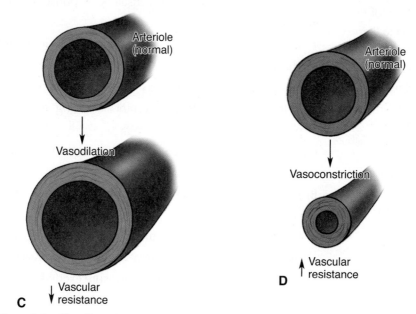

Figure 5-1   **The effect of resistance on pressure. A,** Water flows in large droplets from a wide hose. **B,** If a nozzle is applied to the hose, pressure within the hose increases (*point x*) as evidenced by the squiring water. Arterioles can function like nozzles. **C,** The nozzle is wide open (vasodilation), offering little resistance to flow. Pressure within the vessel decreases as the vessel dilates. **D,** Pressure within the vessel increases as the nozzle is tightened (vasoconstriction) and the resistance to flow increases.

Stroke Volume

- SV is determined by:
  - The degree of ventricular filling during diastole (preload).
  - The resistance against which the ventricle must pump (afterload).
  - The contractile state of the myocardium.

Preload

- **Preload** is the force exerted on the walls of the ventricles at the end of diastole.

  Fluid administration increases preload.

- Preload in the right heart depends on venous return to the heart from the systemic circulation.

- Preload in the left heart depends on venous return from the pulmonary system.
  - The volume of blood returning to the heart influences preload.
  - Frank-Starling mechanism.
    - The greater the preload, the more the ventricles are stretched.
    - To a point, as the greater the stretch of the ventricular fibers, the greater the contractile force.
  - More blood returning to the right atrium increases preload; less blood returning decreases preload.

Afterload

Afterload can be increased by giving vasopressors and can be decreased by giving vasodilators.

- **Afterload** is the pressure or resistance against which the ventricles must pump to eject blood.
- Afterload is influenced by arterial blood pressure, arterial distensibility (ability to become stretched), and arterial resistance.
  - The less the resistance (lower afterload), the more easily blood can be ejected. Increased afterload (increased resistance) results in increased cardiac workload.
  - Vasoconstriction $\rightarrow$ $\uparrow$ resistance $\rightarrow$ $\uparrow$ afterload $\rightarrow$ $\downarrow$ SV.

Cardiovascular Assessment

Scene Safety

On arrival, ensure the scene is safe before proceeding with your assessment of the patient.

Initial Assessment

- From a distance, use the Pediatric Assessment Triangle to form your general impression of the patient. Evaluate the child's appearance, work of breathing, and circulation to determine the severity of the child's illness or injury (Table 5-1) and assist you in determining the urgency for care (Table 5-2).
- If the child appears sick (unstable), proceed immediately with the primary survey and treat problems as you find them.
- If the child appears "not sick" (stable), complete the initial assessment.
- Perform a focused or detailed physical examination, based on the patient's presentation and chief complaint.
- Remember: Your patient's condition can change at any time. A patient who initially appears "not sick" may rapidly deteriorate and appear "sick." Reassess frequently.

Focused History and Physical Examination

Focused History

In addition to the SAMPLE history, consider the following questions when

TABLE 5-1 *General Impression of Cardiovascular Emergencies*

Assessment	Imminent Cardiopulmonary Failure	Cardiopulmonary Failure	Cardiopulmonary Arrest
Mental status	Alert, irritable, anxious, restless	Sleepy, intermittently combative, or agitated	Unresponsive to voice or touch
Muscle tone	Able to maintain sitting position (children older than 4 mo)	Normal or decreased	Limp
Body position	May assume tripod position	May assume tripod position. May need support to maintain sitting position as he/she tires	Unable to maintain sitting position (children older than 4 mo)
Ventilatory rate	Faster than normal for age	Tachypnea with periods of bradypnea; slowing to bradypnea/agonal breathing	Absent
Ventilatory effort	Intercostal retractions. Nasal flaring. Neck muscle use. Seesaw breathing	Nasal flaring. Increased ventilatory effort at sternal notch. Marked use of accessory muscles. Retractions, head bobbing. Inadequate chest excursion. See-saw breathing	Absent
Audible airway sounds	Stridor, wheezing, gurgling	Stridor, wheezing, grunting, gasping	Absent
Skin color	Pink or pale; central cyanosis resolves with oxygen administration	Central cyanosis despite oxygen administration; mottling	Mottling; peripheral and central cyanosis

obtaining a focused history for a condition affecting the cardiovascular system. This list will require modification on the basis of the patient's age and chief complaint.

Shock

History of trauma?

Recent vomiting or diarrhea? Number of diaper changes or trips to the bathroom? Will the child drink?

Has the child had a fever? For how long?

Associated symptoms (e.g., change in mental status, shortness of breath, feeling faint, dizziness)

History of severe asthma or allergic reactions? Previous treatment?

Previous hospitalization for allergic reaction?

Possible bite/sting or ingestion of nuts, shellfish, eggs? New medication?

Dysrhythmias

When did it start/occur (time, sudden, gradual)? What was the child doing when it started/occurred?

TABLE 5-2 *Immediate Interventions for Cardiovascular Emergencies Based on the General Impression*

	Interventions
Imminent cardiopulmonary failure	Approach promptly, but work at a moderate pace Permit the child to assume a position of comfort Correct hypoxia by giving oxygen without causing agitation Provide further interventions based on assessment findings
Cardiopulmonary failure	Move quickly Open the airway and suction if necessary Correct hypoxia by giving supplemental oxygen Begin assisted ventilation if the patient does not improve Provide further interventions based on assessment findings
Cardiopulmonary arrest	Move quickly Perform high–quality chest compressions Defibrillate if indicated Open the airway and use positioning, suctioning, and airway adjuncts as necessary Provide assisted ventilation with oxygen Insert an advanced airway if assisted ventilation is ineffective or the airway cannot otherwise be maintained Administer medications and fluids as indicated Reassess for return of spontaneous breathing and circulation Provide further interventions based on assessment findings

How long did it last? Does it come and go? Is it still present?

Does anything make the symptoms better or worse? (e.g., change in position, rest)

Associated symptoms (e.g., palpitations, change in mental status, shortness of breath, feeling faint, dizziness)

Previous hospitalization for heart related problem?

Chest pain

When did it start/occur (time, sudden, gradual)? What was the child doing when it started/occurred?

Quality (e.g., crushing, tight, stabbing, burning, squeezing)

How long did it last? Does it come and go? Is it still present?

Where is the problem? Describe the character and severity if pain is present (use pain scale) (see Chapter 7).

Associated symptoms (e.g., shortness of breath, feeling faint, dizziness)

Previous history of a similar episode? If yes, what was the diagnosis?

Does anything make the symptoms better or worse? (e.g., change in position)

Heart failure

When did it start/occur (time, sudden, gradual)?

When was the child last well (i.e., without current symptoms)?

History of congenital heart disease?

Poor feeding? Recent weight gain? Decrease in activity?

Does anything make the symptoms better or worse? (e.g., lying down worsens symptoms)

Focused Physical Examination

Assessment of adequate cardiovascular function includes the following objective measurements and clinical parameters:

- Compare the strength and quality of central and peripheral pulses.
  - Pulse quality reflects the adequacy of peripheral perfusion.
  - A weak central pulse may indicate decompensated shock.
  - A peripheral pulse that is difficult to find, weak, or irregular suggests poor peripheral perfusion and may be a sign of shock or hemorrhage.
  - HR is influenced by the child's age, size, and level of activity. A very slow or rapid rate may indicate or may be the cause of cardiovascular compromise.

    Normal HRs by age are listed in Table 5-3.

  - In an adult, a tachycardia is defined as a HR above 100 beats per minute. Because an infant or child's HR can transiently increase during episodes of crying, pain, or in the presence of a fever, the term *tachycardia* is used to describe a significant and persistent increase in HR.
  - The maximum effective HR in infants is 200 beats per minute; in preschool children 150 beats per minute; and in older individuals, 120 beats per minute.[1] In infants, a tachycardia is a HR of more than 200 beats per minute. In a child older than 5 years, a tachycardia is a HR of more than 160 beats per minute.[2]
- Evaluate the cardiac rhythm. Determine if the rate is normal for age, fast, slow, or absent. If the rhythm is pulseless VT or VF, begin CPR and defibrillate with 2 to 4 J/kg as soon as a defibrillator is available.
- Look for visible hemorrhage and control bleeding if present.

TABLE 5-3 *Normal Heart Rates by Age*

Age	Beats/Min[a]
Infant (1 to 12 mo)	100 to 160
Toddler (1 to 3 y)	90 to 150
Preschooler (4 to 5 y)	80 to 140
School-age (6 to 12 y)	70 to 120
Adolescent (13 to 18 y)	60 to 100

[a]Pulse rates for a sleeping child may be 10% lower than the low rate listed in age group.

Decreased skin perfusion is an early sign of shock.

- Evaluate skin color, temperature, moisture.
- Assess skin turgor.
- Evaluate capillary refill in infants and children younger than 6 years of age.
  - If the ambient temperature is warm, color should return within 2 seconds.
  - Capillary refill time of 3 to 5 seconds is delayed and may indicate poor perfusion or exposure to cool ambient temperatures.
  - Capillary refill time above 5 seconds is markedly delayed and suggests shock.
- Blood pressure.
  - Measure blood pressure in children older than 3 years.
  - In children younger than 3 years, a strong central pulse is considered an acceptable sign of adequate blood pressure. Table 5-4 shows the lower limit of normal systolic blood pressure by age.
  - The diastolic blood pressure is usually two thirds of the systolic pressure.
- Pulse pressure.
  - Pulse pressure is the difference between the systolic and diastolic blood pressures and is an indicator of SV.
  - Narrowed pulse pressure is an indicator of circulatory compromise.
- Urine output.
  - Urine output in a well-hydrated infant or child should average 2 mL/kg/hr in a neonate, 1 mL/kg/hr in a child, and 0.5 mL/kg/hr in an adolescent.
  - In general, urine output of less than 1 mL/kg/hr, in the absence of renal disease, is a sign of poor perfusion.
  - Placement of an indwelling urinary catheter assists in determining accurate urine output and kidney perfusion.
  - The rate of urinary flow is a good indicator in evaluating the success of volume expansion.

TABLE 5-4 *Lower Limit of Normal Systolic Blood Pressure by Age*

Age	Lower Limit of Normal Systolic Blood Pressure
Term neonate (0 to 28 days)	More than 60 mm Hg or strong central pulse
Infant (1 to 12 months) central pulse	More than 70 mm Hg or strong
Child (1 to 10 years)	More than 70 + (2 × age in years)
Child (10 years or older)	More than 90 mm Hg

Shock

Shock is inadequate tissue perfusion that results from the failure of the cardiovascular system to deliver sufficient oxygen and nutrients to sustain vital organ function. The underlying cause must be recognized and treated promptly, or cell and organ dysfunction and death may result.

Adequate tissue perfusion requires an intact cardiovascular system. This includes an adequate fluid volume (the blood), a container to regulate the distribution of the fluid (the blood vessels), and a pump (the heart) with sufficient force to move the fluid throughout the container. A malfunction or deficiency of any of these components can affect perfusion.

Overview

- Early (compensated) shock.
  - Compensated shock is inadequate tissue perfusion without hypotension (i.e., shock with a "normal" blood pressure).
  - In compensated shock, the body's defense mechanisms attempt to preserve the vital organs (i.e., the brain, heart, and lungs). The sympathetic division of the ANS is stimulated because of decreased CO.
  - This stage of shock is usually reversible if the cause is promptly identified and corrected. If uncorrected, shock will progress to the next stage.
  - The presence of compensated shock can be identified by the following:
    - Evaluation of HR.
    - Presence and volume (strength) of peripheral pulses.
    - Adequacy of end organ perfusion.
      - Brain: assess mental status.
      - Skin: assess capillary refill, skin temperature.
      - Kidneys: assess urine output.
- Late (decompensated) shock.
  - Decompensated shock begins when compensatory mechanisms begin to fail.
  - At this stage, the "classic" signs and symptoms of shock are evident.
  - Decompensated shock is difficult to treat, but is still reversible if appropriate aggressive treatment is initiated.
  - During this stage of shock:
    - Blood vessels respond to epinephrine and norepinephrine release with maximum constriction.
    - The liver and spleen release stored supplies of red blood cells and plasma.
    - Capillaries become clogged with clumps of red blood cells.

Stages of Shock

Compensated shock is also called reversible shock because at this stage, the shock syndrome is reversible with prompt recognition and appropriate intervention.

Decompensated shock is also called progressive shock.

The presence of hypotension differentiates compensated shock from decompensated shock. Hypotension is a *late* sign of cardiovascular compromise in an infant or child.

PALS Pearl

The initial signs of shock may be subtle in an infant or child. The effectiveness of compensatory mechanisms is largely dependent on the child's previous cardiac and pulmonary health. In the pediatric patient, the progression from compensated to decompensated shock occurs suddenly and rapidly. When decompensation occurs, cardiopulmonary arrest may be imminent.

- ○ Disseminated intravascular coagulopathy (DIC) and other coagulopathies develop.
- Irreversible shock.
  - Compensatory mechanisms fail.
  - Cardiac dysrhythmias may develop as ventricular irritability increases.
  - Cell membranes break down and release harmful enzymes.
  - Irreversible damage to vital organs occurs because of sustained altered perfusion and metabolism, resulting in organ failure and death.

Classification of Shock by Etiology

Inadequate volume

Hypovolemia and sepsis are the most common causes of shock in children.[3]

PALS Pearl

Although the amount and type of information gathered will vary depending on the child's presentation, a history should be obtained as soon as possible from the parent or caregiver. The information obtained may help identify the type of shock present, ascertain the child's previous health, and the onset and duration of symptoms.

Hypovolemic Shock

Etiology

- Hypovolemic shock is a marked reduction in oxygen delivery due to diminished CO secondary to inadequate vascular volume.
  - ↓ Intravascular volume → ↓ venous return (preload) → ↓ ventricular filling → ↓ SV → ↓ CO → inadequate tissue perfusion.
- Hemorrhagic shock (a type of hypovolemic shock) is caused by severe internal or external bleeding. Causes of major blood loss include the following:
  - Vascular injury.
  - Ruptured liver or spleen.
  - Hemothorax.
  - Scalp lacerations.
  - Intracranial hemorrhage (newborn or infant).
  - Fractured femur with vascular laceration.
- Hypovolemic shock may also be caused by a loss of plasma, fluids and electrolytes, dehydration, or endocrine disorders.
- Circulating blood volume.
  - The average circulating blood volume is 80 mL/kg. Average circulating blood volumes by age are listed in Table 5-5.
  - In a healthy child, a loss of 10% to 15% of the circulating blood volume is usually well tolerated and easily compensated (Table 5-6).

TABLE 5-5 *Average Circulating Blood Volume By Age*

Age	Normal Blood Volume (Average)
Preterm infant	90 to 105 mL/kg
Term newborn	85 mL/kg
Infant older than 1 mo to 11 mo	75 mL/kg
Beyond 1 year	67 to 75 mL/kg
Adult	55 to 75 mL/kg

From Barkin RM, Rosen P. *Emergency pediatrics: a guide to ambulatory care,* 5th ed. St. Louis: Mosby, 1999.

Fluid resuscitation is essential in the treatment of all forms of shock. In cardiogenic shock, smaller fluid boluses and a lesser fluid volume is generally used.

TABLE 5-6 *Response to Fluid and Blood Loss in the Pediatric Patient*

	Class I	Class II	Class III	Class IV
Stage of shock		Compensated	Decompensated	Irreversible
Blood volume loss %	Up to 15%	15% to 30%	30% to 45%	More than 45%
Mental status	Slightly anxious	Mildly anxious; restless	Altered; lethargic; apathetic; decreased pain response	Extremely lethargic; unresponsive
Muscle tone	Normal	Normal	Normal to decreased	Limp
Ventilatory rate/effort	Normal	Mild tachypnea	Moderate tachypnea	Severe tachypnea to agonal (preterminal event)
Skin color (extremities)	Pink	Pale, mottled	Pale, mottled, mild peripheral cyanosis	Pale, mottled, central and peripheral cyanosis
Skin turgor	Normal	Poor; sunken eyes and fontanelles in infant/ young child	Poor; sunken eyes and fontanelles in infant/young child	Tenting
Skin temperature	Cool	Cool	Cool to cold	Cold
Capillary refill	Normal	Poor (more than 2 sec)	Delayed (more than 3 sec)	Prolonged (more than 5 sec)
Heart rate	Usually normal if gradual volume loss; increased if sudden loss of volume	Mild tachycardia	Significant tachycardia; possible dysrhythmias; peripheral pulse weak, thready or may be absent	Marked tachycardia to bradycardia (preterminal event)
Blood pressure	Normal	Lower range of normal	Decreased	Severe hypotension
Pulse pressure	Normal or increased	Narrowed	Decreased	Decreased
Urine output	Normal; concentrated	Decreased	Minimal	Minimal to absent

A child may be in shock despite a normal blood pressure.

Reassessment is crucial. Use mental status, blood pressure, HR, peripheral perfusion, capillary refill, and urine output to guide volume replacement.

Assessment Findings

- Compensated shock.
  - Increased HR.
  - Peripheral vasoconstriction: skin mottling, delayed capillary refill, cool extremities.
  - Normal blood pressure.
  - Narrowed pulse pressure.
  - Normal or minimally impaired mental status.
  - Decreased urine output.
- Decompensated shock.
  - Hypotension.
  - Significant tachycardia.
  - Markedly delayed capillary refill.
  - Altered mental status: irritability, lethargy.
  - Minimal urine output.
  - Weak central pulses.
  - Pale, mottled, mild peripheral cyanosis

Acceptable Interventions

- Use personal protective equipment.
- Perform an initial assessment and obtain a focused history. Obtain a history as soon as possible from the parent or caregiver to assist in identifying the cause of shock.
- If trauma is suspected, maintain C-spine stabilization and open the airway with a jaw thrust without head tilt maneuver, if necessary.
- Apply a pulse oximeter and apply supplementary oxygen if indicated; ensure effective oxygenation and ventilation. Titrate oxygen administration to maintain an oxygen saturation level of 94% or higher.
- Begin CPR if a pulse is absent or if the pulse is less than 60 beats per minute with signs of poor perfusion.
- Attach cardiac monitor. Identify the rhythm.
- Obtain vascular access.
  - If immediate vascular access is needed, attempt intravenous (IV) access with two large peripheral IV lines. If unsuccessful, attempt intraosseous (IO) access.
  - Venous access may be difficult to obtain in an infant or child in shock. When shock is present, the most readily available vascular access site is preferred. Peripheral or central venous access is sufficient for fluid resuscitation in most patients.
  - If immediate vascular access is needed and reliable venous access cannot be rapidly achieved, establish IO access. If decompensated shock is present, *immediate* IO access is appropriate.

- If CPR is in progress, attempt vascular access by the route most readily available that will not require interruption of CPR.
- Volume resuscitation.
  - Type and cross emergently if the child has severe trauma and life-threatening blood loss.
  - Administer a bolus of 20 mL/kg of isotonic crystalloid solution (normal saline [NS] or lactated Ringers [LR]) over 5 to 20 minutes. Assess response (i.e., mental status, capillary refill, HR, ventilatory effort, blood pressure).
  - If there is no improvement, give another 20 mL/kg NS or LR fluid bolus and insert a urinary catheter. Assess response.
- Check glucose level. Some children in shock are hypoglycemic because of rapidly depleted carbohydrate stores. If the serum glucose level is less than 60 mg/dL, administer dextrose IV.
- Maintain normal body temperature.
- Insert a urinary catheter. Urine output is a sensitive measure of perfusion status and adequacy of therapy.
- Obtain appropriate laboratory studies.
  - Arterial blood gas to determine pH and cause of pH changes.
  - Electrolytes, glucose, complete blood count (CBC) with differential, coagulation studies.
- Consider the use of vasopressors if poor perfusion persists despite adequate oxygenation, ventilation, and volume expansion.

Unacceptable Interventions
- Failure to use personal protective equipment.
- If trauma is suspected, failure to maintain C-spine stabilization.
- If trauma is suspected, failure to open the airway with a jaw thrust without head tilt maneuver.
- Failure to measure oxygen saturation and give supplemental oxygen, if indicated.
- Failure to assist ventilation with a bag-mask device and supplemental oxygen if signs of inadequate ventilation are present.
- Failure to rapidly establish vascular access.
- Extended attempts to establish IV access in a child with decompensated shock when IO access could be established quickly.
- Failure to rapidly administer a fluid bolus of 20 mL/kg in a child with signs of shock.
- Failure to assess serum glucose level and give dextrose for documented hypoglycemia.
- Administration of hypotonic or glucose-containing solutions for volume resuscitation.

Signs of shock should be treated with a bolus of 20 mL/kg of isotonic crystalloid even if blood pressure is normal.[4]

If severe and prolonged, hypoglycemia may cause brain damage.

- Administering vasopressors or boluses of a nonisotonic fluid in a patient with signs of adequate perfusion.
- Failure to begin CPR if a pulse is absent or less than 60 beats per minute with signs of hypoperfusion.
- Performing tracheal intubation in a child who responds to less invasive interventions.
- If tracheal intubation is required, failure to confirm tracheal tube position using assessment and mechanical methods.
- Treating associated injuries (if present) before stabilization of the airway, oxygenation, ventilation, and circulation.
- Ordering a dangerous or inappropriate intervention.
- Performing any technique resulting in potential harm to the patient.

Cardiogenic Shock

Etiology

Inadequate pump

- Cardiogenic shock occurs because of impaired cardiac muscle function that leads to decreased CO.
- Cardiogenic shock may occur as a primary event in patients who have congenital heart disease or may occur as a complication of shock of any cause.

Signs and symptoms are usually the result of decreased CO.
- **JVD is difficult to assess in infants and young children.**

- Assessment findings.
  - Compensated shock: anxiety, pale skin, cool extremities; diaphoresis, normal or delayed capillary refill; weak, thready peripheral pulses; mild tachycardia, jugular venous distention (JVD) (indicating right ventricular failure), narrowed pulse pressure (rise in diastolic pressure with normal systolic blood pressure), mild basilar crackles, normal or mild decrease in urine output, orthopnea.
  - Decompensated shock: lethargy; pale, mottled, or cyanotic skin; diaphoresis, markedly delayed capillary refill; weak, thready central pulses; peripheral pulses may be absent; hypotension, tachypnea with decreased tidal volume, increasing pulmonary congestion and crackles, oliguria.

The treatment of cardiogenic shock is generally based on increasing contractility, altering preload and afterload, and controlling dysrhythmias if they are present and contributing to shock.

Acceptable Interventions

- Use personal protective equipment.
- Perform an initial assessment and obtain a focused history. Obtain a history as soon as possible from the parent or caregiver to assist in identifying the etiology of shock.
- Apply a pulse oximeter and administer supplemental oxygen if indicated; ensure effective oxygenation and ventilation. Titrate oxygen administration to maintain an oxygen saturation level of 94% or higher.
- Begin CPR if a pulse is absent or if the pulse is less than 60 beats per minute with signs of poor perfusion.
- Attach cardiac monitor. Identify the rhythm.

- Obtain vascular access. If IV access cannot be rapidly established, place an IO needle.
- Check glucose and electrolyte levels. If the serum glucose is below 60 mg/dL, administer dextrose IV/IO.
- Give a small IV/IO fluid bolus of isotonic crystalloid solution (5 to 10 mL/kg of LR or NS). The fluid bolus may be repeated on the basis of the child's response.
  - Repeat the primary survey after *each* fluid bolus. Monitor closely for increased work of breathing and the development of crackles.
  - If the child fails to improve, consider giving an inotrope (e.g., dopamine, dobutamine, or epinephrine) to improve myocardial contractility and increase CO (Table 5-7).
- Vasodilators may be used reduce preload and afterload.
- Treat dysrhythmias if present and contributing to shock.
- Obtain a chest radiograph to help differentiate cardiogenic from non-cardiogenic shock, identify the presence of a pulmonary infection, cardiomegaly, pulmonary edema, or evolving acute respiratory distress syndrome (ARDS).
- Obtain a 12-lead electrocardiogram (ECG) and cardiology consult.

Unacceptable Interventions

- Failure to use personal protective equipment.
- Failure to measure oxygen saturation and give supplemental oxygen, if indicated.
- Failure to assist ventilation with a bag-mask device and supplemental oxygen if signs of inadequate ventilation are present.
- Failure to rapidly establish vascular access.
- Extended attempts to establish IV access in a child with decompensated shock when IO access could be established quickly.

TABLE 5-7 *Medications Used for Cardiopulmonary Resuscitation*

	Positive Inotrope	Positive Chronotrope	Direct Pressor	Indirect Pressor	Vasodilator
Dopamine	++	+	±	++	++[a]
Dobutamine	++	±	−	−	+
Epinephrine	+++	+++	+++	−	−
Isoproterenol	+++	+++	−	−	+++
Norepinephrine	+++	+++	+++	−	−

From Marcdante KJ. The Acutely Ill or Injured Child: Shock. In: Kliegman RM, Marcdante KJ, Jenson HB, Behrman RE, eds. Nelson Essentials of Pediatrics, 5th ed. Philadelphia: Elsevier, 2006.
[a]Primarily splanchnic and renal in low doses (3 to 5 mcg/kg/min)

- Failure to rapidly administer a 5 to 10 mL/kg of LR or NS fluid bolus to a child with signs of decompensated shock.
- Failure to repeat the primary survey after each fluid bolus.
- Failure to assess serum glucose level and give dextrose for documented hypoglycemia.
- Failure to consider the addition of inotropes, vasopressors, or vasodilators if perfusion does not improve with fluid administration.
- Failure to begin CPR if a pulse is absent or slower than 60 beats per minute with signs of poor perfusion.
- Performing tracheal intubation in a child who responds to less invasive interventions.
- If tracheal intubation is required, failure to confirm tracheal tube position using assessment and mechanical methods.
- Ordering a dangerous or inappropriate intervention.
- Performing any technique resulting in potential harm to the patient.

Distributive Shock

Vessel/container problem; increased vascular space

- In distributive shock, a relative hypovolemia occurs when vasodilation increases the size of the vascular space and the available blood volume must fill a greater space (container problem; increased vascular space). This results in an altered distribution of the blood volume (relative hypovolemia) rather than actual volume loss (absolute hypovolemia).
- Distributive shock may be caused by a severe infection (septic shock), severe allergic reaction (anaphylactic shock), spinal cord injury (neurogenic shock), or certain overdoses (e.g., sedatives, narcotics).

Septic Shock

Terminology/Etiology

- **Systemic inflammatory response syndrome (SIRS)** is a response to infection manifested by derangement in two or more of the following: temperature, heart rate, ventilatory rate, and white blood cell count. **Sepsis** is the systemic response to an infection. **Severe sepsis** is sepsis associated with organ dysfunction.
- **Septic shock** is severe sepsis and the persistence of poor perfusion or hypotension for more than 1 hour despite adequate fluid resuscitation or a requirement for inotropic agents or vasopressors.
  - Fever, tachycardia, and vasodilation are common in children with benign infections.
  - Septic shock should be suspected when a child with this inflammatory triad experiences a change in mental status evidenced by inconsolable irritability, lack of interaction with parents, or inability to be aroused.
- Septic shock occurs in two clinical stages.
  - The early (hyperdynamic) phase is characterized by peripheral

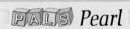

PALS Pearl

Signs and symptoms of distributive shock that are unusual in the presence of hypovolemic shock include warm, flushed skin (especially in dependent areas), and, in neurogenic shock, a normal or slow pulse rate (relative bradycardia).

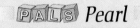

PALS Pearl

If you observe a change in mental status in a febrile child (inconsolable, inability to recognize parents, unarousable), *immediately* consider the possibility of septic shock.

Septic shock is the most common type of distributive shock in children.

vasodilation (warm shock) due to endotoxins that prevent catecholamine-induced vasoconstriction.

- The late (hypodynamic or decompensated) phase is characterized by cool extremities (cold shock) and resembles hypovolemic shock.

- Hypotension is not necessary for the clinical diagnosis of septic shock; however, its presence in a child with clinical suspicion of infection is confirmatory.[5]

Assessment Findings

- Early (hyperdynamic) phase (increased CO).
    - Warm, dry, flushed skin.
    - Blood pressure may be normal or possible widened pulse pressure.
    - Bounding peripheral pulses.
    - Brisk capillary refill.
    - Tachycardia.
    - Tachypnea.
- Late (hypodynamic/decompensated) phase.
    - Mottled, cool extremities.
    - Diminished or absent peripheral pulses.
    - Altered mental status.
    - Tachycardia.
    - Delayed capillary refill.
    - Decreased urine output.

> Late septic shock is usually indistinguishable from other types of shock.

Acceptable Interventions

- Use personal protective equipment.
- Perform an initial assessment and obtain a focused history. Obtain a history as soon as possible from the parent or caregiver to assist in identifying the etiology of shock.
- Apply a pulse oximeter and administer supplemental oxygen if indicated; ensure effective oxygenation and ventilation. Titrate oxygen administration to maintain an oxygen saturation level of 94% or higher.
- Begin CPR if a pulse is absent or if the pulse is less than 60 beats per minute with signs of poor perfusion.
- Attach cardiac monitor. Identify the rhythm.
- Obtain vascular access. If IV access cannot be rapidly established, place an IO needle. Fluid resuscitation with boluses of 20 mL/kg of isotonic crystalloid solution (NS or LR) should be administered and titrated to normalized objective measures such as heart rate (using age-based heart rates), urine output (to at least 1 mL/kg per hour), capillary refill (less than 2 sec), and normal status. If perfusion does not improve, repeat fluid boluses and reassess response, repeating the primary survey after *each* fluid bolus. Monitor closely for increased work of

> Increased work of breathing, hypoventilation, and altered mental status are indications for advanced airway insertion.

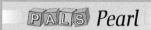 Pearl

Management of septic shock requires aggressive fluid administration. The patient in decompensated septic shock may require significant quantities of fluid. For example, some patients have required 100 to 200 mL/kg in the first few hours of resuscitation. Carefully monitor the patient for crackles and increased work of breathing during rapid fluid administration.

breathing and the development of crackles.

- Check glucose and electrolyte levels. If the serum glucose level is lower than 60 mg/dL, administer dextrose IV.
- If septic shock lasts more than 1 hour despite aggressive fluid resuscitation:[5]
  - Establish central venous access.
  - Establish arterial monitoring.
  - Dopamine is recommended as the first-line vasopressor for fluid-resistant septic shock. Begin the infusion at 5 mcg/kg/min. Continue administration of IV fluid boluses during the dopamine infusion.
- Administer IV antibiotics. Obtain cultures of blood or any other body fluid suspected of being infected before administering antibiotics.

Unacceptable Interventions

- Failure to use personal protective equipment.
- Failure to measure oxygen saturation and give supplemental oxygen, if indicated.
- Failure to assist ventilation with a bag-mask device and supplemental oxygen if signs of inadequate ventilation are present.
- Failure to rapidly establish vascular access.
- Extended attempts to establish IV access in a child with decompensated shock when IO access could be established quickly.
- Failure to rapidly administer a rapid fluid bolus of 20 mL/kg to a child with signs of shock.
- Failure to repeat the primary survey after each fluid bolus.
- Failure to assess serum glucose level and give dextrose for documented hypoglycemia.
- Administration of hypotonic or glucose-containing solutions for volume resuscitation.
- Administering vasopressors or boluses of a non-isotonic fluid in a patient with signs of adequate perfusion.
- Failure to begin CPR if a pulse is absent or below 60 beats per minute with signs of poor perfusion.
- Performing tracheal intubation in a child who responds to less invasive interventions.
- If tracheal intubation is required, failure to confirm tracheal tube position using assessment and mechanical methods.
- Ordering a dangerous or inappropriate intervention.
- Performing any technique resulting in potential harm to the patient.

Anaphylactic Shock

Etiology

Anaphylaxis or anaphylactic shock occurs when the body is exposed to a substance that produces a severe allergic reaction that usually occurs within minutes of the exposure. Common causes include insect stings, medications (e.g., penicillin, sulfa), and some foods (e.g., shellfish, nuts, strawberries).

Assessment Findings

- Swelling of the tongue.
- Stridor, wheezing, coughing, hoarseness, intercostal and suprasternal retractions.
- Tachycardia, hypotension, dysrhythmias.
- Vomiting, diarrhea.
- Anxiety, restlessness.
- Facial swelling and angioedema.
- Urticaria (hives).
- Abdominal pain, cramping.
- Pruritus (itching).

Acceptable Interventions

- Use personal protective equipment.
- Perform an initial assessment and obtain a focused history.
- Remove/discontinue the causative agent.
- Apply a pulse oximeter and administer supplemental oxygen if indicated; ensure effective oxygenation and ventilation. Titrate oxygen administration to maintain an oxygen saturation level of 94% or higher.
- Begin CPR if a pulse if absent or if the pulse is less than 60 beats per minute with signs of poor perfusion.
- Attach a cardiac monitor. Identify the rhythm.
- Give epinephrine 0.01 mg/kg of 1:1000 solution via intramuscular (IM) injection (site of choice is the lateral aspect of the thigh).[6] Maximum single dose of 0.5 mg. May be administered every 15 minutes up to three doses if necessary while attempting IV access.
- Obtain vascular access. If IV access cannot be rapidly established, place an IO needle.
- Rapidly give a 20-mL/kg isotonic crystalloid solution (NS or LR) fluid bolus.
- If perfusion does not improve, repeat one or two fluid boluses and reassess response, repeating the primary survey after *each* fluid bolus. Monitor closely for increased work of breathing and the development of crackles.
- Check glucose level. If the serum glucose level is below 60 mg/dL, administer dextrose IV.
- Consider inhaled bronchodilator therapy (e.g., albuterol).
- Administer other medications to help stop the inflammatory reaction.
- Consider diphenhydramine 1 to 2 mg/kg IM, IV, or orally. Maximum dosage is 50 mg.
- Consider methylprednisolone 1 to 2 mg/kg IV.

Drug Pearl
Diphenhydramine (Benadryl)

- Diphenhydramine is an antihistamine/H_1 receptor antagonist.
- Histamine is released from mast cells following exposure to an antigen to which the body has been previously sensitized. When released into the circulation following an allergic reaction, histamine acts on two different receptors: H_1 and H_2. Stimulation of H_1 receptors causes bronchoconstriction and contraction of the gut. Stimulation of H_2 receptors causes peripheral vasodilation and secretion of gastric acids.
- In anaphylaxis, diphenhydramine is used in conjunction with epinephrine and steroids. Epinephrine causes bronchodilation by stimulating β_2-adrenergic receptors. Diphenhydramine blocks cellular histamine response, but does not prevent histamine release.

Unacceptable Interventions

- Failure to use personal protective equipment.
- Failure to measure oxygen saturation and give supplemental oxygen, if indicated.
- Failure to assist ventilation with a bag-mask device and supplemental oxygen if signs of inadequate ventilation are present.
- Failure to rapidly establish vascular access.
- Extended attempts to establish IV access in a child with decompensated shock when IO access could be established quickly.
- Failure to rapidly administer a rapid fluid bolus of 20 mL/kg to a child with signs of shock.
- Failure to repeat the primary survey after each fluid bolus.
- Failure to assess serum glucose level and give dextrose for documented hypoglycemia.
- Administering vasopressors or boluses of a nonisotonic fluid in a patient with signs of adequate perfusion.
- Failure to begin CPR if a pulse is absent or slower than 60 beats per minute with signs of poor perfusion.
- Performing tracheal intubation in a child who responds to less invasive interventions.
- If tracheal intubation is required, failure to confirm tracheal tube position using assessment and mechanical methods.
- Ordering a dangerous or inappropriate intervention.
- Performing any technique resulting in potential harm to the patient.

Neurogenic Shock

Etiology

- Neurogenic shock is caused by a severe injury to the head or spinal cord (e.g., brain stem injuries, complete transection of the spinal cord) that results in a loss of sympathetic vascular tone below the level of the spinal cord injury.
- The loss of peripheral vascular tone results in widespread vasodilation below the level of the injury → ↓ venous return → ↓ SV → ↓ CO → ↓ tissue perfusion.
  - The total blood volume remains the same, but vessel capacity is increased (relative hypovolemia).
  - Normally, a decrease in blood pressure is accompanied by a compensatory increase in HR. In neurogenic shock, the patient does not become tachycardic because sympathetic activity is disrupted.

Assessment Findings

- Skin is warm and dry.
  - Immediately after the injury, the skin appears flushed due to vaso-

In this type of shock, there is a disruption in the ability of the sympathetic nervous system to control vessel dilation and constriction.

Widespread vasodilation may result in a loss of body heat. Be aware of possible hypothermia.

dilation. Blood eventually pools, leaving the uppermost skin surfaces pale.

- If neurogenic shock occurs with hypovolemia, the extremities often become cool.
- Sweating does not occur below the level of the injury.
- HR within normal limits or bradycardic.
- Hypotension.
- Wide pulse pressure.
- Ventilatory rate/effort and breathing pattern may be affected depending on the location of the injury.
  - Abdominal breathing may result if a high cord injury disrupts the intercostal nerves that control rib movement.
  - If the phrenic nerve is affected, breathing may be shallow, labored, and (possibly) irregular.

Acceptable Interventions

- Use personal protective equipment.
- Perform an initial assessment and obtain a focused history.
- If trauma is suspected, maintain C-spine stabilization and open the airway with a jaw thrust without head tilt maneuver, if necessary.
- Apply a pulse oximeter and administer supplemental oxygen if indicated; ensure effective oxygenation and ventilation. Titrate oxygenation administration to maintain an oxygen saturation level of 94% or higher.
- Begin CPR if a pulse is absent or if pulse is less than 60 beats per minute with signs of poor perfusion.
- Attach a cardiac monitor. Identify the rhythm.
- Obtain vascular access. If IV access cannot be rapidly established, place an IO needle.
  - Rapidly give a 20-mL/kg isotonic crystalloid solution (NS or LR) fluid bolus.
  - If perfusion does not improve, repeat fluid boluses and reassess response, repeating the primary survey after *each* fluid bolus. Monitor closely for increased work of breathing and the development of crackles.
  - Repeat every 20 to 30 minutes as needed until systemic perfusion improves.
- Check glucose level. If the serum glucose level is below 60 mg/dL, administer dextrose IV/IO.
- Maintain normal body temperature.
- Insert a urinary catheter. Urine output is a sensitive measure of perfusion status and adequacy of therapy.
- Consider the use of vasopressors if poor perfusion persists despite adequate oxygenation, ventilation, and volume expansion.

Unacceptable Interventions

- Failure to use personal protective equipment.
- If trauma is suspected, failure to maintain C-spine stabilization.
- If trauma is suspected, failure to open the airway with a jaw thrust without head tilt maneuver.
- Failure to measure oxygen saturation and give supplemental oxygen, if indicated.
- Failure to assist ventilation with a bag-mask device and supplemental oxygen if signs of inadequate ventilation are present.
- Failure to rapidly administer a rapid fluid bolus of 20 mL/kg to a child with signs of shock.
- Failure to repeat the primary survey after each fluid bolus.
- Failure to assess serum glucose level and give dextrose for documented hypoglycemia.
- Administering vasopressors or boluses of a nonisotonic fluid in a patient with signs of adequate perfusion.
- Failure to begin CPR if a pulse is absent or slower than 60 beats per minute with signs of poor perfusion.
- Performing tracheal intubation in a child who responds to less invasive interventions.
- If tracheal intubation is required, failure to confirm tracheal tube position using assessment and mechanical methods.
- Treating associated injuries (if present), before stabilization of the airway, oxygenation, ventilation, and circulation.
- Ordering a dangerous or inappropriate intervention.
- Performing any technique resulting in potential harm to the patient.

Obstructive Shock

Shock that develops from cardiac tamponade, tension pneumothorax, or a massive pulmonary embolism is called obstructive shock because the common pathophysiology in these conditions is obstruction to blood flow from the heart.

Etiology

Ventricular outflow problem

- Tension pneumothorax.
  - A tension pneumothorax can result from blunt or penetrating chest trauma, barotrauma secondary to positive-pressure ventilation (especially when using high amounts of positive end-expiratory pressure [PEEP]), as a complication of central venous catheter placement (usually subclavian or internal jugular), or when a chest tube is clamped or becomes blocked after insertion.
  - In a tension pneumothorax, air enters on inspiration but cannot escape. Intrathoracic pressure increases, the lung collapses, and air under pressure shifts the mediastinum away from the midline,

toward the unaffected side. As intrathoracic pressure increases, the vena cava becomes kinked, decreasing venous return and altering CO.

- Cardiac tamponade.
  - The pericardial sac normally contains less than 1 mL/kg of fluid. In cardiac tamponade, excessive fluid accumulates in the pericardial sac, resulting in reduced ventricular filling, a decrease in SV, and a subsequent decrease in CO.
  - Excess fluid accumulation may occur from pericarditis, after cardiac surgery, after trauma, connective tissue diseases, radiation therapy, and as a complication of central venous catheters.

Assessment Findings

- Tension pneumothorax.
  - Early.
    - Dyspnea.
    - Anxiety.
    - Tachypnea.
    - Tachycardia.
    - Hyperresonance of the chest wall on the affected side.
    - Diminished or absent breath sounds on the affected side.
  - Late.
    - Decreased level of responsiveness.
    - Tracheal deviation toward the unaffected side.
    - Hypotension.
    - Distension of neck veins (may not be present if hypovolemic or in cases of severe hypotension).
    - Cyanosis.
- Cardiac tamponade.
  - Beck's triad: increased jugular venous pressure, hypotension, muffled heart sounds.
  - Dyspnea.
  - Anxiety, restlessness.
  - Cold extremities.
  - Pale, mottled, or cyanotic skin.
  - Tachycardia.
  - Weak or absent peripheral pulses.
  - Narrowed pulse pressure.
  - Pulsus paradoxus.

Acceptable Interventions

- Use personal protective equipment.
- Perform an initial assessment and obtain a focused history. Obtain a history as soon as possible from the parent or caregiver to assist in identifying the etiology of shock.

> Cardiac tamponade and tension pneumothorax present with clear lung sounds however, lung sounds are unequal in a tension pneumothorax.

> Management of obstructive shock depends on the cause.

- If trauma is suspected, maintain C-spine stabilization and open the airway with a jaw thrust without head tilt maneuver, if necessary.
- Apply a pulse oximeter and administer supplemental oxygen if indicated; ensure effective oxygenation and ventilation. Titrate oxygen administration to maintain an oxygen saturation level of 94% or higher.
- Begin CPR if a pulse is absent or the pulse is less than 60 beats per minute with poor perfusion.
- Attach cardiac monitor. Identify the rhythm.
- Obtain vascular access. If immediate vascular access is needed, attempt IV access. If unsuccessful, attempt IO access.
  - Administer a bolus of 20 mL/kg of isotonic crystalloid solution (NS or LR) over 5 to 20 minutes. Assess response (i.e., mental status, capillary refill, HR, respiratory effort, blood pressure).
  - If the child continues to demonstrate signs of inadequate perfusion, give a third 20-mL/kg fluid bolus of NS or LR. Repeat every 20 to 30 minutes as needed until systemic perfusion improves.
- Management of tension pneumothorax.
  - Perform needle decompression of the affected side. Reassess.
  - After needle decompression, insert a thoracostomy tube. Reassess.
  - Obtain a chest radiograph to assess for lung reexpansion and evaluate thoracostomy tube position.
- Management of cardiac tamponade.
  - Volume expansion with isotonic crystalloid solution as necessary to maintain an adequate circulating blood volume.
  - Administration of an inotropic drug such as dobutamine may be useful because it does not increase systemic vascular resistance while increasing CO.
  - Pericardiocentesis is the definitive treatment for cardiac tamponade.
- Check glucose level. If the serum glucose level is less than 60 mg/dL, administer dextrose IV/IO.
- Maintain normal body temperature.
- Obtain appropriate laboratory studies.
- Insert a urinary catheter if necessary.

Unacceptable Interventions

- Failure to use personal protective equipment.
- If trauma is suspected, failure to maintain C-spine stabilization.
- If trauma is suspected, failure to open the airway with a jaw thrust without head tilt maneuver.

PEDIATRIC SHOCK ALGORITHM

Perform an Initial Assessment

If **no** signs of heart failure are present:

- Give a bolus of 20 mL/kg of isotonic crystalloid solution (NS or LR) IV/IO as rapidly as needed (less than 20 minutes) to maintain circulating blood volume.
- Check glucose. Treat if less than 60 mg/dL.
- Maintain normal body temperature
- Correct electrolyte and acid-base disturbances

Assess response (i.e., mental status, capillary refill, heart rate, ventilatory effort, blood pressure).

If inadequate response:

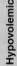

Hypovolemic

Hypovolemic Shock – Nontraumatic: Administer 1 or 2 additional fluid boluses as indicated. Reassess. Consider vasopressors if poor perfusion persists despite adequate oxygenation, ventilation, and volume expansion.
Hemorrhagic Shock: Administer 1 or 2 additional fluid boluses as indicated and reassess. Type and cross emergently if the child has severe trauma and life-threatening blood loss.

Cardiogenic

- Consider giving a small IV/IO fluid bolus of isotonic crystalloid solution (5 to 10 mL/kg of LR or NS). Repeat the primary survey after *each* fluid bolus. The fluid bolus may be repeated based on the child's response. If the child fails to improve, consider giving an inotrope to improve myocardial contractility and increase cardiac output.
- Treat dysrhythmias if present and contributing to shock. Seek expert consultation for additional orders.

Distributive

Anaphylaxis
- Remove/discontinue the causative agent. Give epinephrine 0.01 mg/kg using 1:1000 solution IM. Maximum single dose 0.5 mg. Repeat in 15 min if needed.
- Give 1 or 2 additional fluid boluses as indicated. Reassess. Consider inhaled bronchodilator (albuterol), diphenhydramine 1 to 2 mg/kg IM, IV, or orally; methylprednisolone 1 to 2 mg/kg IV
Septic
- Administer 1 or 2 additional fluid boluses as indicated. Reassess.
- Administer a vasopressor by IV infusion for signs of decompensated shock.
- Give IV antibiotics.
Neurogenic
- Administer 1 or 2 additional fluid boluses as indicated. Reassess.

Obstructive

Tension pneumothorax
- Perform needle decompression followed by chest tube insertion. Reassess.

Cardiac tamponade
- Administer 1 or 2 additional fluid boluses as indicated. Reassess.
- Pericardiocentesis is the definitive treatment for cardiac tamponade.

- Failure to measure oxygen saturation and give supplemental oxygen, if indicated.
- Failure to assist ventilation with a bag-mask device and supplemental oxygen if signs of inadequate ventilation are present.
- Failure to decompress a tension pneumothorax.
- Failure to rapidly establish vascular access.
- Extended attempts to establish IV access in a child with decompensated shock when IO access could be established quickly.
- Failure to rapidly administer a rapid fluid bolus of 20 mL/kg to a child with signs of shock.
- Failure to repeat the primary survey after each fluid bolus.
- Failure to assess serum glucose level and give dextrose for documented hypoglycemia.
- Administration of hypotonic or glucose-containing solutions for volume resuscitation.
- Administering vasopressors or boluses of a nonisotonic fluid in a patient with signs of adequate perfusion.
- Failure to begin CPR if a pulse is absent or slower than 60 beats per minute with signs of poor perfusion.
- Performing tracheal intubation in a child who responds to less invasive interventions.
- If tracheal intubation is required, failure to confirm tracheal tube position using assessment and mechanical methods.
- Treating associated injuries (if present), before stabilization of the airway, oxygenation, ventilation, and circulation.
- Ordering a dangerous or inappropriate intervention.
- Performing any technique resulting in potential harm to the patient.

Cardiopulmonary Failure

Cardiopulmonary failure is a clinical condition identified by deficits in oxygenation, ventilation, and perfusion. Respiratory failure associated with decompensated shock leads to inadequate oxygenation, ventilation, and perfusion, resulting in cardiopulmonary failure. Without prompt recognition and management, cardiopulmonary failure will deteriorate to cardiopulmonary arrest.

Signs of Cardiopulmonary Failure

- Bradypnea with irregular, ineffective ventilations.
- Decreasing work of breathing (tiring).
- Delayed capillary refill time (longer than 5 seconds).
- Bradycardia.

- Weak central pulses and absent peripheral pulses.
- Cool extremities.
- Mottled or cyanotic skin.
- Diminished level of responsiveness.

Cardiopulmonary Arrest

Cardiac arrest is the cessation of cardiac mechanical activity, confirmed by the absence of a detectable pulse, unresponsiveness, and apnea or agonal, gasping breathing. In adults, sudden nontraumatic cardio-pulmonary arrests are usually the result of underlying cardiac disease. In children, cardiac arrests are usually the result of respiratory failure (asphyxia precipitated by acute hypoxia or hypercarbia) or circulatory shock (ischemia from hypovolemia, sepsis, or myocardial dysfunction [cardiogenic shock])[7]. The cause of cardiac arrest in the pediatric patient also varies with age, the underlying health of the child, and the location of the event (Table 5-8).

TABLE 5-8 *Major Causes of Pediatric Cardiac Arrest*

Cardiovascular	
Hypovolemic shock	Septic shock
Congenital heart defect	Cardiogenic shock
Dysrhythmias	Myocarditis
Pericardial effusion	
Respiratory	
Croup/epiglottitis	Foreign body obstruction
Angioedema	Severe asthma
Pneumonia	Respiratory failure
Drowning	Inhalation injury
Bronchiolitis	Bronchopulmonary dysplasia
Neurologic	
CNS infection	Botulism
Ventriculoperitoneal shunt obstruction	Status epilepticus
Trauma	
Head trauma	Hypovolemic shock
Burns	Chest trauma
Other	
Sudden Infant Death Syndrome	Drug toxicity
Metabolic disorders	Poisoning

Rhythm Disturbances

ECG monitoring is an important aspect of pediatric emergency care and is indicated for any pediatric patient who shows signs of significant illness or injury. ECG monitoring may be used to assess the a patient's HR, evaluate the effects of disease or injury on heart function, evaluate the response to medications, or to obtain a baseline recording before, during, and after a medical procedure. Although disorders of HR and rhythm are uncommon in infants and children, when they do occur, they are most often because of hypoxia secondary to respiratory arrest and asphyxia.

A dysrhythmia involves an abnormality in the rate, regularity, or sequence of cardiac activation. In the pediatric patient, dysrhythmias are divided into four broad categories based on HR: (a) normal for age, (b) slower than normal for age (bradycardia), (c) faster than normal for age (tachycardia), or (d) absent/pulseless (cardiac arrest). In children, dysrhythmias are treated only if they compromise CO or have the potential for deteriorating into a lethal rhythm (Table 5-9).

Analyzing a Rhythm Strip

Determine if the rate is normal for age, too fast, too slow, or absent.

- Assess the rate.
  - The values used to define a tachycardia (above 100 beats per minute) and a bradycardia (below 60 beats per minute) in an adult are not the same as those in the pediatric patient.
  - In infants and children, a tachycardia is present if the HR is faster than the upper limit of normal for the patient's age. A bradycardia is present when the HR is slower than the lower limit of normal.

TABLE 5-9 *Summary of the Conduction System*

Structure	Location	Function
Sinoatrial (SA) node	Right atrial wall just inferior to opening of superior vena cava	Primary pacemaker; initiates impulse that is normally conducted throughout the left and right atria
Atrioventricular (AV) node	Posterior septal wall of the right atrium immediately behind the tricuspid valve and near the opening of the coronary sinus	Receives impulse from SA node and delays relay of the impulse to the bundle of His, allowing time for the atria to empty their contents into the ventricles before the onset of ventricular contraction
Bundle of His	Superior portion of interventricular septum	Receives impulse from AV node and relays it to right and left bundle branches
Right and left bundle branches	Interventricular septum	Receives impulse from bundle of His and relays it to Purkinje fibers in ventricular myocardium
Purkinje fibers	Ventricular myocardium	Receives impulse from bundle branches and relays it to ventricular myocardium

- Assess the width of the QRS complex.
  - The duration of the QRS complex is short in an infant and increases with age.
  - If the QRS measures 0.09 seconds or less, the QRS is "narrow," and is presumed to be supraventricular in origin.
  - If the QRS is more than 0.09 seconds in duration, the QRS is "wide" and presumed to be ventricular in origin until proven otherwise.
- Assess rhythm/regularity.
  - To determine if the ventricular rhythm is regular or irregular, measure the distance between two consecutive R-R intervals and compare that distance with the other R-R intervals.
  - To determine if the atrial rhythm is regular or irregular, measure the distance between two consecutive P-P intervals and compare that distance with the other P-P intervals.
- Evaluate the rhythm's clinical significance. How is the patient tolerating the rate and rhythm?
  - Stable: The infant or child is asymptomatic (i.e., normal blood pressure, mental status, and respiratory status).
  - Unstable: Decreased responsiveness, hypotension, or respiratory failure; chest pain due to ischemia may be present in the older child and adolescent.

Determine if the QRS is narrow or wide.

Determine if the rhythm is regular or irregular.

Sick (unstable) or not sick (stable)?

Pediatric dysrhythmias may be transient or permanent, congenital (in a structurally normal or abnormal heart) or acquired (rheumatic fever, myocarditis), caused by a toxin (diphtheria), or by proarrythmic or antiarrhythmic medications, or they may be a consequence of surgical correction of congenital heart disease.[8]

Sinus Rhythm

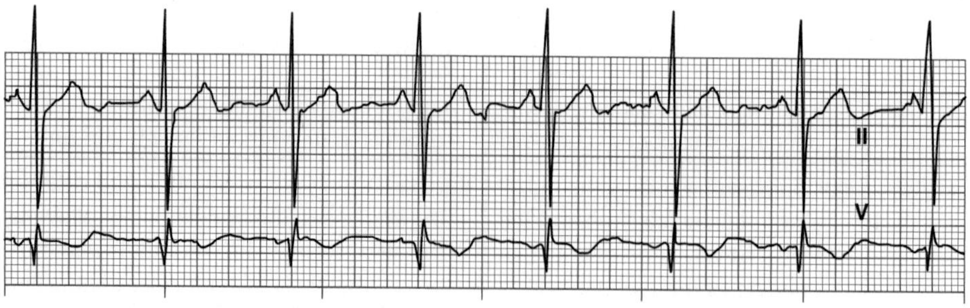

Rhythm Recognition

Many pediatric dysrhythmias are normal variants that do not require treatment.

Figure 5-2   Sinus rhythm.

TABLE 5-10 *Characteristics of Sinus Rhythm*	
Rate	Within normal limits for age
Rhythm	Regular
P waves	Uniform in appearance, positive (upright) in lead II, one precedes each QRS complex
PR interval	Within normal limits for age and constant from beat to beat
QRS duration	0.09 sec or less

Sinus Arrhythmia

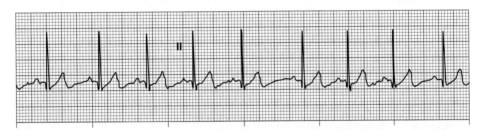

Figure 5-3   Sinus arrhythmia. This rhythm strip is from a 5-year-old girl complaining of abdominal pain. Note the irregular rhythm. The heart rate increases with inspiration (R-R intervals shorten) and decreases with expiration (R-R intervals lengthen).

TABLE 5-11 *Characteristics of Sinus Arrhythmia*	
Rate	Usually within normal limits for age
Rhythm	Irregular, phasic with respiration
P waves	Uniform in appearance, positive (upright) in lead II, one precedes each QRS complex
PR interval	Within normal limits for age and constant from beat to beat
QRS duration	0.09 sec or less
Clinical significance	Normal phenomenon that occurs with respiration and changes in intrathoracic pressure. Heart rate increases with inspiration (R-R intervals shorten) and decreases with expiration (R-R intervals lengthen). Commonly observed in infants and children.

Tachydysrhythmias: Too Fast Rhythms

In infants and children, a tachycardia is present if the HR is faster than the upper limit of normal for the patient's age. A tachycardia may represent either a normal compensatory response to the need for increased CO or oxygen delivery or an unstable dysrhythmia.

Three types of tachycardia are generally seen in children: sinus tachycardia, SVT, and VT with a pulse. Sinus tachycardia is the most common of these rhythms. As its name implies, SVT originates above the ventricles, while VT arises from within the ventricles, below the bifurcation of the bundle of His. SVT and VT can produce ventricular rates so rapid that ventricular filling time is reduced, SV decreases, and CO falls. Tachydysrhythmias seen in adults such as atrial flutter, ectopic atrial tachycardia, and junctional tachycardia are rare in children unless primary cardiac disease is present.

Sinus Tachycardia

Sinus tachycardia (Figure 5-4) is a normal compensatory response to the need for increased CO or oxygen delivery. In sinus tachycardia, the HR is usually less than 220 beats per minute in infants or 180 beats per minute

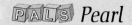
PALS *Pearl*

The initial emergency management of pediatric dysrhythmias requires a response to four important questions:
1. Is a pulse (and other signs of circulation) present?
2. Is the rate within normal limits for age, too fast, too slow, or absent?
3. Is the QRS wide (ventricular in origin) or narrow (supraventricular in origin)?
4. Is the patient sick (unstable) or not sick (stable)?

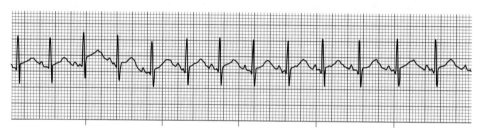

Figure 5-4   Sinus tachycardia.

TABLE 5-12 *Characteristics of Sinus Tachycardia*

Rate	Faster than the upper limit of normal for age; rate usually slower than 220 bpm in infants and slower than 180 bpm in children
Rhythm	Regular
P waves	Uniform in appearance, positive (upright) in lead II, one precedes each QRS complex
PR interval	Within normal limits for age and constant from beat to beat
QRS duration	0.09 sec or less
Cause	Anxiety, fear, fever, crying, hypovolemia, hypoxemia, pain, congestive heart failure, respiratory distress, toxins/poisonings/drugs, myocardial disease
Clinical significance	Compensatory response to the body's need for increased cardiac output or oxygen delivery. Increased myocardial workload is usually well tolerated by the infant or child with a healthy heart.
Treatment	Identify and treat the underlying cause

bpm, beats per minute.

in children. Onset of the rhythm occurs gradually. The ECG shows a regular, narrow QRS complex rhythm that often varies in response to activity or stimulation. P waves are present before each QRS complex. The history given typically explains the rapid HR (i.e., pain, fever, volume loss due to trauma, vomiting, or diarrhea).

Patient management includes treatment of the underlying cause that precipitated the rhythm (e.g., administering medications to relieve pain, administration of fluids to correct hypovolemia due to diarrhea). Electrical therapy and antiarrhymics are *not* used in the treatment of sinus tachycardia.

Supraventricular Tachycardia

SVT (Figures 5-5 and 5-6) is the most common tachydysrhythmia that necessitates treatment in the pediatric patient.

Unlike sinus tachycardia, SVT is not a normal compensatory response to physiologic stress. In SVT, the HR is usually more than 220 beats per minute in infants or 180 beats per minute in children. Onset of the rhythm occurs abruptly. The ECG shows a regular, narrow QRS complex rhythm that does not vary in response to activity or stimulation. P waves are often indiscernible due to the rapid rate and may be lost in the T wave of the preceding beat. If P waves are visible, they differ in appearance from P waves that originate in the sinoatrial (SA) node. In the absence of known congenital heart disease, the history obtained is usually nonspecific (i.e., the history does not explain the rapid HR).

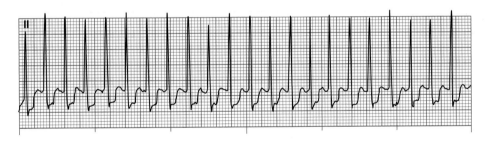

Figure 5-5   Supraventricular tachycardia (SVT) in a child complaining of chest pain.

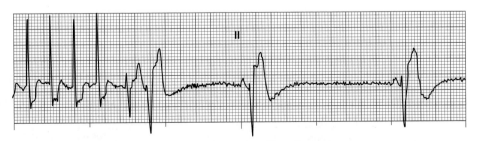

Figure 5-6   The same child (as shown in Figure 5-5) after administration of one intravenous dose of adenosine.

TABLE 5-13 *Characteristics of Supraventricular Tachycardia*

Rate	240 ± 40 bpm; may be as high as 300 bpm in infants
Rhythm	Regular
P waves	Often indiscernible due to rapid rate; may be lost in the T wave of the preceding beat. If P waves are visible, they differ in appearance from P waves that originate in the sinoatrial node and there is a 1:1 relationship to the QRS.
PR interval	Usually not measurable because P waves are not visible
QRS duration	0.09 sec or less unless an intraventricular conduction delay exists
Cause	Most often due to a reentrant mechanism that involves the atrioventricular junction or an accessory pathway
Clinical significance	Onset and termination of the rhythm are often abrupt (paroxysmal); tachydysrhythmias may result in decreased cardiac output (↑ heart rate → ↓ ventricular filling time → ↓ stroke volume → ↓ cardiac output)
Treatment	Vagal maneuvers, antiarrhythmics, or synchronized cardioversion depending on the stability of the patient (see Tachycardia Algorithm)

bpm, beats per minute.

TABLE 5-14 *Differentiation of Sinus Tachycardia and Supraventricular Tachycardia*

	Sinus Tachycardia	Supraventricular Tachycardia
Rate	Usually slower than 220 bpm in infants and 180 bpm in children	Usually 220 bpm or more in infants and 180 bpm or more in children
Ventricular rate and regularity	Varies with activity/stimulation	Constant with activity/stimulation
Onset and termination	Gradual	Abrupt
P waves	Visible; normal appearance	Often indiscernible; if visible, differ in appearance from sinoatrial node P waves
History	History given explains rapid heart rate; pain, fever, volume loss due to trauma, vomiting, or diarrhea	In the absence of known congenital heart disease, history is usually nonspecific (i.e., history given does not explain rapid heart rate)
Physical examination	May be consistent with volume loss (blood, diarrhea, vomiting), possiblefever, clear lungs, liver of normal size	Signs of poor perfusion including diminished peripheral pulses, delayed capillary refill, pallor, increased work of breathing, possible crackles, enlarged liver

bpm, beats per minute.

Rapid ventricular rates may be associated with lightheadedness, syncope, dyspnea, weakness, nervousness, and complaints of palpitations and chest pain or pressure in the older child. Signs of shock may be evident depending on the duration and rate of the tachycardia and the presence of primary cardiac disease. A child with normal cardiovascular function

Infants with SVT often present with heart failure because the tachycardia goes unrecognized for a long time.

may tolerate a rapid ventricular rate for several hours before signs of heart failure or shock will develop. Infants may tolerate the rapid ventricular rate associated with SVT for hours or days before developing signs of poor CO, heart failure, and cardiogenic shock.

Vagal maneuvers (see Chapter 6) are used to slow conduction through the atrioventricular (AV) node, resulting in slowing of the HR. Success rates with vagal maneuvers vary and depend on the presence of underlying conditions in the patient, the patient's age, and the patient's level of cooperation.

Ventricular Tachycardia

VT is a serious cardiac dysrhythmia that originates in the ventricles (Figure 5-7). Because the rhythm originates below the AV junction, the ventricles may be depolarized without receiving the additional 10% to 30% of ventricular filling produced by atrial contraction. The inadequate ventricular filling and rapid ventricular rate associated with this rhythm results in decreased SV and CO.

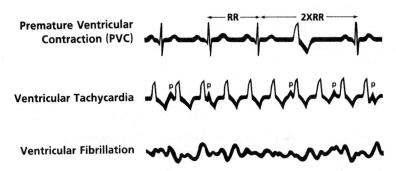

Figure 5-7   Examples of dysrhythmias originating in the ventricles.

Order a bedside glucose and toxicology screen for any child that presents with unexplained VT.

VT is uncommon in infants and children unless an underlying cardiovascular disorder exists. This dysrhythmia may be seen in children who have had open-heart surgical repair for tetralogy of Fallot or other anomalies or who have a cardiomyopathy, myocarditis, or myocardial tumor. VT may occur in an infant or child with a preexisting conduction abnormality such as long QT syndrome (see sidebar), and may be seen in the end stages of acidosis, hypoxemia, hypovolemia, or hypothermia. Secondary causes of VT include electrolyte imbalance (as seen in hyperkalemia or hypomagnesemia) and ingestion of certain toxins (such as tricyclic antidepressants).

When the QRS complexes of VT are of the same shape and amplitude, the rhythm is termed *monomorphic VT* (Figure 5-8). When the QRS complexes of VT vary in shape and amplitude, the rhythm is termed *polymorphic VT* (Figure 5-9).

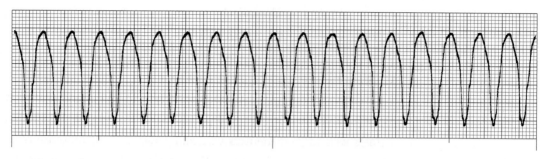

Figure 5-8   Monomorphic ventricular tachycardia (VT).

TABLE 5-15 *Characteristics of Monomorphic Ventricular Tachycardia*

Rate	120 to 250 bpm
Rhythm	Essentially regular
P waves	Usually not seen; if present, they have no set relationship to the QRS complexes appearing between them at a rate different from that of the ventricular tachycardia.
PR interval	None.
QRS duration	Greater than 0.09 sec; may be difficult to differentiate between the QRS and T wave.
Cause	May be caused by acute hypoxemia, acidosis, electrolyte imbalance, reactions to medications, toxins/poisons/drugs, myocarditis.
Clinical significance	Slower rates may be well tolerated. Rapid rates often result in decreased ventricular filling time and decreased cardiac output; may degenerate into ventricular fibrillation.
Treatment	If no pulse, defibrillation. Pulse present, antiarrhythmics or synchronized cardioversion depending on the stability of the patient (see Tachycardia Algorithm).

bpm, beats per minute.

Polymorphic Ventricular Tachycardia

Polymorphic VT (Figure 5-9) is a rapid ventricular dysrhythmia with beat-to-beat changes in the shape and amplitude of the QRS complexes. Polymorphic VT associated with a long QT interval is called torsades de pointes (TdP). Polymorphic VT associated with a normal QT interval is simply called polymorphic VT.

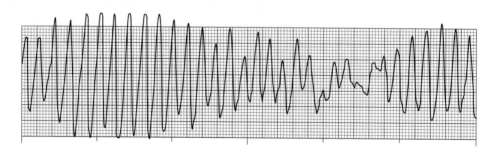

Figure 5-9   Polymorphic ventricular tachycardia.

TABLE 5-16 *Characteristics of Polymorphic Ventricular Tachycardia*

Rate	150 to 300 bpm, typically 200 to 250 bpm
Rhythm	May be regular or irregular
P waves	None
PR interval	None
QRS duration	Greater than 0.09 sec; gradual alteration in amplitude and direction of the QRS complexes
Causes	May be precipitated by slow heart rates; associated with medications or electrolyte disturbances that prolong the QT interval; a prolonged QT interval may be congenital or acquired; lengthening of the QT interval may be the only warning sign suggesting impending torsades de pointes.
Clinical significance	Symptoms are usually related to the decreased cardiac output that occurs because of the fast ventricular rate; signs of shock are often present; patient may experience a syncopal episode or seizures; may occasionally terminate spontaneously and recur after several seconds or minutes; may deteriorate to ventricular fibrillation
Treatment	If no pulse, defibrillation. Pulse present, magnesium sulfate is drug of choice (see Tachycardia Algorithm)

bpm, beats per minute.

Acceptable Interventions: Tachycardia with Adequate Perfusion

- Use personal protective equipment.
- Perform an initial assessment and obtain a focused history.
- If the child is stable (i.e., normal blood pressure for age, alert with palpable distal pulses, and normal breathing):
  - Apply a pulse oximeter and administer supplemental oxygen if indicated; ensure effective oxygenation and ventilation. Titrate oxygen administration to maintain an oxygen saturation level of 94% or higher.
  - Attach a cardiac monitor and identify the rhythm.
  - Establish vascular access.
- If the rhythm is SVT:
  - Ensure the patient's history does not indicate causes of *sinus* tachycardia (i.e., dehydration, fever).
  - Attempt vagal maneuvers.
    - Obtain a 12-lead ECG before and after a vagal maneuver and monitor the ECG continuously during the maneuver.
  - If the rhythm persists, give adenosine IV.
    - Initial dose: Adenosine 0.1 mg/kg rapid IV bolus (maximum initial dose 6 mg). Follow immediately with a rapid normal saline IV flush of at least 5 mL. Reassess.
    - Second dose: If there is no response after 1 to 2 minutes, give adenosine 0.2 mg/kg IV to a maximum individual dose of 12 mg, using the same technique. Reassess.

In stable patients with SVT, adenosine is the drug of choice because of its rapid onset of action and minimal effects on cardiac contractility.

Long QT Syndrome

Long QT syndrome (LQTS) is an abnormality of the heart's electrical system. The mechanical function of the heart is entirely normal. The electrical problem is thought to be due to defects in cardiac ion channels that affect repolarization. These electrical defects predispose affected persons to torsades de pointes (TdP) that leads to a sudden loss of consciousness (syncope) and may result in sudden cardiac death.

LQTS may be acquired or inherited. The acquired form of LQTS is more common and usually caused by medications that prolong the QT interval. Inherited LQTS is caused by mutations of genes that encode the cardiac ion channels. Some cases of LQTS are associated with congenital deafness.

Symptoms of LQTS vary and range from no dysrhythmias to recurrent syncope, cardiac arrest, and sudden death. Actual seizures are uncommon in LQTS, but epilepsy is one of the common errors in diagnosis.

Cases in which LQTS should be considered include a sudden loss of consciousness during physical exertion or during emotional excitement, sudden and unexplained loss of consciousness during childhood and teenage years, a family history of unexplained syncope, any young person who has an unexplained cardiac arrest, and epilepsy in children. Common triggers of LQTS include swimming, running, startle (e.g., an alarm clock, a loud horn, a ringing phone), anger, crying, test taking, or other stressful situations.

The diagnosis of LQTS is commonly suspected or made from the ECG. β-Blockers are frequently used in the management of patients with LQTS. Implantation of an implantable cardioverter-defibrillator along with use of β-blockers is recommended for LQTS patients with previous cardiac arrest and who have reasonable expectation of survival with a good functional status for more than 1 year.

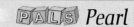 **Pearl**

SVT with abnormal (aberrant) conduction through the bundle branches produces a wide QRS complex. Differentiation of supraventricular tachycardia (SVT) with abnormal conduction (also called wide-QRS SVT) from ventricular tachycardia is often difficult. Wide-QRS SVT is relatively uncommon, occurring in less than 10% of children with SVT. Since almost all wide-QRS tachycardias are ventricular tachycardia, any wide-QRS tachycardia in an infant or child should be presumed to be ventricular in origin and treated as ventricular tachycardia.

- If the rhythm is VT:
  - Consult a pediatric cardiologist.
  - Obtain a 12-lead ECG.
  - Obtain a focused history, including family history for ventricular dysrhythmias or sudden death.
  - If the rhythm is regular and the QRS monomorphic, consider giving adenosine IV to help differentiate SVT from VT.
  - If the rhythm persists, seek expert consultation before attempting pharmacologic conversion with amiodarone or procainamide.
- Identify and treat possible reversible causes of the dysrhythmia:
  - Hypovolemia—replace volume
  - Hypoxia—give oxygen
  - Hydrogen ion—correct acidosis

Amiodarone and procainamide should not be administered together because both prolong the QT interval.

Drug Pearl
Adenosine

- Adenosine is found naturally in all body cells and is rapidly metabolized in the blood vessels. Adenosine slows the rate of the SA node, slows conduction time through the AV node, can interrupt reentry pathways that involve the AV node, and can restore sinus rhythm in SVT.
- Reentry circuits are the underlying mechanism for most episodes of SVT in infants and children. Adenosine acts at specific receptors to cause a temporary block of conduction through the AV node, interrupting these reentry circuits.
- Adenosine has a half-life of less than 10 seconds. It has an onset of action of 10 to 40 seconds and a duration of 1 to 2 minutes. Because of its short half-life, and to enhance delivery of the drug to its site of action in the heart, select the injection port on the IV tubing that is nearest the patient and administer the drug using a two-syringe technique. Prepare one syringe with the drug, and the other with a normal saline flush of at least 5 mL. Insert both syringes into the injection port in the IV tubing. Administer the drug medication IV or IO as rapidly as possible (i.e., over a period of seconds) and *immediately* follow with the saline flush.
- Adenosine may cause facial flushing because the drug is a mild cutaneous vasodilator and may cause coughing, dyspnea, and bronchospasm because it is a mild bronchoconstrictor.

Drug Pearl
Amiodarone

- Amiodarone directly depresses the automaticity of the SA and AV nodes, slows conduction through the AV node and in the accessory pathway of patients with Wolff-Parkinson-White syndrome, inhibits α-adrenergic and β-adrenergic receptors, and possesses both vagolytic and calcium-channel blocking properties. Because of these properties, amiodarone is used for a wide range of both atrial and ventricular dysrhythmias in adults and children.
- Amiodarone prolongs the PR, QRS, and QT intervals, and has an additive effect with other medications that prolong the QT interval (e.g., procainamide, phenothiazines, some tricyclic antidepressants, thiazide diuretics, sotalol).
- Seek expert consultation before giving amiodarone to an infant or child with a perfusing rhythm.
- Hypotension, bradycardia, and AV block are adverse effects of amiodarone administration. Slow the infusion rate or discontinue if seen.

Drug Pearl
Procainamide

- Procainamide is used for both atrial and ventricular dysrhythmias because it suppresses automaticity in the atria and ventricles and depresses conduction velocity within the conduction system.
- During administration, carefully monitor the patient's ECG and blood pressure. Observe the ECG closely for increasing PR and QT intervals, widening of the QRS complex, heart block, and/or onset of TdP. If the QRS widens to more than 50% of its original width or hypotension occurs, slow or discontinue the infusion.
- Procainamide should not be used in patients with a prolonged QRS duration or QT interval because of the potential for heart block or in patients with preexisting QT prolongation/TdP.
- Procainamide should not be used with other medications that prolong the QT interval (e.g., amiodarone).

Drug Pearl
Lidocaine

- Lidocaine depresses spontaneous ventricular depolarization but does not affect SA or AV node depolarization and is used in the treatment of ventricular dysrhythmias (e.g., ventricular tachycardia, ventricular fibrillation).
- Lidocaine toxicity may be seen in patients with persistently poor cardiac output and hepatic failure. Signs and symptoms of lidocaine toxicity are primarily central nervous system (CNS)–related including drowsiness, disorientation, muscle twitching, or seizures.

- Hypo-/hyperkalemia–correct electrolyte disturbances
- Hypoglycemia–give dextrose if indicated
- Hypothermia–rewarming measures
- Toxins/poisons/drugs–antidote/specific therapy
- Tamponade (cardiac)–pericardiocentesis
- Tension pneumothorax–needle decompression, chest tube insertion
- Thrombosis (coronary or pulmonary)–anticoagulation? Surgery?

Unacceptable Interventions: Tachycardia with Adequate Perfusion

- Failure to use personal protective equipment.
- Failure to adequately assess the patient.
- Inability to quickly determine if the child is sick or not sick (i.e., unstable or stable).
- Failure to measure oxygen saturation and give supplemental oxygen, if indicated.
- Failure to correctly identify the ECG rhythm.

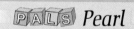

PALS Pearl

Be sure to obtain ECG tracings before, during, and after interventions for any patient experiencing a cardiac dysrhythmia.

- Failure to establish vascular access.
- Administration of verapamil to an infant.
- Failure to administer adenosine rapidly IV bolus.
- Medication errors.
- Attempting synchronized cardioversion or defibrillation for an infant or child in SVT or VT with signs of adequate perfusion.
- Failure to correctly differentiate sinus tachycardia from SVT.
- Ordering a dangerous or inappropriate intervention.
- Performing any technique resulting in potential harm to the patient.

Acceptable Interventions: Tachycardia with Poor Perfusion

Do not delay cardioversion to establish vascular access if the child is unresponsive or hypotensive.

- Use personal protective equipment.
- Perform an initial assessment and obtain a focused history.
- If the child is unstable ("sick") (i.e., acutely altered mental status, signs of shock, or hypotension) immediate treatment with electrical or pharmacologic cardioversion is warranted (see Tachycardia Algorithm).
- Apply a pulse oximeter and administer supplemental oxygen if indicated; ensure effective oxygenation and ventilation. Titrate oxygen administration to maintain an oxygen saturation level of of 94% or higher.
- Attach a cardiac monitor and identify the rhythm.
- Establish vascular access.

If the child is responsive, sedate if possible but do not delay cardioversion.

- If the rhythm is SVT:
  - If vascular access is already available, adenosine may be administered before synchronized cardioversion, but do not delay cardioversion if establishment of vascular access (IV or IO) will take more than 20 to 30 seconds to accomplish.
  - If vascular access is immediately available, give adenosine 0.1 mg/kg rapidly IV or IO (maximum initial dose 6 mg), immediately followed by a rapid normal saline IV flush of at least 5 mL. If there is no response in 1 to 2 minutes, give adenosine 0.2 mg/kg IV/IO to a maximum individual dose of 12 mg, using the same technique.
  - If vascular access has not been established, or if the child fails to respond to adenosine, perform synchronized cardioversion starting with 0.5 to 1 J/kg. If cardioversion does not terminate the dysrhythmia, increase the energy level to 2 J/kg. If the dysrhythmia persists despite a second shock or the tachycardia recurs quickly, consider amiodarone or procainamide before delivering a third shock.
- If the rhythm is VT:
  - Perform synchronized cardioversion. Begin with 0.5 to 1 J/kg. If the dysrhythmia persists, increase the energy level to 2 J/kg.
- Identify and treat possible reversible causes of the dysrhythmia

PEDIATRIC TACHYCARDIA ALGORITHM

Assess ABCs, ensure effective oxygenation and ventilation
Attach pulse oximeter and monitor/defibrillator
If pulseless, begin CPR - go to cardiac arrest algorithm

Narrow-QRS (0.09 sec or less)
Probable sinus tachycardia or
supraventricular tachycardia (SVT)

Algorithm assumes
serious signs and
symptoms persist.

R H Y T H M

Probable Sinus Tachycardia:
*History explains rapid rate
*Gradual rhythm onset
*P waves present/normal
*Ventricular rate/regularity varies
with activity/stimulation
*Variable R to R interval with
constant PR interval
*Rate usually slower than 220
beats/min in infant and slower
than 180 beats/min in child

R H Y T H M

Probable SVT:
*History does not explain rapid rate
*P waves absent/abnormal
*Rhythm onset - abrupt
*Ventricular rate/regularity constant
with activity/stimulation
*Abrupt rate changes
*Rate usually 220 beats/min
or more in infant and 180 beats/min
or more in child

Identify and treat underlying
cause

S T A B L E

Obtain 12-lead ECG, consult
pediatric cardiologist
Try vagal maneuvers
Start IV, identify/treat causes
Give adenosine IV
If rhythm persists, consider
amiodarone or procainamide

U N S T A B L E

Consider vagal maneuvers
If IV/IO in place,
give adenosine
If no vascular access or adenosine
ineffective, sedate if needed and
perform synchronized cardioversion
with 0.5 to 1 J/kg; use 2 J/kg for a
second shock if rhythm persists. If
rhythm persists despite second shock
or tachycardia recurs quickly, consider
amiodarone or procainamide before
delivering a third shock

Wide-QRS (more than 0.09 sec)
Probable ventricular tachycardia

S T A B L E

Obtain 12-lead ECG, consult
pediatric cardiologist
Start IV, identify/treat causes
Consider adenosine IV if
rhythm regular and QRS
monomorphic

U N S T A B L E

If hypotension, acutely altered
mental status, or signs of
shock, sedate if needed
(but do not delay cardioversion)
and perform synchronized
cardioversion with 0.5 to 1 J/kg;
use 2 J/kg if rhythm persists

C O N S I D E R   C A U S E S

*Hypovolemia – replace volume
*Hypoxia – give oxygen
*Hydrogen ion – correct acidosis
*Hypo-/hyperkalemia – correct
electrolyte disturbances
*Hypoglycemia – give dextrose if
indicated
*Hypothermia – rewarming
measures
*Toxins/poisons/drugs –
antidote/specific therapy
*Tamponade (cardiac) –
pericardiocentesis
*Tension pneumothorax – needle
decompression, chest tube
insertion
*Thrombosis (coronary or
pulmonary) – anticoagulation?
Surgery?

D R U G S

Adenosine IV/IO: 0.1 mg/kg rapid IV bolus (maximum first dose 6 mg); if no
effect, may double and repeat dose once (max second dose 12 mg)
Amiodarone 5 mg/kg IV over 20 to 60 min*
Procainamide 15 mg/kg IV over 30 to 60 min*
*Do not routinely give amiodarone and procainamide together

Unacceptable Interventions: Tachycardia with Poor Perfusion

- Failure to use personal protective equipment.
- Failure to adequately assess the patient.
- Inability to quickly determine if the child is sick or not sick (i.e., unstable or stable).
- Failure to measure oxygen saturation and give supplemental oxygen, if indicated.
- Failure to assist ventilation with a bag-mask device and supplemental oxygen if signs of inadequate ventilation are present.
- Failure to correctly identify the ECG rhythm.
- Failure to establish vascular access.
- Extended attempts to establish IV access in a child with decompensated shock when IO access could be established quickly.
- Medication errors.
- Attempting synchronized cardioversion or defibrillation for an infant or child in SVT or VT and signs of adequate perfusion.
- Failure to correctly differentiate sinus tachycardia from SVT.
- Failure to deliver the correct energy level(s) for the specific dysrhythmia.
- Failure to identify and treat potentially reversible causes of the dysrhythmia.
- Performing tracheal intubation in a child who responds to less invasive interventions.
- If tracheal intubation is required, failure to confirm tracheal tube position using assessment and mechanical methods.
- Ordering a dangerous or inappropriate intervention.
- Performing any technique resulting in potential harm to the patient.

Bradydysrhythmias: Too Slow Rhythms

In infants and children, a bradycardia is present if the HR is slower than the lower limit of normal for the patient's age. Bradycardias can be classified as either primary or secondary. A **primary bradycardia** is usually caused by structural heart disease. An infant or child with structural cardiac disease may develop bradycardia because of AV block or sinus node dysfunction. Physical examination of these children may reveal a mid-line sternal scar and they may have an implanted pacemaker to treat the bradycardia.

A sinus rate below 90 beats per minute in neonates and below 60 beats per minute thereafter is considered a sinus bradycardia.[8]

A **secondary bradycardia** is a slow HR due to a noncardiac cause. Causes of secondary bradycardias include increased vagal (parasympathetic) tone (vomiting, increased intracranial pressure, vagal maneuvers, suctioning, or tracheal intubation procedure), hypothermia, hyperkalemia, and ingestion of medications such as calcium channel blockers (verapamil, diltiazem), digoxin, and β-blockers (propranolol).

Remember that CO = SV × HR. Therefore, a decrease in either SV or HR may result in a decrease in CO. A bradycardia can produce significant symptoms unless SV increases to compensate for the decrease in HR. Unless corrected promptly, decreasing CO will eventually produce hemodynamic compromise.

In the pediatric patient, most slow rhythms occur secondary to hypoxia and acidosis.

Sinus Bradycardia

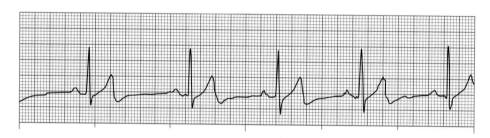

Figure 5-10 Sinus bradycardia.

TABLE 5-17 *Characteristics of Sinus Bradycardia*

Rate	Slower than the lower range of normal for age
Rhythm	Essentially regular
P waves	Uniform in appearance, positive (upright) in lead II, one precedes each QRS complex
PR interval	Within normal limits for age and constant from beat to beat
QRS duration	0.09 sec or less
Cause	Hypoxemia, acidosis, increased vagal tone (e.g., suctioning, tracheal intubation)
Clinical significance	May be normal in conditioned adolescent athletes and in some children during sleep. In other patients, decreased cardiac output may occur because of slow rate, despite normal stroke volume.
Treatment	Search for treatable cause. Ensure good oxygenation and ventilation. Begin chest compressions if the heart rate is slower than 60 bpm in an infant or child with poor systemic perfusion despite oxygenation and ventilation. Establish vascular access. Epinephrine, atropine, possible pacing (see Bradycardia Algorithm).

bpm, beats per minute.

Atrioventricular Blocks

AV blocks are divided into three main types: first-, second-, and third-degree AV block (Figure 5-11). The clinical significance of an AV block depends on the degree (severity) of the block, the rate of the escape pacemaker (junctional vs. ventricular), and the patient's response to that ventricular rate.

- First-degree AV block.
  - In first-degree AV block, all impulses from the SA node are conducted, but the impulses are delayed before they are conducted to the ventricles.
  - This delay in AV conduction results in a PR interval that is longer than normal, but constant.
- Second-degree AV block.
  - In second-degree AV block, some impulses are not conducted to the ventricles.
  - In second-degree AV block type I (also known as Wenckebach or Mobitz type I), P waves appear at regular intervals, but the PR interval progressively lengthens until a P wave is not conducted.
  - In second-degree AV block type II (also known as Mobitz type II), P waves appear at regular intervals, and the PR interval is constant before each conducted QRS. However, impulses are periodically blocked, appearing on the ECG as a P wave with no QRS after it (dropped beat). This type of AV block may progress to third-degree AV block without warning.
- Third-degree AV block.
  - In third-degree AV block (also known as complete heart block), the atria and ventricles beat independently of each other because impulses generated by the SA node are blocked before reaching the ventricles.

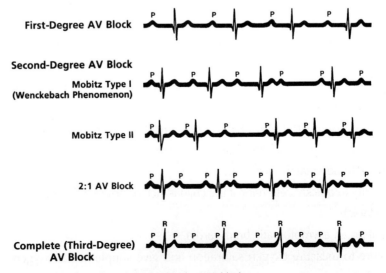

Figure 5-11 Examples of atrioventricular (AV) blocks.

- A secondary pacemaker (either junctional or ventricular) stimulates the ventricles; therefore, the QRS may be narrow or wide depending on the location of the escape pacemaker and the condition of the intraventricular conduction system.

Acceptable Interventions: Symptomatic Bradycardia

Interventions for a slow rhythm are unnecessary if the patient is asymptomatic. For example, adolescent athletes at rest or children who are sleeping may demonstrate no symptoms with a slow HR. If an infant or child is symptomatic because of a bradycardia, initial interventions focus on assessment of the airway and ventilation rather than administration of epinephrine, atropine, or other drugs because problems with adequate oxygenation and ventilation are more common in children than cardiac causes of bradycardia (see Bradycardia Algorithm).

- Use personal protective equipment.
- Perform an initial assessment and obtain a focused history.
- If the child is unstable ("sick") (i.e., acutely altered mental status, hypotension, or signs of shock) immediate intervention is necessary.
- Apply a pulse oximeter and administer supplemental oxygen if indicated; ensure effective oxygenation and ventilation. Titrate oxygen administration to maintain an oxygen saturation level of 94% or higher.
- Attach a cardiac monitor and identify the rhythm. Establish vascular access.
- If the HR is slower than 60 beats per minute with signs of hypoperfusion, begin CPR. Reassess the patient after 2 minutes to determine if bradycardia and signs of hemodynamic compromise persist.
- Identify and treat possible reversible causes of the dysrhythmia.
- Give epinephrine 0.01 mg/kg (1:10,000 solution) IV/IO; if vascular access is not available, give tracheally 0.1 mg/kg (1:1,000 solution). Maximum dose 1 mg IV/IO; 2.5 mg tracheally.
- Give atropine IV/IO 0.02 mg/kg or a tracheal dose of 0.04 to 0.06 mg/kg if the bradycardia is due to suspected increased vagal tone or primary AV block. Minimum dose 0.1 mg, maximum single dose 0.5 mg.
- Consider pacing.

Unacceptable Interventions: Symptomatic Bradycardia

- Failure to use personal protective equipment.
- Failure to adequately assess the patient.
- Inability to quickly determine if the child is sick or not sick (i.e., unstable or stable).
- Treating an asymptomatic bradycardia.
- Failure to measure oxygen saturation and give supplemental oxygen, if indicated.

SYMPTOMATIC BRADYCARDIA ALGORITHM

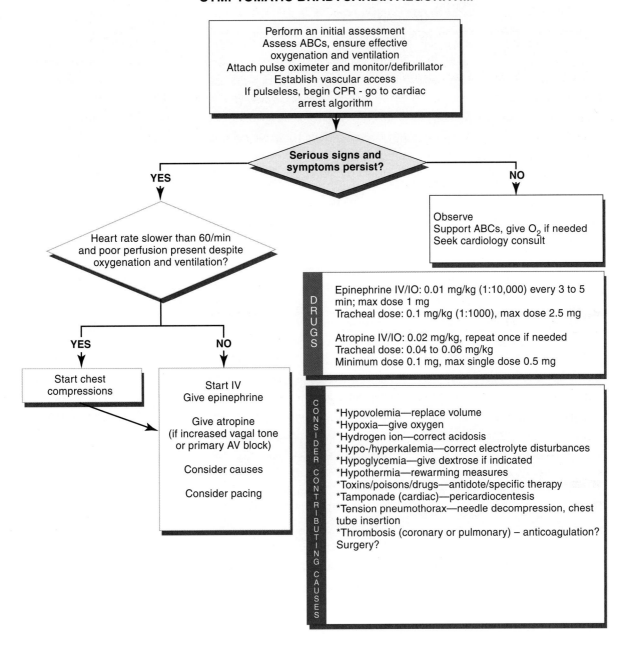

Perform an initial assessment
Assess ABCs, ensure effective oxygenation and ventilation
Attach pulse oximeter and monitor/defibrillator
Establish vascular access
If pulseless, begin CPR - go to cardiac arrest algorithm

Serious signs and symptoms persist?

YES

NO

Observe
Support ABCs, give O_2 if needed
Seek cardiology consult

Heart rate slower than 60/min and poor perfusion present despite oxygenation and ventilation?

YES

NO

Start chest compressions

Start IV
Give epinephrine

Give atropine
(if increased vagal tone or primary AV block)

Consider causes

Consider pacing

DRUGS

Epinephrine IV/IO: 0.01 mg/kg (1:10,000) every 3 to 5 min; max dose 1 mg
Tracheal dose: 0.1 mg/kg (1:1000), max dose 2.5 mg

Atropine IV/IO: 0.02 mg/kg, repeat once if needed
Tracheal dose: 0.04 to 0.06 mg/kg
Minimum dose 0.1 mg, max single dose 0.5 mg

CONSIDER CONTRIBUTING CAUSES

*Hypovolemia—replace volume
*Hypoxia—give oxygen
*Hydrogen ion—correct acidosis
*Hypo-/hyperkalemia—correct electrolyte disturbances
*Hypoglycemia—give dextrose if indicated
*Hypothermia—rewarming measures
*Toxins/poisons/drugs—antidote/specific therapy
*Tamponade (cardiac)—pericardiocentesis
*Tension pneumothorax—needle decompression, chest tube insertion
*Thrombosis (coronary or pulmonary) – anticoagulation? Surgery?

Drug Pearl
Atropine

- Atropine enhances AV conduction and increases heart rate (positive chronotropic effect) by accelerating the SA node discharge rate and blocking the vagus nerve. Atropine has little or no effect on the force of contraction (inotropic effect).
- Epinephrine is the drug of choice if bradycardia is due to hypoxia and oxygenation and ventilation do not correct the bradycardia.

- Give atropine before epinephrine if the bradycardia is due to increased vagal tone or if AV block is present.
- Do not give atropine slowly or in smaller than recommended doses (0.1 mg) because paradoxic slowing of the heart rate can occur. Paradoxic slowing may last 2 minutes.

Drug Pearl
Dopamine

- Dopamine is an endogenous catecholamine with dose-related actions (there is some "overlap" of effects). At low doses (0.5 to 5 mcg/kg/min), dopamine acts on dopaminergic receptors that are located mainly in mesenteric, renal, and coronary vessels, causing vasodilation. At moderate doses (5 to 10 mcg/kg/min), dopamine stimulates the β_1-adrenergic receptors on the myocardium

increasing myocardial contractility and stroke volume, thereby increasing cardiac output. At high doses (10 to 20 mcg/kg/min), dopamine acts on vascular α-adrenergic receptors, producing systemic vasoconstriction. Because of the extreme variation in dosages required to activate receptor sites in patients, it is impossible to predict the infusion rate required for an individual patient.

Drug Pearl
Epinephrine

- Epinephrine is a direct-acting endogenous catecholamine with moderate β_2-adrenergic (bronchodilation) and potent α-adrenergic (vasoconstriction) and β_1-adrenergic ($\uparrow$ heart rate, $\uparrow$ force of contraction) properties.
- Although epinephrine's β_1 effects increase myocardial oxygen consumption, it is generally well tolerated in the pediatric patient.
- In cardiac arrest, epinephrine produces beneficial effects primarily because of its α-adrenergic stimulating effects: $\uparrow$ peripheral vascular resistance (vasoconstriction) $\rightarrow \uparrow$ diastolic pressure $\rightarrow \uparrow$ myocardial and cerebral blood flow during CPR.

- Failure to assist ventilation with a bag-mask device and supplemental oxygen if signs of inadequate ventilation are present.
- Failure to correctly identify the ECG rhythm.
- Failure to begin CPR if the HR is slower than 60 beats per minute and accompanied by signs of inadequate perfusion despite adequate oxygenation and ventilation.
- Failure to establish vascular access.
- Extended attempts to establish IV access in a child with decompensated shock when IO access could be established quickly.
- Failure to administer epinephrine for a symptomatic bradycardia unresponsive to basic life support interventions.
- Failure to give atropine before epinephrine if the bradycardia is due to suspected increased vagal tone or primary AV block.
- Medication errors.
- Failure to correctly perform transcutaneous pacing.

- Performing tracheal intubation in a child who responds to less invasive interventions.
- If tracheal intubation is required, failure to confirm tracheal tube position using assessment and mechanical methods.
- Ordering a dangerous or inappropriate intervention.
- Performing any technique resulting in potential harm to the patient.

Absent/Pulseless Rhythms

In cardiopulmonary arrest, central pulses and the work of breathing are absent and the patient is unresponsive. Absent/pulseless rhythms include the following:

- Pulseless VT, in which the ECG displays a wide QRS complex at a rate faster than 120 beats per minute.
- VF, in which irregular chaotic deflections that vary in shape and amplitude are observed on the ECG but there is no coordinated ventricular contraction.
- Asystole, in which no cardiac electrical activity is present.
- Pulseless electrical activity (PEA), in which electrical activity is visible on the ECG but central pulses are absent.

Ventricular Fibrillation

VF is a chaotic rhythm that originates in the ventricles. In VF, there is no organized depolarization of the ventricles. The ventricular myocardium quivers and, as a result, there is no effective myocardial contraction and no pulse. The resulting rhythm is irregularly irregular with chaotic deflections that vary in shape and amplitude. No normal-looking waveforms are visible.

VT and VF are uncommon in children. When these rhythms are seen, it usually signifies serious myocardial pathology or dysfunction due to congenital heart disease, cardiomyopathies, or an acute inflammatory injury to the heart (e.g., myocarditis), or due to a reversible cause including drug toxicity (e.g., recreational drugs, tricyclic antidepressants, digoxin overdose), metabolic causes (e.g., hyperkalemia, hypermagnesemia, hypocalcemia, or hypoglycemia), or hypothermia.

Commotio cordis (VF due to a blunt, nonpenetrating blow to the chest) is an underappreciated cause of sudden cardiac death in young patients. It most frequently occurs in males at a mean age of 13.6. Sports that place athletes at risk for commotion cordis are those that involve a blow to the chest from an opponent, a stick, or a ball; baseball, lacrosse, hockey, and the martial arts are the most common.[9] Although most patients who sustain commotion cordis do not survive, CPR and defibrillation within 3 minutes of the event have resulted in favorable outcomes in some cases (Figure 5-12).

Defibrillation and CPR are the most effective treatments for pulseless VT and VF.

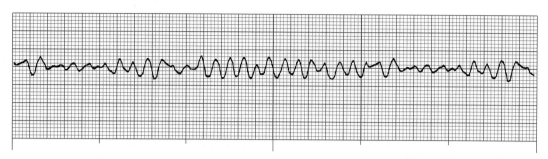

Figure 5-12 Ventricular fibrillation (VF). The patient in VF is unresponsive, apneic, and pulseless.

TABLE 5-18 *Characteristics of Ventricular Fibrillation*

Rate	Cannot be determined because there are no discernible waves or complexes to measure
Rhythm	Rapid and chaotic with no pattern or regularity
P waves	Not discernible
PR interval	Not discernible
QRS duration	Not discernible
Causes	Hypoxia, acidosis, hypo-/hyperkalemia, hypoglycemia, hypothermia, hypovolemia, tablets/toxins (drug overdose), cardiac tamponade, tension pneumothorax, thrombosis (coronary or pulmonary), and trauma (among other causes)
Significance	Terminal rhythm
Treatment	Confirm patient is unresponsive, has absent (or only gasping) breathing, and no pulse. Begin CPR until a defibrillator is available. (see Cardiac Arrest Algorithm, p. 216).

Asystole (Ventricular Standstill)

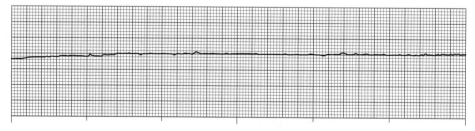

Figure 5-13 Asystole.

Pulseless Electrical Activity

PEA is a clinical situation, not a specific dysrhythmia. PEA exists when organized electrical activity (other than VT) is observed on the cardiac monitor, but the patient is pulseless (Figure 5-14).

Many conditions may cause PEA. PEA has a poor prognosis unless the underlying cause can be rapidly identified and appropriately managed.

TABLE 5-19 *Characteristics of Asystole*

Rate	Ventricular activity not discernible but atrial activity may be observed ("P wave" asystole)
Rhythm	Ventricular not discernible, atrial may be discernible
P waves	Usually not discernible
PR interval	Not measurable
QRS duration	Absent
Causes	Hypoxia, acidosis, hypo-/hyperkalemia, hypoglycemia, hypothermia, hypovolemia, tablets/toxins (drug overdose), cardiac tamponade, tension pneumothorax, thrombosis (coronary or pulmonary), and trauma (among other causes). Ventricular asystole may occur temporarily following termination of a tachydysryhthmia following medication administration, defibrillation, or synchronized cardioversion.
Clinical significance	Absence of cardiac output; terminal rhythm. Patient is unresponsive, apneic, and pulseless.
Treatment	See Cardiac Arrest Algorithm, p. 216

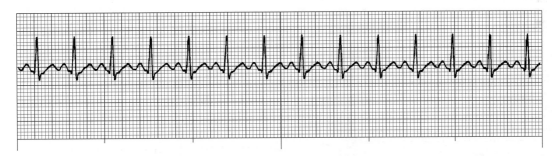

Figure 5-14 Pulseless electrical activity (PEA)—organized electrical activity without a palpable pulse.

Acceptable Interventions: Absent/Pulseless Rhythms

- Use personal protective equipment.
- After confirming patient is nonresponsive, apneic, and pulseless, call for help, send for a defibrillator, and begin CPR. As soon as they are available, attach a ECG monitor or defibrillator pads to the patient's bare chest and identify the rhythm.
- If a "nonshockable rhythm" is present (the rhythm is PEA or aystole):
  - Continue CPR and establish vascular access without interrupting chest compressions
  - Give epinephrine 0.01 mg/kg (1:10,000 solution) IV/IO, maximum of 1 mg (10 mL) every 3 to 5 minutes as long as the patient does not have a pulse
  - Attempt to identify and treat reversible causes of the arrest
  - Consider placement of an advanced airway, confirm tube position with primary and secondary techniques
  - Recheck the patient's cardiac rhythm every 2 minutes with minimal interruptions in chest compressions

CARDIAC ARREST ALGORITHM

Confirm patient is unresponsive,
apneic, pulseless
Call for help, send for defibrillator
Begin CPR; attach ECG monitor or
defibrillator pads to patient's bare
chests and identify rhythm

Assess ECG rhythm Shockable?

NO

YES

Electrical activity present?
Check pulse.
No pulse or asystole:
Resume CPR for about 2 min
During CPR, give vasopressor
Consider advanced airway
placement, consider reversible
cause of arrest.
Recheck rhythm after 2 min CPR.

Pulse present?
Assess vital signs,
begin post-cardiac arrest care.

Continue CPR until defibrillator ready.
Initial shock 2 to 4 J/kg, resume CPR
starting with chest compressions.
Start IV/IO without interrupting CPR,
give vasopressor.
Recheck rhythm after 2 min CPR.
If shockable rhythm, second shock
4 J/kg, resume CPR.
Consider advanced airway placement,
consider reversible cause of arrest.
Recheck rhythm after 2 min CPR.
If shockable rhythm, third shock 4 J/kg
or higher (max energy dose 10 J/kg or
adult dose, whichever is lower),
resume CPR.
Without interrupting CPR,
give antiarrythmic.
Recheck rhythm after 2 min of CPR.

D R U G S

Vasopressors
Epinephrine IV/IO: 0.01 mg/kg
(1:10,000) every 3 to 5 min;
max dose 1 mg
Tracheal dose: 0.1 mg/kg
(1:1000), max 2.5 mg

Antiarrhythmics
Amiodarone IV/IO 5 mg/kg
Lidocaine IV/IO 1 mg/kg (if
amiodarone is not available)
Magnesium IV/IO (if the rhythm is
torsades) 25 to 50 mg/kg,
max single dose 2 g

Algorithm assumes previous
step was unsucccessful

M O N I T O R

Attempt/verify:
*Advanced airway placement
*Vascular access
Monitor and treat:
*Glucose
*Electrolytes
*Temperature
*CO_2

R E V E R S I B L E   C A U S E S

*Hypovolemia—replace volume
*Hypoxia—give oxygen
*Hydrogen ion—correct
acidosis
*Hypo-/hyperkalemia—correct
electrolyte disturbances
*Hypoglycemia—give dextrose
if indicated
*Hypothermia—rewarming
measures
*Toxins/poisons/drugs—
antidote/specific therapy
*Tamponade (cardiac)—
pericardiocentesis
*Tension pneumothorax—
needle decompression, chest
tube insertion
*Thrombosis (coronary or
pulmonary) – anticoagulation?
Surgery?

R E A S S E S S

*Airway
*Oxygenation/ventilation
*Paddle/pad position/contact
*Effectiveness of CPR
*No O_2 flowing over patient
during shocks

- Reassess advanced airway position, electrode position and contact, effectiveness of CPR, equipment in use is functioning properly, confirm appropriate interventions, consider alternative medications and special resuscitation circumstances
- If a shockable rhythm is present (the rhythm is pulseless VT or VF):
  - Continue CPR until the defibrillator is ready to deliver a shock. Clear the area around the patient and deliver one shock using an initial dose of 2 to 4 J/kg. Immediately resume CPR, starting with chest compressions for about 2 minutes.
  - Establish vascular access without interrupting chest compressions and then give epinephrine every 3 to 5 minutes as long as the patient does not have a pulse.
  - After 2 minutes of CPR, recheck the rhythm. If a shockable rhythm is present, clear the patient, and defibrillate using 4 J/kg. Immediately resume CPR, starting with chest compressions.
  - Consider placement of an advanced airway; confirm tube position with primary and secondary techniques. Search for possible reversible causes of the arrest.
  - After 2 minutes of CPR, recheck the rhythm. If a shockable rhythm is present, clear the patient, and defibrillate using 4 J/kg or more, maximum energy dose not to exceed 10 J/kg or the adult dose (whichever is lower). Immediately resume CPR, starting with chest compressions.
  - Without interrupting CPR, give amiodarone (or lidocaine if amiodarone is not available). Give magnesium sulfate if the rhythm is torsades.
    - Amiodarone 5 mg/kg IV/IO bolus; may be repeated up to 2 times for refractory pulseless VT/VF
    - Lidocaine 1 mg/kg IV/IO bolus
    - Magnesium sulfate 25 to 50 mg.kg IV/IO; maximum single dose 2 g
  - Check a pulse if an organized rhythm is present on the monitor. If there is an organized rhythm on the monitor and a pulse is present, check the patient's blood pressure and other vital signs and begin post-cardiac arrest care.

  ### Unacceptable Interventions: Absent/Pulseless Rhythms
- Failure to use personal protective equipment.
- Failure to adequately assess the patient.
- Administration of oxygen by a means other than positive-pressure ventilation.
- Failure to correctly identify the ECG rhythm.
- Failure to begin CPR.

- Unsafe operation of defibrillator (failure to clear self or others before shocking).
- Failure to recognize rhythm change.
- Failure to establish vascular access.
- Extended attempts to establish IV access when IO access could be established quickly.
- Medication errors.
- Failure to confirm tracheal tube position using assessment and mechanical methods.
- Failure to search for possible reversible causes of the arrest.
- Ordering a dangerous or inappropriate intervention.
- Performing any technique resulting in potential harm to the patient.

Case Study Resolution

This child is sick. Further assessment reveals a ventilatory rate of 40, HR of 136 beats per minute, and capillary refill of 4 seconds. His blood pressure is 62/44 mm Hg. The child's presentation suggests anaphylaxis. Move quickly. Ensure a patent airway. Apply a pulse oximeter and administer supplemental oxygen as indicated; ensure effective oxygenation and ventilation. Be prepared to intubate if necessary. Attach a cardiac monitor. Check a glucose level. This child was given epinephrine 0.01 mg/kg of 1:1000 solution IM and diphenhydramine mg/kg IM with prompt resolution of his symptoms.

References

1. Barkin RM, Rosen P. *Emergency pediatrics: a guide to ambulatory care*, 5th ed. St. Louis: Mosby, 1999.

2. Hazinski MF. Manual of pediatric critical care. St. Louis: Mosby, 1999.

3. Frankel LR, Kache S. Shock. In: Kliegman RM, Behrman RE, Jenson HB, Stanton BF, eds. *Nelson textbook of pediatrics*, 18th ed. Philadelphia: WB Saunders, 2007.

4. Kleinman ME, Chameides L, Schexnayder SM, et al. Part 14: Pediatric advanced life support: 2010 American Heart Association Guidelines for Cardiopulmonary Resuscitation and Emergency Cardiovascular Care. Circulation 2010;122(suppl 3):S876–S908.

5. Carcillo JA, Fields AI, American College of Critical Care Medicine Task Force Committee Members. Clinical practice parameters for hemodynamic support of pediatric and neonatal patients in septic shock. Crit Care Med 2002;30:1365–1378.

6. Susil G. Allergic emergencies (anaphylaxis). In: Custer JW, Rau RE, eds. *The Harriet Lane handbook: a manual for pediatric house officers*, 18th ed. Philadelphia: Mosby, 2009.

7. Berg MD, Nadkarni VM, Zuercher M, Berg RA. In-hospital pediatric cardiac arrest. *Pediatr Clin North Am* 2008 Jun;55(3):589-604, x. Review.

8. Dubin A. Cardiac Arrhythmias. In: Kliegman RM, Behrman RE, Jenson HB, Stanton BF, eds. Nelson textbook of pediatrics, 18th ed. Philadelphia: WB Saunders, 2007.

9. Lawless C, Best T. Sudden death in athletes: causes, screening strategies, use of participation guidelines, and treatment of episodes. In DeLee JC, Drez Jr D, Miller MD, eds. DeLee and Drez's orthopaedic sports medicine, 3rd ed. Philadelphia: Elsevier, 2009.

Chapter Quiz

1. For the infant or child in early shock, the body attempts to compensate by:
   A) Increasing contractility.
   B) Decreasing capillary refill time.
   C) Increasing the heart rate.
   D) Decreasing the ventilatory rate.

2. In the pediatric patient, cardiac arrest is most often due to:
   A) Myocardial trauma
   B) Respiratory failure
   C) Drug intoxication
   D) Severe electrolyte or acid-base imbalance

3. List the four essential questions to ask in the initial emergency management of a pediatric patient with a dysrhythmia.
   A) _____
   B) _____
   C) _____
   D) _____

4. True or False: Afterload is the force or resistance against which the heart must pump to eject blood.

5. Which of the following dysrhythmias is a normal phenomenon that occurs with breathing and changes in intrathoracic pressure?
   A) Supraventricular tachycardia
   B) Sinus arrhythmia
   C) Ventricular tachycardia
   D) Complete AV block

6. Identify the following rhythm. (Lead II):

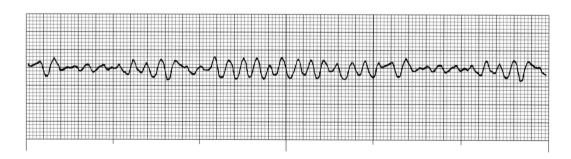

Identification: _____

7. Identify the following rhythm. (Lead II):

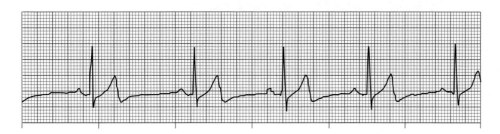

Identification: _____

8. Identify the following rhythm. (Lead II):

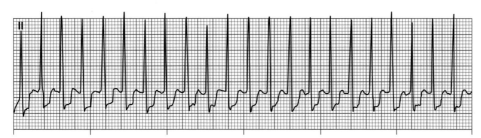

Identification: _____

9. Identify the following rhythm. (Lead II):

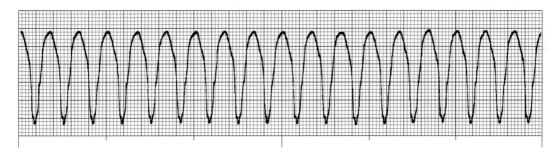

Identification: _____

10. Identify the following rhythm. (Lead II):

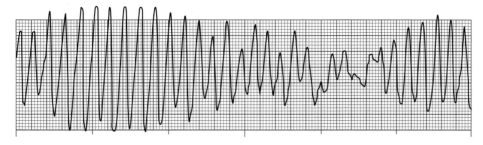

Identification: _____

11. Identify the following rhythm:

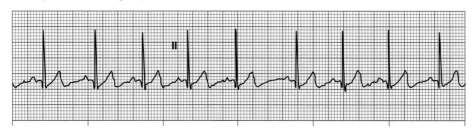

Identification: _____

12. Identify the following rhythm. (Lead II):

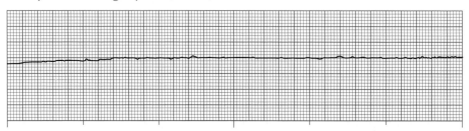

Identification: _____

13. Which of the following is the first medication administered in the management of a patient in cardiopulmonary arrest?
    A) Amiodarone
    B) Magnesium
    C) Lidocaine
    D) Epinephrine

14. The heart's primary pacemaker is the _____ , which is located in the _____ .
    A) SA node; right atrium
    B) SA node; left atrium
    C) AV node; right atrium
    D) AV node; left atrium

Questions 15–18 pertain to the following scenario.

You are called to see an 18-month-old child with difficulty breathing. Mom reports the child has had a cough and cold for the past two days and appears worse today. You note the child is cyanotic and appears limp in his mother's arms. His ventilatory rate is rapid and shallow. Intercostal retractions are visible and wheezing is audible without a stethoscope.

15. From the information provided, complete the following documentation regarding the Pediatric Assessment Triangle.

    Appearance:

    Breathing:

    Circulation:

16. Your initial assessment reveals a patent airway. The child's ventilatory rate is 60/min. Auscultation of the chest reveals wheezes bilaterally. A weak brachial pulse is present at a rate of 194 beats/min. The skin is cyanotic. Capillary refill is 2 to 3 seconds; temperature is 101.8 F; and the pulse oximeter reveals a SpO_2 of 80%. This child's presentation is most consistent with:

    A) Respiratory distress

    B) Respiratory failure

    C) Respiratory arrest

    D) Cardiopulmonary arrest.

17. Is this child sick or not sick? Describe your approach to the initial management of this patient.

18. The child's condition worsens. Central cyanosis persists despite administration of 100% oxygen. The child's ventilatory rate is now 8 to 14/min and shallow. The cardiac monitor reveals narrow QRS complexes at a rate of 32/min. You are unable to palpate a peripheral pulse, but a weak central pulse is present. An IV has been established. You should now:

    A) Begin chest compressions and give epinephrine.

    B) Give atropine.

    C) Continue to monitor the child closely for signs of deterioration.

    D) Give adenosine.

Chapter Quiz Answers

1. C. For the infant or child in early shock, the body attempts to compensate by increasing the heart rate. Because of the immaturity of sympathetic innervation to the ventricles, infants and children have a relatively fixed stroke volume and are therefore dependent on an adequate heart rate to maintain adequate cardiac output.

2. B. In children, cardiopulmonary arrest is usually the result of respiratory failure or shock that progresses to cardiopulmonary failure with profound hypoxemia and acidosis, and eventually cardiopulmonary arrest.

3. The initial emergency management of pediatric dysrhythmias requires a response to four important questions:
   A) Is a pulse (and other signs of circulation) present?
   B) Is the rate within normal limits for age, too fast, too slow, or absent?
   C) Is the QRS wide (ventricular in origin) or narrow (supraventricular in origin)?
   D) Is the patient sick (unstable) or not sick (stable)?

4. True. Afterload is the force or resistance against which the heart must pump to eject blood.

5. B. Sinus arrhythmia is a normal phenomenon that occurs with ventilation and changes in intrathoracic pressure. The heart rate increases with inspiration (R–R intervals shorten) and decreases with expiration (R–R intervals lengthen). Sinus arrhythmia is commonly observed in infants and children.

6. Ventricular fibrillation (VF)

7. Sinus bradycardia

8. Supraventricular tachycardia (SVT)

9. Monomorphic ventricular tachycardia (VT)

10. Polymorphic ventricular tachycardia

11. Sinus arrhythmia

12. Asystole

13. D. Epinephrine (a vasopressor) is the first drug given in cardiac arrest. Amiodarone is the preferred antiarrhythmic in cardiac arrest due to pulseless VT or VF. Lidocaine may be used if amiodarone is not available. Magnesium is given only if the rhythm is Torsades de Pointes.

14. A. The heart's primary pacemaker is the SA node, which is located in the right atrium.

15. Pediatric Assessment Triangle (first impression) findings:
    Appearance: Awake but appears limp
    Breathing: Ventilations are rapid and shallow; audible wheezing is present; increased work of breathing evident
    Circulation: Skin is cyanotic; no evidence of bleeding

16. B. This child's presentation is most consistent with respiratory failure. The presence of tachypnea and tachycardia reflects compensatory mechanisms that are attempting to increase cardiac output. However, these mechanisms will fail (signifying the onset of cardiopulmonary failure) as oxygen demand increases and the child tires. Aggressive treatment is essential.

17. This child is sick. Move quickly. Open the airway and suction if necessary. Correct hypoxia by giving supplemental oxygen. Begin assisted ventilation if the patient does not improve. Provide further interventions based on assessment findings.

18. A. If there is no improvement after approximately 30 seconds of effective assisted ventilation and the child's heart rate is less than 60 beats/min with signs of poor perfusion, begin CPR and give epinephrine. If the bradycardia persists, consider pacing. Adenosine is contraindicated in this situation because the patient is bradycardic. Adenosine is used to *slow* the heart rate in supraventricular tachycardia (SVT).

6 Cardiovascular Interventions

Case Study

On a warm summer day in mid-June, a 3-year-old boy is found floating face down in the swimming pool of an apartment complex. The baby-sitter pulled the child from the pool. She states the child was last seen 10 to 15 minutes ago. She does not know how to perform cardiopulmonary resuscitation (CPR). Your general impression reveals a pale, motionless child with no obvious signs of breathing or circulation. Further assessment reveals the child is unresponsive, apneic, and pulseless. The child's chest is pale and his extremities are blue. CPR is started and a cardiac monitor is applied. The monitor reveals asystole.

What should you do next?

Objectives

1. State the proper ventilation and compression rates for infants and children when performing CPR.
2. Describe the indications for vascular access.
3. Discuss age-appropriate vascular access sites for infants and children.
4. State the indications for intraosseous infusion (IOI).
5. Identify the landmarks for IOI.
6. Describe the advantages and disadvantages of peripheral venous, central venous, and intraosseous vascular access.
7. Define defibrillation and synchronized cardioversion.
8 Describe proper placement of hand-held defibrillator paddles or self-adhesive monitoring/defibrillation pads.
9. Identify indications for defibrillation and synchronized cardioversion.
10. Describe the procedure for defibrillation and synchronized cardioversion.
11. For each of the following dysrhythmias, identify the energy levels currently recommended and indicate if the shock should be delivered using synchronized cardioversion or defibrillation.
    a. Pulseless ventricular tachycardia (VT)/ventricular fibrillation (VF).
    b. Supraventricular tachycardia (SVT).

12. Discuss the indications and procedure for transcutaneous pacing (TCP).

13. List examples of vagal maneuvers that may be used in the pediatric patient.

Basic Life Support

Assess Scene Safety:

An infant is less than 1 year of age. A child is considered 1 year of age until puberty. For resuscitation training purposes puberty is defined as breast development in females and the presence of axillary hair in males.

Assess Responsiveness

Assess Breathing

- Assess the scene for safety. Is it safe to approach the victim? If the scene is not safe, alert Emergency Medical Services (EMS) for help and make sure other bystanders are aware of the existing danger.

- Assess the victim for life-threatening conditions and shout for help if necessary. For example "I need help here!

- Assess and make a quick determination regarding the nature of the emergency and the approximate age of the victim.

- Simultaneously establish the patient's mental status and his ability to maintain an open airway. Determine level of responsiveness using AVPU:
  - **A**=Alert
  - **V**=Responds to verbal stimuli
  - **P**=Responds to painful stimuli
  - **U**=Unresponsive

- Quickly assess the child's level of responsiveness by gently tapping the child and speaking loudly, "Are you OK?" Use the child's name if you know it. Do not shake the child.

- If the child is unresponsive but breathing, activate the emergency response system and reassess the child often until additional help arrives and patient care is transferred to advanced life support personnel.

- The child with respiratory distress should be permitted to remain in the position he/she finds most comfortable in order to maintain airway patency.

- If the child is unresponsive, quickly look to see if he is breathing. If normal breathing is present, CPR is not needed.

- Positioning or moving a victim may be necessary if:
  - You find an unresponsive victim lying face down.
  - You must momentarily leave a breathing victim unattended.
  - The victim is breathing but unresponsive.
  - The victim is vomiting or has debris in his or her mouth.
  - The victim's life is in immediate danger in his or her current location.

- The following techniques are suggested for repositioning or moving a victim:
  - If you are alone, the victim is an unresponsive child, and trauma to the head or neck is suspected:
    - Kneel at the victim's waist.
    - Attempt to roll the victim as a single unit. Grasp the victim's opposite shoulder and opposite hip and roll the victim toward you.
    - As soon as movement begins, remove your hand from the victim's shoulder and support his or her head and neck until the victim is flat on his or her back on a flat, hard surface, such as a sturdy table, the floor, or the ground.
  - If an assistant is available, one person should stabilize the head and neck while the other rescuer rolls the victim's body. Roll the victim's body as a single unit.
  - If the victim is an infant and trauma is not suspected, carry the infant with his or her head in your hand, torso supported by your forearm, and the infant's legs straddling your elbow.
- If the child is unresponsive but has normal breathing and trauma to the head or neck is not suspected, place the child in the recovery position.
  - Kneel at the child's waist.
  - Position the child's arm that is closest to you up and away from the child's side.
  - Bend the child's leg that is opposite you upward.
  - Grasp the child's hip and shoulder and roll him or her toward you, resting the child's head on his or her extended arm. The child's bent leg should help keep him or her from rolling.
  - If the child is to be left in this position for an extended period, alternate the child's position to the opposite side every 30 minutes. Continue to monitor airway, breathing, and circulation.

Assess Circulation

- If the child is unresponsive and is not breathing (or only gasping), sending someone to activate the emergency response system and then check for a pulse for up to 10 seconds. Feel for a brachial pulse in an infant. Feel for a carotid or femoral pulse in a child.
- If a pulse is present and the rate is 60 beats per minute or faster but breathing is inadequate, begin rescue breathing at a rate of 1 breath every 3 to 5 seconds (12 to 20 ventilations per minute) until breathing resumes. Recheck the pulse about every 2 minutes.
- If there is no pulse (or you are unsure if there is a pulse) or a pulse is present but the rate is slower than 60 beats per minute with signs of poor perfusion (i.e, pallor, mottling, cyanosis), begin chest compressions.

- If two or more rescuers are present, one should start CPR immediately and another should activate the emergency response system and obtain an AED.
- A lone rescuer who finds a patient unresponsive should perform CPR for about 2 minutes (about 5 cycles), briefly leave the patient to phone for help and get an AED, and then return to the patient to resume CPR and use the AED.

- In cardiac arrest, compressing the chest compresses the heart and increases intrathoracic pressure, creating blood flow and enabling the delivery of oxygen to the brain and heart. When performing chest compressions, systole is the chest compression phase and diastole is the release phase.[1] Myocardial blood flow is dependent on coronary perfusion pressure, which is generated when performing external chest compressions. Coronary perfusion pressure is a key determinant of success in resuscitation and adequate cerebral and coronary perfusion pressure is critical to neurologically normal survival.[1] Because it takes time to build up cerebral and coronary perfusion pressures, stopping chest compressions for even a few seconds causes cerebral and coronary perfusion pressures to fall quickly and dramatically, reducing blood flow to the brain and heart. When chest compressions are stopped during cardiac arrest, no blood flow is generated and is referred to as "no flow time." Even after compressions are resumed, several chest compressions are needed to restore coronary perfusion pressure. Because the only source of coronary and cerebral perfusion comes from the blood pressure generated from high-quality chest compressions in a cardiac arrest, push hard, push fast, allow full chest recoil, do not over-ventilate, and minimize interruptions to perform procedures, analyze rhythms, check for pulses, or change rescuer position for ventilation.

Lone Rescuer Chest Compressions: Infant

- A lone rescuer should use the 2-finger technique to perform chest compression in infants. Imagine a line between the nipples (intermammary line). Place the flat part of your middle and ring fingers about one finger's width below this imaginary line (Figure 6-1).
- Press down on the sternum and deliver compressions at a rate of at least 100 per minute. Apply firm pressure, depressing the sternum at least 1/3 the depth of the chest (about 1.5 inches or 4 cm). Do not apply pressure over the ribs, bottom tip of the sternum (xiphoid process), or over the upper abdomen.
- Release pressure on the chest after each compression and allow the chest to recoil completely (enabling the heart to refill with blood).

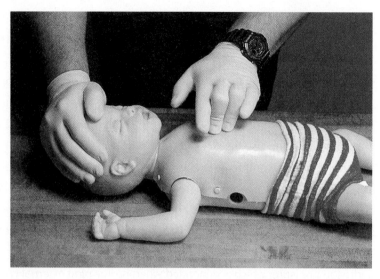

Figure 6-1   Locating finger position for infant chest compression.

Lone Rescuer Chest Compressions: Child

- Find the lower half of the sternum (center of the chest between the nipples) and place the heel of one hand there (Figure 6-2). Using the heel of one hand with the rescuer's other hand on top (adult CPR technique) is also acceptable.
- Position yourself directly over the child's chest. With your arms straight and your elbows locked, press down on the sternum and deliver compressions at a rate of at least 100 per minute. Apply firm pressure, depressing the sternum about 1/3 the depth of the chest (about 2 inches or 5 cm). Do not apply pressure over the ribs, bottom tip of the sternum, or over the upper abdomen.

Infant and Child CPR: Two Rescuers

- If two or more rescuers are present, one should start CPR immediately while the other activates the emergency response system and retrieves an AED.
- The 2-thumb-encircling hands technique is recommended when performing 2-rescuer CPR for an infant. One rescuer encircles the chest with both hands and compresses the sternum between his opposing thumbs at a rate of at least 100 per minute. The rescuer's thumbs should be positioned about 1 finger's width below the nipple line (Figure 6-3). This technique is preferred over the two-finger technique because it produces higher coronary artery perfusion pressure and, results more consistently in appropriate depth or force of compression, and may generate higher systolic and diastolic pressures during

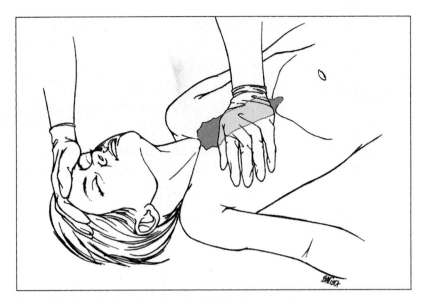

Figure 6-2   Locating hand position for child chest compression.

cardiac arrest.[2] If a rescuer cannot physically encircle a victim's chest, use the two finger technique as previously described. The second rescuer is responsible for keeping the airway open and ventilating the patient at the rate of 15 compressions to 2 ventilations.

- When performing 2-rescuer CPR for a child, one rescuer provides chest compressions using the same technique described for a lone-rescuer child CPR at the rate of at least 100 per minute. The second rescuer keeps the child's airway open and ventilates the patient at a ratio of 15 compressions to 2 ventilations (see Airway and Breathing section below).

- Because performing chest compressions is tiring and rescuer fatigue can lead to inadequate compression rate, depth, and recoil, the compressor role should be alternated between rescuers about every 2 minutes to prevent compressor fatigue.[2] To minimize interruptions in chest compressions, the switch in rescuer roles should be accomplished as quickly as possibly (ideally in less than 5 seconds).

- Assess the pulse after about 2 minutes of CPR. If there is still no pulse, continue CPR with cycles of 15 compressions to 2 breaths.

Airway and Breathing

- After delivering 30 compressions (15 compressions if 2 rescuers are present), open the airway using the head tilt-chin lift and give 2 breaths. If you suspect a neck or spinal injury, use a jaw thrust without the head tilt maneuver to open the airway.

- Each ventilation should take about 1 second. Make sure the breaths are effective (the chest rises). If the chest does not rise, reposition the head, make a better seal, and try again. Avoid excessive ventilation (too many breaths or too large a volume). Resume chest compressions immediately after giving two breaths.

- Once an advanced airway is in place, do not pause chest compressions for a breath. The rate of ventilations should then change to 8 to 10 breaths/minute (a breath every 6 to 8 seconds).

- Upon arrival of an AED, apply the adhesive pads to the patient's chest, turn the AED on, and follow the machine's prompts. If a shock is advised, clear the patient, give 1 shock, immediately resume CPR for 5 cycles, then reanalyze rhythm. Shock delivery should ideally occur as soon as possible after compressions. If no shock is advised, immediately resume CPR. About every 2 minutes, the AED will prompt rescuers to re-analyze the rhythm. AEDS are discussed in more detail later in this chapter. A summary of basic ,life support interventions is shown in Table 6-1.

Defribrillation

Vascular Access

- Maintain hydration.
- Restore fluid and electrolyte balance.
- Provide fluids for resuscitation.
- Administration of medications, volume expanders, blood and blood components, maintenance solutions.
- Obtain venous blood specimens for laboratory analysis.

Indications for Vascular Access

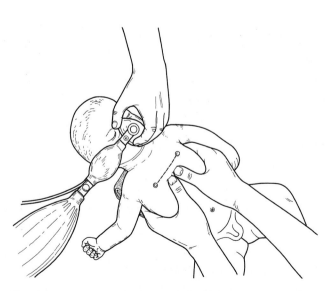

Figure 6-3 Two-rescuer infant cardiopulmonary resuscitation, two thumb–encircling hands technique.

TABLE 6-1 *Summary of Basic Life Support Interventions*

	Infant	**Child**	**Adult**
Age	Younger than 1 y	1 yr to puberty (about 12 to 14 yr)	Older than 12 to 14 y
Ventilation rate	One breath every 3 to 5 sec (12 to 20 breaths/min)	One breath every 3 to 5 sec (12 to 20 breaths/min)	One breath every 5 to 6 sec (10 to 12 breaths/min)
Assess pulse	Brachial	Carotid or femoral	Carotid
Compress with	Two fingers (one rescuer) or two thumb-encircling hands (two rescuers)	Heel of 1 hand or as for adult	Heel of one hand, the other hand on top
Compression depth	At least 1/3 the depth of the chest (about 1.5 in [4 cm])	At least 1/3 the depth of the chest (about 2 in [5 cm])	At least 2 in (5 cm)
Compression rate	At least 100/min	At least 100/min	At least 100/min
Compression to ventilation ratio	1 rescuer = 30:2 2 rescuers = 15:2	1 rescuer = 30:2 2 rescuers = 15:2	1 or 2 rescuers = 30:2

General Principles

- In the management of cardiopulmonary arrest and decompensated shock, the preferred vascular access site is the largest, most readily accessible vein. If no IV is in place at the onset of cardiac arrest, the intraosseous route is useful as the initial means of vascular access.[3]
- The preferred IV solutions in cardiac arrest are normal saline or lactated Ringer's solution. Large volumes of dextrose-containing solutions should not be infused because hyperglycemia may induce osmotic diuresis, produce or aggravate hyperkalemia, and worsen ischemic brain injury.

Peripheral Venous Access

Advantages

- Effective route for fluid and medication administration.
- Does not require interruption of resuscitation efforts.
- Easier to learn than central venous access techniques.
- If IV attempt unsuccessful, site easily compressible to reduce bleeding.
- Fewer complications than central venous access.

Disadvantages

- In circulatory collapse, peripheral veins may be absent or difficult to access.
- Small vessel diameter.
- Greater distance from the central circulation.
- Should be used only for administration of isotonic solutions; hypertonic or irritating solutions may cause pain and phlebitis.

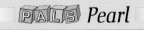 *Pearl*

Medications administered via a peripheral vein during CPR should be followed with a saline flush of 5 to 10 mL to facilitate delivery of the medication to the central circulation.

Venipuncture Sites

Preferred sites for venous access in infants are shown in Figure 6-4.

- Scalp veins (infants).
  - Very small veins found close to the surface and more easily seen than extremity veins.
  - Rarely useful during resuscitation efforts.
  - May be useful for fluid and medication administration after patient stabilization.
- Upper extremity veins (Figure 6-5).
  - Forearm veins (may be difficult to locate in chubby babies).
    - Cephalic.
    - Median basilic.
    - Median antecubital.
  - Dorsal hand veins.
    - Tributaries of the cephalic and basilic veins.

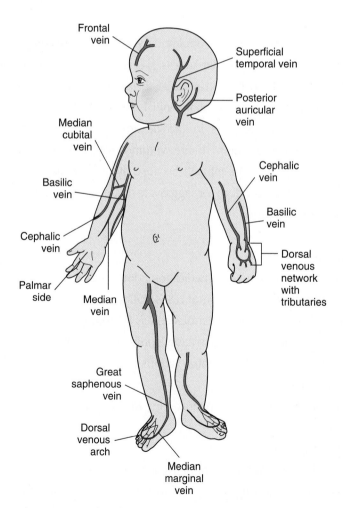

Figure 6-4   Preferred sites for venous access in infants.

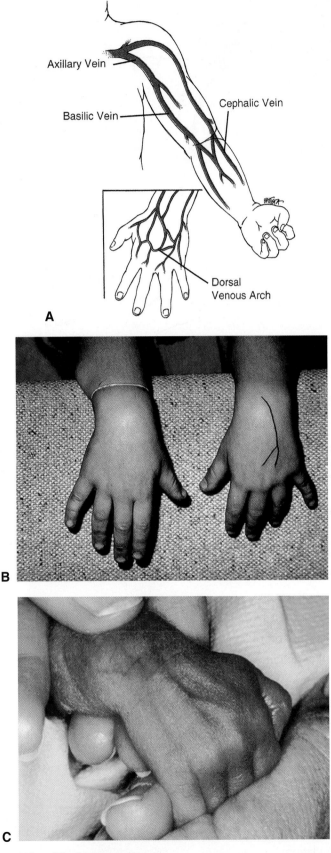

Figure 6-5   Veins of the forearm and hand.

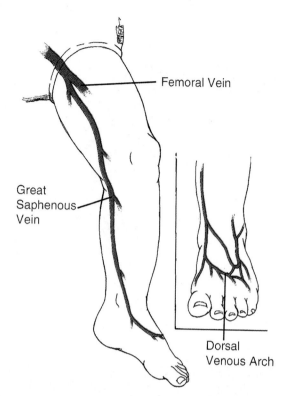

Figure 6-6   Lower extremity veins.

- ∘ Dorsal venous arch.
- Lower extremity veins (Figure 6-6).
  - Saphenous.
  - Median marginal.
  - Dorsal venous arch.

Indications

Central Venous Access

- Emergency access to venous circulation when peripheral sites are not readily accessible.
- Need for long-term IV therapy.
- Administration of large volumes of fluid.
- Administration of blood products, hypertonic solutions, caustic medications, or parenteral feeding solutions.
- Plasmapheresis, exchange transfusion, or dialysis.
- Placement of transvenous pacemaker electrodes.
- Central venous pressure monitoring or central venous blood sampling.

Advantages

- Rapid volume expansion.
- Delivery of medications closer to their sites of action.
- More reliable route of venous access than peripheral venous cannulation.
- Central venous pressure measurement.

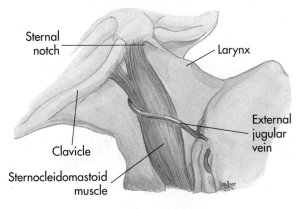

Figure 6-7   Anatomy of the external jugular vein.

Disadvantages

- Special equipment (syringe, catheter, needle) required.
- Excessive time may be required for placement.
- Higher complication rate than with peripheral venipuncture.
- Skill deterioration.
- Inability to initiate procedure while other patient care activities in progress.

Sites

External Jugular Vein

- The external jugular (EJ) vein lies superficially along the lateral portion of the neck (Figure 6-7). It extends from behind the angle of the jaw and passes downward across the sternocleidomastoid muscle until it enters the thorax at a point just above the middle third of the clavicle. It joins the subclavian vein just behind the clavicle.
- Advantages.
  - Usually easy to cannulate because the vein is superficial and easy to visualize.
  - Provides rapid access to the central circulation.
- Disadvantages.
  - May not be readily accessible during an arrest situation due to rescuers working to manage the airway.
  - May be easily dislodged.
  - May be positional with head movement.
  - May be difficult to thread a guidewire or catheter into the central circulation because of the tortuous angle of entry into the sub-clavian vein.
- Procedure.
  - Use body substance isolation precautions.
  - Auscultate and document bilateral breath sounds to establish a baseline.

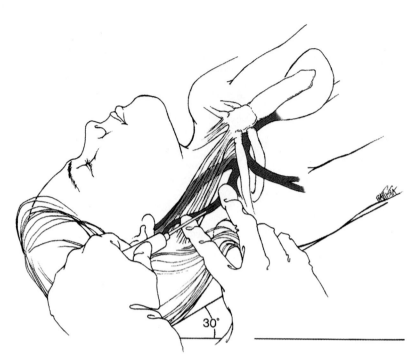

Figure 6-8   Cannulating the external jugular vein.

- Restrain the child in a supine, head-down position of 30 degrees.
- If no head or neck trauma is suspected, turn the child's head to the left (the right side is preferred for venipuncture), away from the venipuncture site. Cleanse the site. If time permits, use local anesthesia with 1% lidocaine.
- For peripheral cannulation, insert a short over-the-needle catheter into the vein. For central venous cannulation, insert a through-the-needle catheter or catheter-over-guidewire.
- Apply pressure to the external jugular vein just above the clavicle (Figure 6-8). This temporarily occludes the vessel and causes it to distend, making cannulation easier.
- Apply slight traction to the vein to stabilize it. Advance the needle at a small angle from the skin plane (about 10 degrees) until a "pop" is felt as the needle enters the lumen of the vein. Advance the needle or catheter slightly after feeling the pop to ensure placement within the vessel lumen. Attach a prepared IV infusion set.
- Reassess breath sounds. If central venous cannulation was attempted, obtain a chest radiograph to verify that the tip of the catheter is correctly positioned at or above the junction of the superior vena cava and right atrium and rule out pneumothorax.

Internal Jugular Vein

- The internal jugular (IJ) vein runs from the base of the skull downward along the carotid artery and then through the triangle formed by the clavicle and the two heads of the sternocleidomastoid muscle before it meets the subclavian vein behind the clavicle.

- Cannulation of the right side of the neck is preferred because of the following:
  - The dome of the right lung and pleura are lower than on the left side.
  - There is more or less a straight course to the right atrium.
  - The thoracic duct is not in the way (empties on the LEFT side).
- Advantages
  - Less risk of pneumothorax with this technique versus subclavian.
  - Hematomas in the neck are visible and more easily compressible.
  - Easier access during CPR than subclavian.
  - Usually remains patent even when peripheral veins are collapsed.
- Disadvantages.
  - Adjacent structures easily damaged.
  - More training required than peripheral venipuncture.
  - May interrupt resuscitation efforts.
  - Higher complication rate than with peripheral venipuncture.
  - Limits patient neck movement.
- Procedure: central (middle) approach.
  - Use personal protective equipment.
  - Auscultate and document bilateral breath sounds to establish a baseline.
  - Restrain the child in a supine, head-down position of 30 degrees. If no head or neck trauma is suspected, turn the child's head to the left (the right side is preferred for venipuncture), away from the venipuncture site.
  - Attach a 3-mL syringe to a large-gauge catheter, lining up the bevel of the needle with the numbers on the syringe.
  - Identify landmarks by observation and palpation (clavicle and the triangle formed by the two lower heads of the sternocleidomastoid

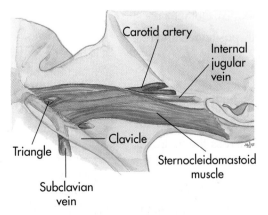

Figure 6-9   Anatomy of the internal jugular vein.

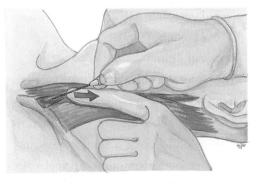

Figure 6-10   Cannulation of the internal jugular vein—central approach.

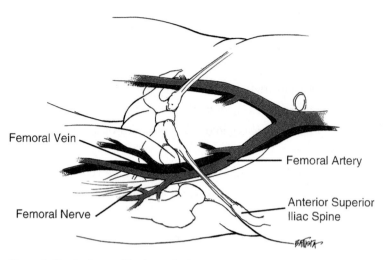

Figure 6-11   Anatomy of the femoral vein.

muscle) (Figure 6-9). Cleanse the site. If time permits, use local anesthesia with 1% lidocaine.

- Insert the needle at a 30- to 45-degree angle, bevel up, into the center of the triangle formed by the two heads of sternomastoid muscle and the clavicle. With the needle directed toward the feet, slowly advance the needle aiming toward the ipsilateral nipple, while applying gentle negative pressure to the syringe (Figure 6-10).

- When a free flow of blood appears in the syringe, remove the syringe and occlude the needle hub with a gloved finger to prevent air embolism. (Newer catheter packaging makes this step unnecessary because the guidewire is advanced through the syringe or from a Y port.)

- Advance a guidewire through the needle. Remove the needle and advance the appropriate central venous catheter over the guidewire to the junction of the superior vena cava and right atrium during exhalation. Remove the guidewire and connect the catheter to a prepared IV infusion set.

- Secure the catheter in place. Reassess breath sounds. Obtain a chest radiograph to ensure the catheter tip is correctly positioned and rule out pneumothorax.

Femoral Vein

- The femoral vein lies directly medial to the femoral artery (Figure 6-11). If a line is drawn between the anterior superior iliac spine and the symphysis pubis, the femoral artery runs directly across the midpoint. Medial to that point is the femoral vein.

- If the femoral artery pulse is palpable, the artery can be located with a finger and the femoral vein will lie immediately medial to the pulsation.

- Advantages.

If bright red blood forcibly fills the syringe, it is probable that the carotid artery has punctured. Remove the needle and apply firm pressure for at least 10 minutes.

PALS Pearl

Inadvertent puncture of the carotid artery can occur when attempting cannulation of the jugular vein. If a hematoma occurs on one side of the neck, it is hazardous to attempt venipuncture on the opposite side because of the possibility of bilateral hematomas severely compromising the airway.

An acronym used to recall relevant anatomy is NAVEL = **N**erve, **A**rtery, **V**ein, **E**mpty space, **L**igament.

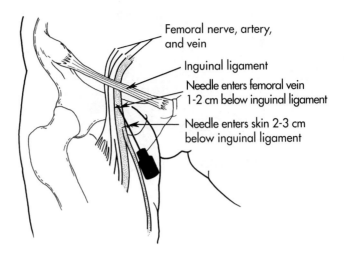

Femoral nerve, artery, and vein

Inguinal ligament

Needle enters femoral vein 1-2 cm below inguinal ligament

Needle enters skin 2-3 cm below inguinal ligament

Figure 6-12   Cannulation of the femoral vein.

- Distant from major sites of activity during resuscitation efforts.
- Vein does not collapse like peripheral veins.
- Once cannulated, easy access to the central circulation.
- In case of bleeding, the neck of the femur and pelvis provide hard surfaces against which direct pressure may be applied.
- Disadvantages.
  - If a pulse is absent, the vein may be hard to locate.
  - Injury to the femoral artery, femoral nerve, and hip capsule may occur; however, injury is unlikely if proper technique is used.
- Procedure.
  - Use personal protective equipment.
  - Restrain the patient's lower extremities with slight external rotation.
  - Attach a 3-mL syringe to a large-gauge catheter, lining up the bevel of the needle with the numbers on the syringe.
  - Identify the femoral vein medial to the femoral artery. Cleanse the site thoroughly. If time permits, use local anesthesia with 1% lidocaine.
  - Insert the needle 2 to 3 cm below the inguinal ligament and just medial to the femoral artery (Figure 6-12). Slowly advance the needle parallel to the femoral artery while gently withdrawing the plunger of the syringe. When a free flow of blood appears in the syringe, remove the syringe and occlude the needle hub with a gloved finger to prevent air embolism.
  - Advance a guidewire through the needle. Remove the needle and advance the appropriate central venous catheter over the guidewire. Remove the guidewire and connect the catheter to a prepared IV infusion set.
  - Secure the catheter in place. Obtain a radiograph to ensure the catheter tip is correctly positioned.

The right femoral vein may be easier to cannulate than the left because of a straighter path to the inferior vena cava.

A finger should remain on the artery to assist in landmark identification and avoid insertion of the catheter into the artery.

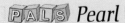 **PALS** *Pearl*

During CPR, pulsations may be palpable in the femoral area that may originate from either the femoral vein or femoral artery. If CPR is in progress and femoral vein cannulation is attempted, insert the needle directly over the pulsations.

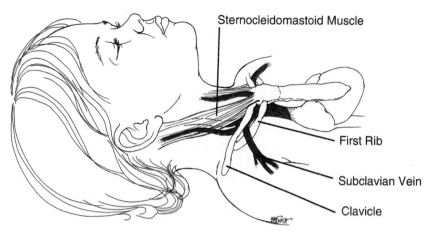

Figure 6-13   Anatomy of the subclavian vein.

Subclavian Vein

- The subclavian vein is a continuation of the axillary vein at the outer border of the first rib. It joins the IJ vein behind the medial end of the clavicle to form the brachiocephalic (innominate) vein (Figure 6-13). The subclavian vein is immobilized by small attachments to the first rib and clavicle. It lies anterior to the subclavian artery and is separated from it by the anterior scalene muscle.
- Advantages.
  - Usually remains patent even when peripheral veins are collapsed.
  - More subsequent patient neck movement with prolonged cannulation.
- Disadvantages.
  - Significant risk of pneumothorax, hemothorax, subclavian artery puncture.
  - More training required than peripheral venipuncture.
  - May interrupt resuscitation efforts.
  - Higher complication rate than with peripheral venipuncture.
- Procedure: infraclavicular approach.
  - Use personal protective equipment.
  - Auscultate and document bilateral breath sounds to establish a baseline.
  - Restrain the child in a supine, head-down position of 30 degrees. If no head or neck trauma is suspected, turn the child's head to the left (the right side is preferred for venipuncture), away from the venipuncture site. Attach a 3-mL syringe to a large-gauge catheter, lining up the bevel of the needle with the numbers on the syringe.
  - Identify landmarks: the suprasternal notch and the junction of the middle and medial thirds of the clavicle. Cleanse the site. If time permits, use local anesthesia with 1% lidocaine.
  - Firmly press a fingertip into the suprasternal notch to establish a

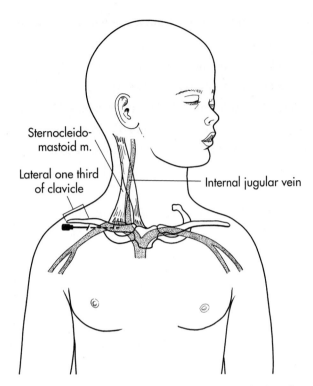

Figure 6-14 Cannulation of the subclavian vein—infraclavicular approach.

Sternocleido-mastoid m.

Lateral one third of clavicle

Internal jugular vein

point of reference. Introduce the needle, bevel up, just under the clavicle at the junction of the middle and medial thirds of the clavicle.

- Holding the syringe and needle parallel to the frontal plane, slowly advance the needle while applying gentle negative pressure to the syringe, aiming the needle at the suprasternal notch (Figure 6-14). When a free flow of blood appears in the syringe, remove the syringe and occlude the needle hub with a gloved finger to prevent air embolism. (Newer catheter packaging makes this step unnecessary because the guidewire is advanced through the syringe or from a Y port.)

- Advance a guidewire through the needle. Remove the needle and advance the appropriate central venous catheter over the guidewire to the junction of the superior vena cava and right atrium during exhalation. Remove the guidewire and connect the catheter to a prepared IV infusion set.

- Secure the catheter in place. Reassess breath sounds. Obtain a chest radiograph to ensure the catheter tip is correctly positioned and rule out pneumothorax.

Atrial or ventricular dysrhythmias may be observed on the cardiac monitor if the guidewire or catheter enters the right atrium. If a dysrhythmia is observed, withdraw the guidewire or catheter a few centimeters and reassess.

Intraosseous Infusion

IOI is the process of infusing medications, fluids, and blood products into the bone marrow cavity. Because the marrow cavity is continuous with the venous circulation, fluids and medications administered by the IO route are subsequently delivered to the venous circulation.

In the presence of cardiac arrest or decompensated shock, an IOI should be established in any patient when IV access cannot be rapidly achieved. IOI is a temporary means of vascular access. The duration of the infusion should be limited to a few hours. Venous access is often easier to obtain after initial fluid and medication resuscitation via the intraosseous route.

Indications

- Cardiopulmonary arrest or decompensated shock where vascular access is essential and venous access is not readily achieved.
- Multi-system trauma with associated shock and/or severe hypovolemia.
- Unresponsive patient in need of immediate medications or fluid resuscitation (e.g., burns, sepsis, near-drowning, anaphylaxis, status epilepticus).
- Presence of burns or a traumatic injury preventing access to the venous system at other sites.

Advantages

- Skill is easily mastered, even if done infrequently; healthcare professionals experienced in the technique can often establish IO access in 60 seconds or less.
- Preferred access sites are distant from major sites of activity during resuscitation efforts.
- Low incidence of complications.
- Medications and fluids administered IV can be administered IO.
- Absorption of medications administered via the IO route is more rapid than medications administered via the subcutaneous or rectal routes.
- Blood sampling for laboratory studies is possible.
- Venous access is often easier to obtain after initial fluid resuscitation via the intraosseous route.

Disadvantages

- Short term intervention until venous access can be obtained.
- Causes extreme pain in the responsive patient.

Contraindications

- Femoral fracture on the ipsilateral side.
- Osteopetrosis (high fracture potential).
- Osteogenesis imperfecta (high fracture potential).
- Fracture at or above the insertion site.
- Severe burn overlying the insertion site (unless this is the *only* available site).
- Infection at insertion site (unless this is the *only* available site).
- Use of the same bone in which an unsuccessful IO attempt was made.

PALS Pearl

- Infusion pumps should be used for all IV infusions in infants and children to avoid inadvertent circulatory overload unless large volumes of fluid are deliberately administered as part of the resuscitation effort.
- Minidrip infusion sets should be used and closely monitored if infusion pumps are not available.

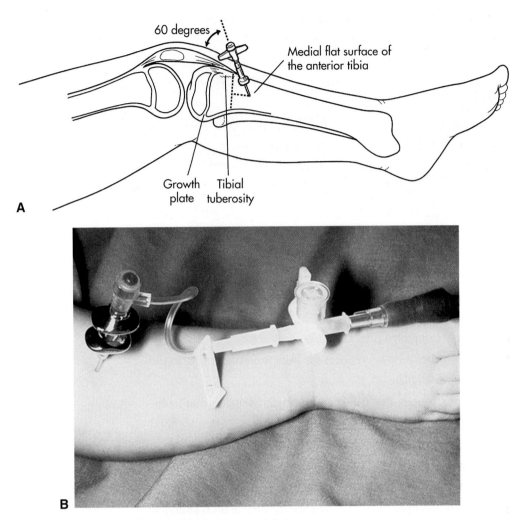

Figure 6-15 Anterior tibial approach for intraosseous infusion.

Procedure

The preferred site for IOI is the anteromedial surface of the proximal tibia. This site is preferred because of the broad flat surface of the bone, the thin layer of skin that covers it, the ease of palpation of this bony landmark, and use of the proximal tibia does not interfere with airway management and CPR.

- Use personal protective equipment.
- Place the infant or child in a supine position. Place a towel roll or small sandbag in the popliteal fossa to provide support, optimize positioning, and minimize the risk of fractures (Figure 6-15).
- Identify the landmarks for needle insertion. Palpate the tibial tuberosity. The site for IOI insertion lies 1 to 3 cm (one finger's width) below this tuberosity on the medial flat surface of the anterior tibia.
- Cleanse the intended insertion site. If the child is responsive and time permits, use local anesthesia with 1% lidocaine.
- Stabilize the patient's leg. With the needle angled away from the joint,

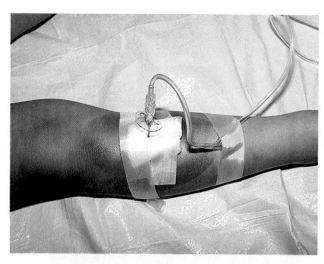

Figure 6-16 Secure the intraosseous needle and tubing in place with a sterile dressing and tape. Observe the site every 5 to 10 minutes for the duration of the infusion. Monitor for signs of infiltration and assess distal pulses.

insert the needle using firm pressure.

- Angling away from the joint reduces the likelihood of damage to the epiphyseal growth plate.
- Firm pressure pushes the needle through the skin and subcutaneous tissue.

• Advance the needle using a twisting motion at an angle of 60 to 90 degrees away from the epiphyseal plate (i.e., toward the toes). A twisting or boring motion is necessary to advance the needle through the periosteum of the bone. Advance the needle until a sudden decrease in resistance or a "pop" is felt as the needle enters the marrow cavity.

• Unscrew the cap, remove the stylet from the needle, attach a 10-mL saline-filled syringe to the needle, and attempt to aspirate bone marrow into the syringe.

- If aspiration is successful, slowly inject 10 to 20 mL of saline to clear the needle of marrow, bone fragments, and/or tissue. Observe for any swelling at the site.
- If aspiration is unsuccessful, consider other indicators of correct needle position:
  - The needle stands firmly without support.
  - A sudden loss of resistance occurred on entering the marrow cavity (this is less obvious in infants than in older children because infants have soft bones).
  - Fluid flows freely through the needle without signs of significant swelling of the subcutaneous tissue.
- If signs of infiltration are present, remove the IO needle and attempt the procedure at another site.

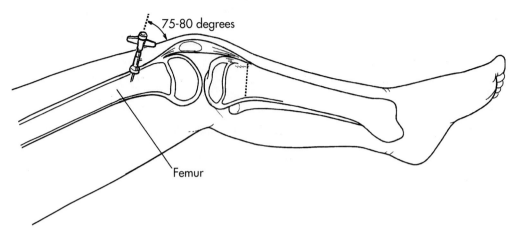

Figure 6-17 Distal femur approach. Insert the intraosseous needle 2 to 3 cm proximal to the external condyle in the midline and direct it superiorly at a 75- to 80-degree angle.

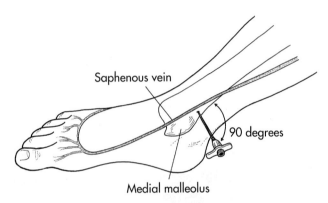

Figure 6-18 Distal tibia approach. Insert the intraosseous needle at a 90-degree angle, just proximal to the medial malleolus and posterior to the saphenous vein.

- If no signs of infiltration are present, attach standard IV tubing. A syringe, pressure infuser, or IV infusion pump may be needed to infuse fluids.
- Secure the needle and tubing in place with a sterile dressing and tape (Figure 6-16). Observe the site every 5 to 10 minutes for the duration of the infusion. Monitor for signs of infiltration and assess distal pulses.
- Attempt to establish venous access as soon as possible and discontinue the IOI. After the IO needle is removed, hold manual pressure for at least 5 minutes and then apply a sterile dressing to the site.

Alternate Intraosseous Infusion Sites

- Distal femur, 2 to 3 cm above the lateral condyle in the midline (Figure 6-17).
- Medial surface of the distal tibia 1 to 2 cm above the medial malleolus (may be a more effective site in older children) (Figure 6-18).
- Anterior superior iliac spine (may be a more effective site in older children) (Figure 6-19).

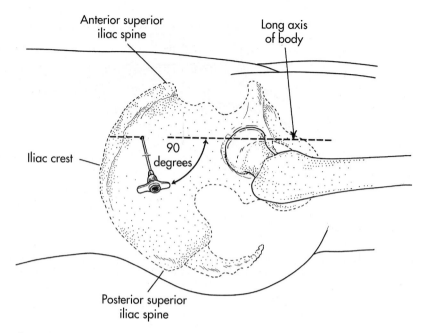

Figure 6-19   Anterior superior iliac spine approach. Insert the intraosseous needle at a 90-degree angle to the long axis of the body.

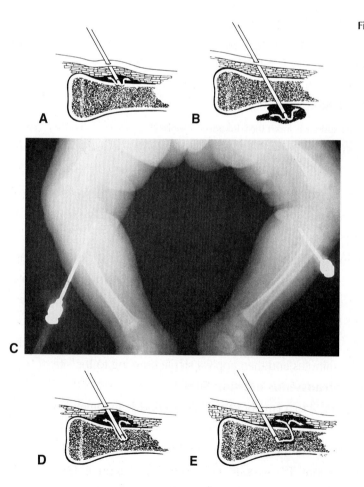

Figure 6-20   Possible problems encountered with intraosseous (IO) infusion. A, Incomplete penetration of the bony cortex. **B,** Penetration of the posterior cortex. **C,** Radiograph of bilaterally misplaced IO needles with penetration through the posterior tibial cortices. **D,** Fluid or medications escaping around the needle through the puncture site. **E,** Fluid leaking through a nearby previous cortical puncture site.

Possible Problems Encountered with Intraosseous Infusion

- Incomplete penetration of the bony cortex (Figure 6-20A).
- Penetration of the posterior cortex (Figures 6-20B and 6-20C).
- Fluid or medications escaping around the needle through the puncture site (Figure 6-20D).
- Fluid leaking through a nearby previous cortical puncture site (Figure 6-20E).
- Fracture of the tibia.
- Local abscess or cellulitis.
- Lower extremity compartment syndrome.
- Osteomyelitis.
- Loss of vascular access site may occur due to needle obstruction by marrow, bone fragments, or tissue.

Electrical Therapy

Defibrillation

Definition and Purpose

Defibrillation is the therapeutic delivery of an unsynchronized electrical current (the delivery of energy has no relationship to the cardiac cycle) through the myocardium over a very brief period to terminate a cardiac dysrhythmia.

Defibrillation does not "jump start" the heart. The shock attempts to deliver a uniform electrical current of sufficient intensity to simultaneously depolarize ventricular cells, including fibrillating cells, briefly "stunning" the heart. This provides an opportunity for the heart's natural pacemakers to resume normal activity. The pacemaker with the highest degree of automaticity should then assume responsibility for pacing the heart.

A **defibrillator** is a device used to administer an electrical shock at a preset voltage to terminate a cardiac dysrhythmia (Figure 6-21). A defibrillator consists of a **capacitor** that stores energy, an adjustable high-voltage power supply that allows the operator to select an energy level, a charge switch/button that allows the capacitor to charge, discharge switches/buttons that allow the capacitor to discharge, and hand-held paddles (Figure 6-22A) or self-adhesive monitoring/defibrillator pads (Figure 6-22B) that deliver the energy from the defibrillator to the patient.

Self-adhesive pads record and monitor the cardiac rhythm and are used to deliver the shock. These pads are used during "hands-free" or "hands-off" defibrillation and consist of a flexible metal "paddle," a layer of conductive gel, and an adhesive ring that holds them in place on the patient's chest. "Hands-free" defibrillation enhances operator safety by

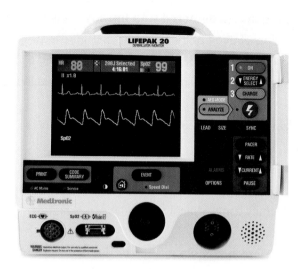

Figure 6-21 Medtronic PhysioControl LIFEPAK 20 monitor/defibrillator.

physically separating the operator from the patient. Instead of leaning over the patient with hand-held paddles, the operator delivers a shock to the patient by means of discharge buttons located on a remote cable, an adapter, or on the defibrillator itself.

Defibrillators deliver energy or current in "waveforms" that flow between two electrode patches (or paddles). Waveforms are classified by whether the current flow delivered is in one direction, two directions, or multiple directions. Monophasic waveforms use energy delivered in one (mono) direction through the patient's heart. With biphasic waveforms, energy is delivered in two (bi) phases—the current moves in one direction, stops, and then passes through the heart a second time in the opposite direction in a very short period (milliseconds). Most defibrillators sold today use biphasic waveform technology.

The strength of the electrical shock delivered is expressed in joules (J). **Transthoracic impedance** refers to the natural resistance of the chest wall to the flow of current.

Factors Known to Affect Transthoracic Resistance

Paddle Size

Paddles and self-adhesive pads appear to be equally effective.[3] Optimum pad size for defibrillation and pacing based on patient age and weight vary by manufacturer. Carefully follow all manufacturer instructions.

Studies have shown that adults paddles/pads should be used for patients weighing more than 10 kg (22 lbs) (older than 1 year).[3-7] Use infant size paddles/pads for infants weighing less than 10 kg (22 lbs) or those whose chests are too small to accommodate standard paddles/pads. Generally, use the largest paddles or pads that will fit the

Combination pads have multiple names, including "combo pads," "multi-purpose pads," "multi-function electrode pads," "combination electrodes," "therapy electrodes," and "self-adhesive monitoring/defibrillation pads". Not all combination pads are alike. Some pads can be used for defibrillation, synchronized cardioversion, ECG monitoring, and pacing. Others can be used for defibrillation, synchronized cardioversion, and ECG monitoring, but not for pacing. Be sure you are familiar with the capabilities of the pads you are using.

Energy (joules) = Current (amperes) × Voltage (volts) × Time (seconds)

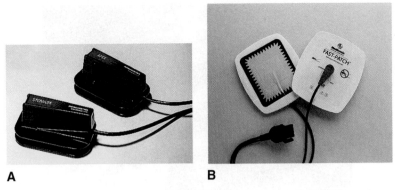

Figure 6-22 **A**, Hand-held paddles. **B**, Self-adhesive monitoring/defibrillation pads.

patient's chest without overlapping with at least 1 inch (3 cm) separating the pads.[3]

Use of Conductive Material

When using hand-held paddles, the use of gels, pastes, or pregelled defibrillation pads aids the passage of current at the interface between the defibrillator paddles/electrodes and the body surface. Failure to use conductive material results in very high transthoracic impedance, a lack of penetration of current, and burns to the skin surface. Combination pads are pregelled and do not require the application of additional gel to the patient's chest. Use of improper pastes, creams, gels, or pads can cause burns or sparks and pose a risk of fire in an oxygen-enriched environment.[8] Use of excessive gel may result in spreading of the material across the chest wall during resuscitation, leading to arcing of the current between paddles and an insufficient delivery of current to the heart. Damp skin and air pockets beneath hand-held paddles or self-adhesive defibrillation pads increase transthoracic resistance and may cause an uneven delivery of current.[9]

Selected Energy

Defibrillation is the definitive treatment for pulseless VT or VF. When treating cardiac dysrhythmias using electrical therapy, selecting the appropriate energy level (joules) is important. It is acceptable to use an initial energy dose for pulseless VT or VF of 2 to 4 J/kg.[3] If the dysrhythmia persists, it is reasonable to increase the dose to 4 J/kg. If the dysrhythmia persists subsequent energy levels should be at least 4 J/kg. Higher energy levels may be considered but should not exceed 10 J/kg or the adult maximum dose.[3]

Paddle/Pad Position

Follow the manufacturer's instructions regarding placing proper placement of self-adhesive pads, hand-held paddles, and pregelled adhesive pads. Hand-held paddles or self-adhesive defibrillator pads may

---

Do not use alcohol-soaked pads for defibrillation—they may ignite!

Never use ultrasound gel for defibrillation.

When biphasic waveform defibrillation is used, the waveforms compensate for transthoric impedance to allow uniform delivery of energy. The patient's transthoracic impedance is measured through the paddles or combination pads in contact with the patient's chest.

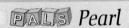 *Pearl*

If one of the shocks delivered successfully terminates pulseless VT/VF but the dysrhythmia recurs, begin defibrillation at the last energy level used that resulted in successful defibrillation.

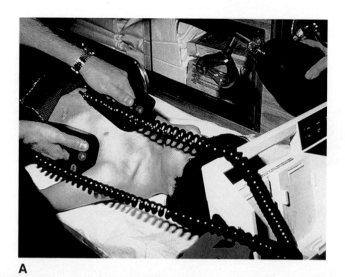

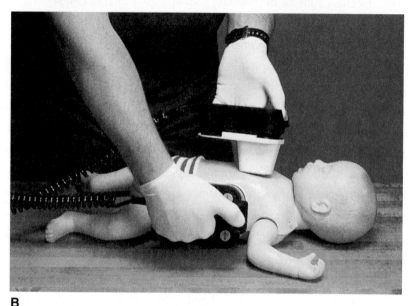

Figure 6-23 A, Sternum-apex (anterolateral) paddle position for a child using adult paddles. **B**, Sternum-apex paddle position using infant paddles.

be placed in one of the following positions for transthoracic defibrillation:

- Sternum-apex (anterolateral) position. Place the sternum paddle over the right side of the patient's upper chest below the clavicle. Place the other (apex) paddle to the left of the patient's left nipple over the left lower ribs (Figure 6-23). This paddle position is most commonly used during resuscitation because the anterior chest is usually readily accessible.

- Anterior-posterior position. Place one paddle (or self-adhesive monitoring/defibrillation pad) immediately to the left of the sternum and the other on the back behind the heart (Figure 6-24).

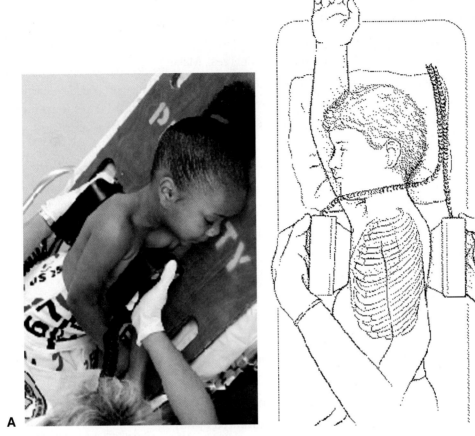

Figure 6-24 Anterior-posterior paddle position.

Paddle Pressure

When using hand-held paddles for defibrillation, firm paddle-to-chest contact pressure lowers transthoracic resistance by improving contact between the skin surface and the paddles and decreasing the amount of air in the lungs. No pressure is applied when using self-adhesive monitoring/defibrillation pads.

Defibrillation: Indications

- Pulseless VT
- Ventricular fibrillation

Defibrillation Procedure

- Turn the power on to the monitor/defibrillator
- If hand-held paddles are used, apply conductive gel to the paddles or place disposable pre-gelled defibrillator pads to the patient's bare torso. Place the defibrillator paddles on the patient's torso and apply firm pressure. If adhesive pads are used, place them in proper position on the patient's bare torso.
- Verify the presence of VT or VF on the monitor.
- While the defibrillator is readied, instruct the IV/medication team

member to prepare the initial drugs that will be used and start an IV after the first shock is delivered.

- Select 2 J/kg on the defibrillator, charge the defibrillator, and recheck the ECG rhythm.

- If the rhythm is unchanged, call "Clear!" and look (360-degrees). Make sure everyone is clear of the patient, bed, and any equipment connected to the patient. If the area is clear, press the SHOCK buttons to discharge energy to the patient. After the shock has been delivered, release the buttons.

- Instruct the resuscitation team to immediately resume CPR, beginning with chest compressions. Instruct the IV/medications team member to start an IV and give a vasopressor (epinephrine). *CPR should not be interrupted to start an IV or give medications.* Give epinephrine every 3 to 5 minutes as long as the patient does not have a pulse. After 5 cycles of CPR (about 2 minutes), recheck the rhythm.

- If a shockable rhythm is present:

  - Select 4 J/kg on the defibrillator, charge the defibrillator and then call "Clear!" Check to be certain everyone is clear of the patient, defibrillate, and then immediately resume CPR, starting with chest compressions. Next, give an antiarrhythmic. Give amiodarone or lidocaine if amiodarone is not available. Give magnesium sulfate if the rhythm is torsades. Consider placement of an advanced airway and possible causes of the arrest. After 5 cycles of CPR (about 2 minutes), recheck the rhythm.

  - If VT/VF persists, defibrillate with 4 J/kg or more (maximum energy dose not to exceed 10 J/kg or the adult dose, whichever is lower). Resume CPR, and give epinephrine.

- If a shockable rhythm is not present:

  - Check a pulse if an organized rhythm is present on the monitor. If there is an organized rhythm on the monitor and a pulse is present, check the patient's blood pressure and other vital signs and begin post-cardiac arrest care.

  - If there is an organized rhythm on the monitor but there is no pulse (pulseless electrical activity) or if the rhythm is asystole, resume CPR, consider possible causes of the arrest, and give medications and other emergency care as indicated.

An **automated external defibrillator** (AED) is an external defibrillator that has a computerized cardiac rhythm analysis system. AEDS are easy to use. Voice prompts and visual indicators guide the user through a series of steps that may include defibrillation. When the adhesive electrodes are attached to the patient's chest, the AED examines the

Remove supplemental oxygen sources (masks, nasal cannulae, resuscitation bags, and ventilator tubing) from the area of the patient's bed before defibrillation and cardioversion attempts and place them at least 3 1/2 to 4 feet away from the patient's chest.

In cardiac arrest due to pulseless VT/VF, defibrillation and CPR are more important than starting an IV, inserting an advanced airway, and giving drugs.

If the defibrillator's lowest dose exceeds the calculated dose, use the lowest dose available. When the calculated dose is between two available energy levels, choose the higher level.

If defibrillation terminates pulseless VT/VF and then recurs, begin defibrillation at the last energy setting that resulted in an ECG rhythm change.

If the patient's rhythm changes, run a rhythm strip for placement in the patient's medical record.

Automated External Defibrillation

patient's cardiac rhythm and analyzes it. Some AEDs require the operator to press an "analyze" control to initiate rhythm analysis whereas others automatically begin analyzing the patient's cardiac rhythm when the electrode pads are attached to the patient's chest. Safety filters check for false signals such as radio transmissions, poor electrode contact, 60-cycle interference, and loose electrodes.

When the AED analyzes the patient's cardiac rhythm, it "looks" at multiple features of the rhythm, including QRS width, rate, and amplitude. If the AED detects a shockable rhythm, it then charges its capacitors. In addition to VF, AEDs will recommend a shock for monomorphic VT and polymorphic VT.

Use a standard AED for a patient who is unresponsive, apneic, pulseless, and 8 years of age or older (about 55 pounds or more than 25 kg) (Figure 6-25A). Several AED manufacturers have designed pediatric attenuators (pad/cable systems) for use with standard AEDs for infants and children up to about 25 kg (8 years of age) (Figure 6-25B). When the pediatric cable is attached to the AED, the machine recognizes the pediatric cable connection and automatically adjusts its defibrillation energy to pediatric levels. Use an AED equipped with a pediatric attenuator, if available, for an unresponsive, apneic, pulseless child who weighs less than 55 pounds (25 kg)[3]. If unavailable, use a standard AED. For infants, use of a manual defibrillator is preferred. If a manual defibrillator is not available, an AED equipped with a pediatric attenuator is desirable. If neither is available, use a standard AED.[3]

> If an AED with a special pediatric pad/cable system is not available, use a standard AED.

AED Operation

- Use personal protective equipment.
- Confirm the patient is unresponsive, apneic (or only has gasping breathing), and pulseless. Begin chest compressions until the AED is ready.
- Turn the power on to the AED. Depending on the brand of AED, this is accomplished by either pressing the "on" button or lifting up the monitor screen or lid. Open the package containing the adhesive pads. Connect the pads to the AED cables (if not preconnected), and then apply the pads to the patient's bare chest in the locations specified by the AED manufacturer. Most models require connection of the AED cable to the AED before use.
- Analyze the ECG rhythm.
  - If several "looks" confirm the presence of a shockable rhythm, the AED will signal a shock is indicated. Listen for the voice prompts. Artifact due to motion or 60-cycle interference may simulate VF and interfere with accurate rhythm analysis. While the AED is analyzing the patient's cardiac rhythm, all movement (including chest

compressions, artificial ventilations, and movement associated with patient transport) must stop.

- Clear the area surrounding the patient. Be sure to look around you.
  - Ensure everyone is clear of the patient, bed, and any equipment connected to the patient.

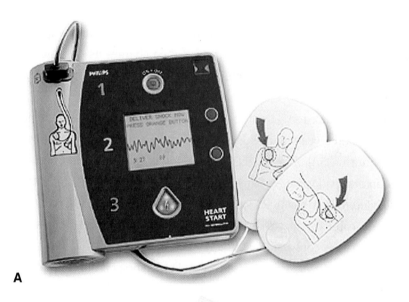

A

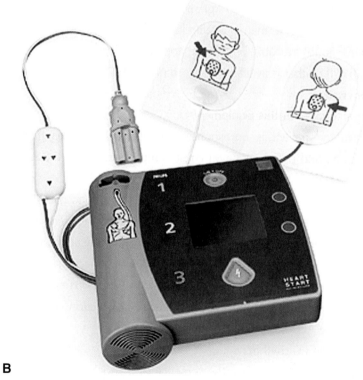

B

Figure 6-25 **A,** A standard automated external defibrillator (AED) should be used for patients who are apneic, pulseless, and 8 years of age or older (approximately 25 kg body weight or more). **B,** This defibrillation pad and cable system reduces the energy delivered by a standard AED to that appropriate for a child.

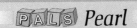 *Pearl*

Always follow the AED manufacturer's guidelines for the application, use, and maintenance of the AED.

- If the area is clear, press the shock control to defibrillate the patient.
- After delivering the shock, immediately resume CPR, beginning with chest compressions.

AED: Advantages

- Voice prompts the user.
- Easy to learn; memorizing treatment protocol is easier than recalling the steps of CPR.
- Less training required to operate and maintain skills than conventional defibrillators.
- Promotes rescuer safety by permitting remote, "hands-free" defibrillation.

AED: Special Considerations

- If the patient has a pacemaker or implantable cardioverter-defibrillator (ICD) an AED may be used; but the AED pads should be placed at least 1 inch from the implanted device. If the ICD is in the process of delivering shocks to the patient, allow it about 30 to 60 seconds to complete the cycle.
- If the patient's chest is dirty or covered with water, quickly wipe the chest before applying the AED pads.

Synchronized Cardioversion

When discussing synchronized cardioversion, the QRS complex is often simply referred to as the "R wave."

Description and Purpose

Synchronized cardioversion is a type of electrical therapy in which a shock is "timed" or "programmed" for delivery during ventricular depolarization (QRS complex). When the "sync" control is pressed, a synchronizing circuit searches for the highest (R wave deflection) or deepest (QS deflection) part of the QRS complex and delivers the shock a few milliseconds after this portion of the QRS. Delivery of a shock during this portion of the cardiac cycle reduces the potential for the delivery of current during ventricular repolarization, which includes the vulnerable portion of the T wave. When a QRS complex is detected, the monitor places a "flag" or "sync marker" on that complex that may appear as an oval, square, line, or highlighted triangle on the ECG display, depending on the monitor used. When the shock controls are pressed while the defibrillator is charged in "sync" mode, the machine will discharge energy only if both discharge buttons are pushed and the monitor tells the defibrillator that a QRS complex has been detected.

Indications

Because the machine must be able to detect a QRS complex in order to "sync," synchronized cardioversion is used to treat rhythms in the "sick" (unstable) patient who has a clearly identifiable QRS complex and a rapid ventricular rate such as SVT due to reentry, atrial fibrillation, atrial flutter, atrial tachycardia, and monomorphic VT with pulse. Signs of hemodynamic compromise include poor perfusion, hypotension, or heart failure. Synchronized cardioversion is not used to treat disorganized rhythms (such as polymorphic VT) or those that do not have a clearly identifiable QRS complex (such as VF).

Procedure

- Turn the monitor/defibrillator on and identify the rhythm on the cardiac monitor. Print an ECG strip to document the patient's rhythm. Make sure suction and emergency medications are available.

- If using standard paddles, you must use defibrillation gel or defibrillation gel pads between the paddle electrode surface and the patient's skin. Place pregelled defibrillation pads on the patient's bare chest at this time. If using multipurpose adhesive electrodes, place them in proper position on the patient's bare chest.

Place ECG electrodes away from defibrillator paddle sites.

- Press the "sync" control on the defibrillator. Select a lead with an optimum QRS complex amplitude (positive or negative) with no artifact. If using adhesive electrodes, select the "paddles" lead. Make sure the machine is marking or flagging each QRS complex and no artifact is present. The sense marker should appear near the middle of each QRS complex. If sense markers do not appear or are seen in the wrong place (such as on a T wave,) adjust the ECG size or select another lead.

- If the patient is awake and time permits, administer sedation per physician's orders unless contraindicted. Make sure the machine is in "sync" mode and then select the appropriate energy level on the defibrillator (0.5 to 1 J/kg) for the initial shock. Charge the defibrillator and recheck the ECG rhythm. If using standard paddles, place the paddles on the pregelled defibrillator pads on the patient's chest and apply firm pressure. If the rhythm is unchanged call "Clear!" and look around you. Make sure everyone is clear of the patient, bed, and any equipment connected to the patient. A slight delay may occur while the machine detects the next QRS complex. Release the shock control after the shock has been delivered.

- Reassess the ECG rhythm and the patient. If the tachycardia persists, ensure the machine is in sync mode before delivering another shock. The energy dose may be increased to 2 J/kg for the second and subsequent attempts if necessary.

- If the dysrhythmia persists despite a second shock or the tachycardia recurs quickly, consider administering amiodarone or procainamide before delivering a third shock.

- If the rhythm changes to VF, confirm that the patient has no pulse while another team member quickly verifies that all electrode and cable connections are secure, turn off the sync control, and defibrillate.

Some defibrillators revert to defibrillation (unsynchronized) mode after the delivery of a synchronized shock. This is done to allow immediate defibrillation in case synchronized cardioversion produces VF. Other defibrillators remain in sync mode after a synchronized shock. If VF occurs during synchronized cardioversion, make sure the sync button is off before attempting to defibrillate.

Transcutaneous Pacing (TCP)

Transcutaneous pacing (TCP) is the use of electrical stimulation through pacing pads positioned on a patient's torso to stimulate contraction of the heart. TCP is also called *temporary external pacing* or *noninvasive pacing*. Although TCP is a type of electrical therapy, the current delivered is considerably less than that used for cardioversion or defibrillation. The energy levels selected for cardioversion or defibrillation are indicated in joules. The stimulating current selected for TCP is measured in milliamperes (mA). The range of output current of a transcutaneous pacemaker varies depending on the manufacturer. You must be familiar with the equipment before you need to use it.

Indications

TCP may be used for the patient with profound symptomatic bradycardia refractory to basic and advanced life support therapy.

Procedure

Do not place the pads over open cuts, sores, or metal objects.

Sedation or analgesia may be needed to minimize the discomfort associated with this procedure.

Mechanical capture occurs when pacing produces a measurable hemodynamic response (e.g., palpable pulse, measurable blood pressure).

- Pacer pad positioning varies by manufacturer. Follow the manufacturer's recommendations for proper pad placement (Figures 6-26 and 6-27).
- Connect the patient to an ECG monitor and obtain a rhythm strip. Connect the pacing cable to the pacemaker and to the adhesive pads on the patient.
- Turn the power on to the pacemaker and set the pacing rate to the desired number of paced pulses per minute (ppm). After the rate has been regulated, start the pacemaker (Figure 6-28).
  - Increase the stimulating current (output or mA) slowly but steadily until pacer spikes are visible before each QRS complex (capture).
  - Observe the cardiac monitor for electrical capture (usually evidenced by a wide QRS and broad T wave). Evaluate mechanical capture by assessing the patient's femoral pulse.
  - Once capture is achieved, continue pacing at an output level slightly higher (approximately 2 mA) than the threshold of initial electrical capture.
- Assess the patient's blood pressure, pulse oximetry, and level of responsiveness. Monitor the patient closely, including assessment of the skin for irritation where the pacing pads have been applied. Document and record the ECG rhythm.

Complications
- Skin burns
- Interference with sensing due to patient agitation or muscle contractions
- Pain from electrical stimulation of the skin and muscles
- Failure to recognize the pacemaker is not capturing

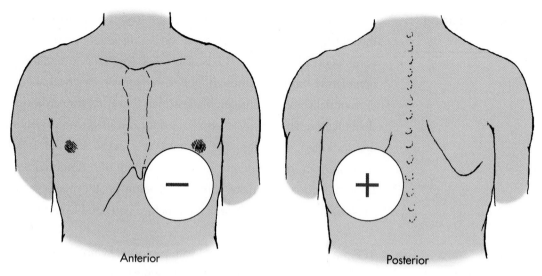

Figure 6-26   Anterior-posterior positioning of transcutaneous electrodes.

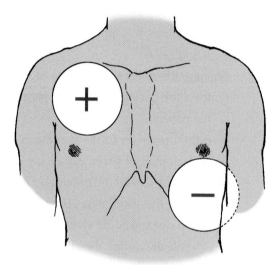

Figure 6-27   Anterolateral positioning of transcutaneous electrodes.

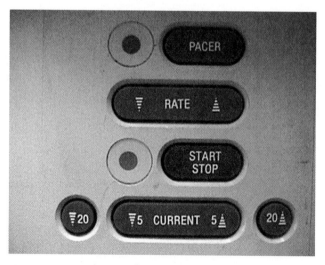

Figure 6-28   Transcutaneous pacemaker controls.

TABLE 6-2 *Electrical Therapy: Summary*

Intervention	Dysrhythmia	Recommended Energy Levels
Defibrillation	Pulseless VT/VF	2 J/kg initially, then 4 J/kg for second shock; at least 4 J/kg and higher may be considered for the third and subsequent shocks, not to exceed 10 J/kg or the adult maximum dose, whichever is lower
Synchronized cardioversion	SVT due to reentry Atrial fibrillation Atrial flutter Atrial tachycardia Monomorphic VT with a pulse	0.5 to 1 J/kg initially, then 2 J/kg for subsequent shocks
Transcutaneous pacing	Severe bradycardia (e.g., complete AV block)	Set initial rate Increase the output (mA) until pacer spikes are visible before each QRS complex. Verify capture.

AV, atrioventricular; SVT, supraventricular tachycardia; VT, ventricular tachycardia; VF, ventricular fibrillation.

- Failure to recognize the presence of underlying treatable VF
- Tissue damage, including third degree burns, has been reported in patients with improper or prolonged TCP
- When pacing is prolonged, pacing threshold changes, leading to capture failure

Contraindications

- Major chest trauma that precludes placement of the pacing pads.

A summary of the electrical therapy discussed in this chapter appears in Table 6-2.

Vagal Maneuvers

Vagal maneuvers are methods used to stimulate baroreceptors located in the internal carotid arteries and the aortic arch. Stimulation of these receptors results in reflex stimulation of the vagus nerve and release of acetylcholine. Acetylcholine slows conduction through the AV node, resulting in slowing of the heart rate.

Indications

Vagal maneuvers may be tried in the stable but symptomatic child in SVT or during preparation for cardioversion or drug therapy for this dysrhythmia. Success rates with vagal maneuvers vary and depend on the patient's age, level of cooperation, and the presence of underlying conditions.

Vagal maneuvers that may be used in the pediatric patient include the following:

- Application of a cold stimulus to the face (e.g., a washcloth soaked in iced water, cold pack, or crushed ice mixed with water in a plastic bag or glove) for up to 10 seconds. This technique is often effective in infants and young children. When using this method, do not obstruct the patient's mouth or nose or apply pressure to the eyes.
- Valsalva maneuver. Instruct the child to blow through a straw or take a deep breath and bear down as if having a bowel movement for 10 seconds. This strains the abdominal muscles and increases intra-thoracic pressure. In the younger child, abdominal palpation may be used to create the same effect. Abdominal palpation causes the child to bear down in an attempt to resist the pressure.
- Gagging. Use a tongue depressor or culturette swab to briefly touch the posterior oropharynx.
- Carotid sinus massage may be used in older children. This procedure is performed with the patient's neck extended. Firm pressure is applied just under the angle of the jaw for up to 5 seconds. Simultaneous, bicarotid pressure should *never* be peformed.

Techniques

When using vagal maneuvers, keep the following points in mind:

- Ensure oxygen, suction, a defibrillator, and crash cart are available before attempting the procedure.
- Obtain a 12-lead ECG before and after the vagal maneuver.
- Continuous monitoring of the patient's ECG is essential. Note the onset and end of the vagal maneuver on the ECG rhythm strip.
- In general, a vagal maneuver should not be continued for more than 10 seconds.
- Application of external ocular pressure may be dangerous and should not be used because of the risk of retinal detachment.

Special Considerations

Hemodynamically unstable tachycardia when immediate synchronized cardioversion is imperative.

Contraindications

- Syncope.
- Bradydysrhythmias (e.g., sinus arrest, AV block, asystole).
- Ventricular dysrhythmias.

Complications

Case Study Resolution

Continue CPR. Consider insertion of an advanced airway and then confirm its position using assessment and mechanical methods. Establish vascular access and give epinephrine. Provide further interventions based on the child's response to therapy.

References

1. Ewy GA: Cardiocerebral resuscitation: the new cardiopulmonary resuscitation, *Circulation* 2005;111(16):2134–2142.

2. Berg MD, Schexnayder SM, Chameides L, et al. Part 13: Pediatric basic life support: 2010 American Heart Association Guidelines for Cardiopulmonary Resuscitation and Emergency Cardiovascular Care. *Circulation* 2010;122(suppl 3):S862–S875.

3. Kleinman ME, Chameides L, Schexnayder SM, et al. Part 14: Pediatric advanced life support: 2010 American Heart Association Guidelines for Cardiopulmonary Resuscitation and Emergency Cardiovascular Care. *Circulation* 2010;122(suppl 3):S876 –S908.

4 Atkins DL, Sirna S, Kieso R, et al. Pediatric defibrillation: importance of paddle size in determining transthoracic impedance, *Pediatrics* 1988;82(6):914–918.

5. Atkins DL, Kerber RE. Pediatric defibrillation: current flow is improved by using "adult" electrode paddles, *Pediatrics* 1994;94(1):90–93.

6. Samson RA, Atkins DL, Kerber RE. Optimal size of self-adhesive preapplied electrode pads in pediatric defibrillation, *Am J Cardiol* 1995;75(7):544–545.

7. Killingsworth CR, Melnick SB, Chapman FW, et al. Defibrillation threshold and cardiac responses using an external biphasic defibrillator with pediatric and adult adhesive patches in pediatric-sized piglets, *Resuscitation* 2002;55(2):177–185.

8. Hummell RS, Ornato JP, Wienberg SM, et al. Spark-generating properties of electrode gels used during defibrillation: a potential fire hazard. *JAMA* 1988;260:3021–3024.

9. Crockett PJ, Droppert BM, Higgins SE, et al. *Defibrillation: what you should know.* Redmond, WA:Physio-Control Corp, 1996.

Chapter Quiz

Questions 1–12 refer to the following scenario:

A 6-year-old boy is complaining of stomach pain. The child's father says his son has had frequent vomiting and diarrhea for the past 72 hours. He is seeking medical care because his son vomited immediately on awakening this morning and then had diarrhea. Dad put his son in the shower to wash him and his son "collapsed" for about 10 to 15 seconds. You observe the child sitting in a chair with his hand over his stomach. He appears uncomfortable and restless, but is aware of your presence. The child has listened intently to the conversation between you and his father. His face and lips appear pale. Some mottling of the extremities is present. His breathing is unlabored at a rate that appears normal for his age.

1. Which of the following statements is true of your interactions with a child of this age?
   A) Speak to the child in a respectful, friendly manner, as if speaking to an adult.
   B) When speaking with the caregiver, include the child.
   C) Avoid frightening or misleading terms such as shot, deaden, germs, etc.
   D) Establish a contract with the child - tell him that if he does not cooperate with you, you are certain he will have to have surgery.

2. From the information provided, complete the following documentation regarding the Pediatric Assessment Triangle.
   Appearance:
   Breathing:
   Circulation:

3. Your initial assessment reveals a patent airway. The child's ventilatory rate is 20/min. Auscultation of the chest reveals clear breath sounds bilaterally. A radial pulse is easily palpated at a rate of 157 beats/min. The skin is pale and dry. The child's capillary refill is 3 seconds, temperature is 99.4° F, and his blood pressure is 82/56. The normal heart rate range for a 6-year-old child at rest is _____ beats/min.
   A) 60 to 100.
   B) 70 to 120.
   C) 80 to 140.
   D) 90 to 150.

4. You have applied the cardiac monitor and observe the ECG shown below.

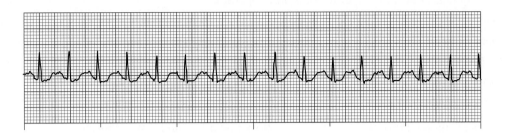

This rhythm is:

A) Atrial flutter.

B) Supraventricular tachycardia.

C) Sinus tachycardia.

D) Ventricular tachycardia.

5. Assessment of the child's skin turgor reveals an elapsed time of 4 1/2 seconds for the skin to return to normal. You estimate the child's degree of dehydration to be:

A) Less than 5% of the child's body weight.

B) 5% to 8% of the child's body weight.

C) 9% to 10% of the child's body weight.

D) More than 10% of the child's body weight.

6. The lower limit of a normal systolic blood pressure for a child of this age is:

A) About 60 mm Hg.

B) About 70 mm Hg.

C) About 80 mm Hg.

D) About 90 mm Hg.

7. This child's history and presentation are consistent with:

A) Compensated hypovolemic shock.

B) Irreversible cardiogenic shock.

C) Decompensated anaphylactic shock.

D) Preterminal distributive shock.

8. Select the **incorrect** statement.

A) Hypotension is an early sign of shock in a child.

B) The diastolic blood pressure is usually two-thirds of the systolic pressure.

C) A child may be in shock despite a normal blood pressure.

D) Blood pressure is one of the least sensitive indicators of adequate circulation in children.

9. The presence of compensated shock can be identified by:
   A) Assessment of heart rate, ECG rhythm, and skin temperature.
   B) Assessment of the presence and strength of peripheral pulses, mental status, and pupil response to light.
   C) Assessment of heart rate, presence and strength of peripheral pulses, and the adequacy of end-organ perfusion.
   D) Assessment of end-organ perfusion, ECG rhythm, and pupil response to light.

10. Which of the following methods of vascular access should be attempted first in this child?
    A) Establish an intraosseous infusion.
    B) Establish an internal jugular intravenous (IV) line.
    C) Establish an IV using the saphenous vein.
    D) Establish an IV in the antecubital fossa.

11. True or False: As you prepare to establish vascular access, the child becomes uncooperative. A reasonable approach in this situation would be to ask the child's father to assist in restraining his son in order to accomplish the procedure as quickly as possible.

12. Vascular access has been successfully established. You should begin volume resuscitation with a fluid bolus of:
    A) 10 mL/kg.
    B) 20 mL/kg.
    C) 30 mL/kg.
    D) 50 mL/kg.

Questions 13–19 refer to the following scenario:

A 2-year-old drowning victim is apneic and pulseless. CPR is in progress.

13. The cardiac monitor reveals the rhythm below.

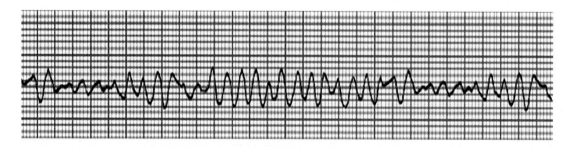

This rhythm is:
A) Ventricular tachycardia.
B) Atrial fibrillation.
C) Ventricular fibrillation.
D) Asystole.

14. CPR is in progress. Your next intervention should be to:
    A) Establish vascular access, insert a tracheal tube, and then perform synchronized cardioversion followed by immediate defibrillation.
    B) Insert a tracheal tube, establish vascular access, and then prepare to defibrillate.
    C) Perform synchronized cardioversion followed by immediate defibrillation.
    D) Prepare to defibrillate.

15. The initial energy dose used for defibrillation should be:
    A) 0.5 joules/kg.
    B) 1 joule/kg.
    C) 2 joules/kg.
    D) 3 joules/kg.

16. After delivery of the shock, you should:
    A) Attempt a vagal maneuver.
    B) Establish vascular access.
    C) Attempt transcutaneous pacing.
    D) Resume CPR immediately, starting with chest compressions.

17. A tracheal tube has been inserted. To confirm proper positioning of the tube, you should first listen:
    A) Over the epigastrium.
    B) Over the posterior chest.
    C) Over the left lateral chest in the axilla.
    D) Over the right lateral chest in the axilla.

18. A 6-year-old is found unresponsive, not breathing, and pulseless. A standard AED can be used if an AED with a pediatric pad/cable system is not available.
    A) True
    B) False

Chapter Quiz Answers

1. B. When the patient is a school-age child (6 to 12 years of age), include the child when speaking with the caregiver. If the patient is an adolescent, speak to him in a respectful, friendly manner, as if speaking to an adult. Although it is reasonable to make a contract with a child of this age ("I promise to tell you everything I am going to do if you will help me by cooperating"), it is inappropriate and unprofessional to threaten him.

2. Pediatric Assessment Triangle (first impression) findings:
   Appearance: Awake and restless; aware of surroundings; listening intently
   Breathing: Respirations appear normal for age; normal ventilatory effort
   Circulation: Pale face and lips. Some mottling of the extremities is present.

3. B. The normal heart rate for a 6 to 12 year old at rest is 70 to 120 beats/min.

4. C. The rhythm shown is sinus tachycardia at 157 beats/min.

5. D. When evaluating skin turgor to estimate dehydration, if it takes less than 2 seconds for the skin to return to normal, suspect the approximate degree of dehydration to be less than 5% of the child's body weight. 2-3 seconds = 5% to 8% of the child's body weight; 3-4 seconds = 9% to 10% of the child's body weight; and longer than 4 seconds = more than 10% of the child's body weight.

6. C. The lower limit of a normal systolic blood pressure for a child between 1 and 10 years of age can be estimated using the formula 70 + (2 × age in years). This child's minimum systolic blood pressure should be about 82 mm Hg.

7. A. This child's history and presentation is consistent with compensated hypovolemic shock.

8. A. Hypotension is a late sign of shock in a child. Tachycardia and signs of poor perfusion such as pale, cool, mottled skin occur earlier and are more reliable indicators than hypotension.

9. C. The presence of compensated shock can be identified by evaluation of heart rate, the presence and volume (strength) of peripheral pulses, and the adequacy of end-organ perfusion (Brain - assess mental status, skin - assess capillary refill, skin temperature, and kidneys - assess urine output).

10. D. In this situation, you should first attempt to establish a peripheral IV line in the antecubital fossa. If the child was in decompensated shock or cardiac arrest, intraosseous access could be attempted if IV access was not rapidly achieved.

11. False. Because a child expects his or her caregiver to protect them, do not ask a caregiver to restrain a child or participate in any way other than to comfort the child.

12. B. Administer a bolus of 20 mL/kg of isotonic crystalloid solution (NS or LR) over 5 to 20 minutes. Assess response (i.e., mental status, capillary refill, heart rate, ventilatory effort, blood pressure).

13. C. The rhythm shown is ventricular fibrillation.

14. D. Defibrillation is the definitive treatment for pulseless VT/VF. Defibrillation takes priority over establishing vascular access and placement of a tracheal tube. Synchronized cardioversion is used to shock hemodynamically compromising tachycardias with a pulse.

15. C. The initial energy dose used to defibrillate pulseless VT/VF is 2 J/kg.

16. D. After delivery of a shock, immediately resume CPR, starting with chest compressions. A vagal maneuver may be tried in the stable but symptomatic child in supraventricular tachycardia or during preparation for cardioversion or drug therapy for SVT. Transcutaneous pacing may be used for the patient with profound symptomatic bradycardia refractory to basic and advanced life support therapy.

17. A. To confirm proper positioning of the tube, listen first over the epigastrium. The presence of bubbling or gurgling sounds during auscultation of the epigastrium suggests the tube is incorrectly positioned in the esophagus. To correct this problem, deflate the tracheal tube cuff (if a cuffed tube was used), remove the tube, and preoxygenate before reattempting intubation. In infants, breath sounds may be heard over the stomach but should not be louder than midaxillary sounds.

18. A. If an AED with a pediatric pad/cable system is not available, a standard AED may be used.

Fluids and Medications

Case Study

An 11-year-old boy arrives at the hospital with shoulder pain. The child's wrestling coach states the boy was taken down hard by his opponent in a wrestling match and complained of a sudden, severe pain in his right shoulder. Your first impression reveals the boy is awake and alert. He is holding his right extremity close to his chest. There is no evidence of respiratory distress. His skin is pink. Deformity of the right shoulder is visible.

How will you assess the intensity of this child's pain?

Objectives

1. Define the following terms: chronotrope, dromotrope, inotrope, pain, sedation, analgesia, amnesia, and anesthesia.
2. Describe the location and effects of stimulation of alpha, beta, and dopaminergic receptors.
3. Describe advantages and disadvantages associated with pediatric medication administration routes.
4. Describe two tools that may be used to assess pain in the pediatric patient.
5. Explain the importance of pain management.
6. Describe techniques for nonpharmacologic management of pain in infants and children.
7. Discuss common pharmacologic agents used in pain management and sedation.
8. Describe the levels of sedation/analgesia.
9. Identify factors that may increase the risk of complications during sedation/analgesia.
10. Explain the importance of postsedation monitoring.

Pharmacology Review

Review of the Autonomic Nervous System

The autonomic nervous system (ANS) consists of sympathetic and parasympathetic divisions. The sympathetic division mobilizes the body, allowing the body to function under stress ("fight or flight" response). The parasympathetic division is responsible for the conservation and restoration of body resources ("feed and breed" or "resting and digesting" response) (Table 7-1).

Stimulation of sympathetic nerve fibers results in the release of norepinephrine. Norepinephrine binds to receptor sites located in the plasma membrane of cells. Sympathetic (adrenergic) receptor sites are divided into alpha, beta, and dopaminergic receptors (Table 7-2).

TABLE 7-1 *Overview of the Divisions of the Autonomic Nervous System*

	Sympathetic Division	**Parasympathetic Division**

	"Fight or flight" response
	    Mobilizes the body
	    Allows the body to function under stress
		"Feed and breed" or "resting and digesting" response
		    Conservation of body resources
		    Restoration of body resources

Neurotransmitter	Norepinephrine	Acetylcholine
Synonymous terms	Adrenergic, sympathomimetic, catecholamine, anticholinergic, parasympatholytic, cholinergic blocker	Cholinergic, parasympathomimetic, sympathetic blocker, cholinomimetic, sympatholytic, adrenergic blocker
Opposite terms	Sympatholytic, antiadrenergic, sympathetic blocker, adrenergic blocker	Parasympatholytic, anticholinergic, cholinergic blocker, vagolytic

TABLE 7-2 *Sympathetic (Adrenergic) Receptors*

	α_1	α_2	β_1	β_2	**Dopaminergic**
Location	Vascular smooth muscle	Skeletal blood vessels	Myocardium	Predominantly in bronchiolar and arterial smooth muscle	Coronary arteries, renal, mesenteric, and visceral blood vessels
Effects of stimulation	Vasoconstriction ↑ peripheral vascular resistance	Inhibits norepinephrine release	↑ heart rate ↑ myocardial contractility ↑ oxygen consumption	Relaxation of bronchial smooth muscle; arteriolar dilation	Dilation

Dopaminergic receptor sites are located in the coronary arteries, renal, mesenteric, and visceral blood vessels. Stimulation of dopaminergic receptor sites results in dilation.

Different body tissues have different proportions of α- and β-receptors. In general, α-receptors are more sensitive to norepinephrine and β-receptors are more sensitive to epinephrine. Stimulation of α-receptor sites results in constriction of blood vessels in the skin, cerebral, and splanchnic circulation.

β-receptor sites are divided into β_1 and β_2. β_1-receptors are found in the heart. Stimulation of β_1-receptors results in an increased heart rate, contractility, and, ultimately, irritability of cardiac cells. β_2-receptor sites are found in the lungs and skeletal muscle blood vessels. Stimulation of these receptor sites results in dilation of the smooth muscle of the bronchi and blood vessel dilation.

Important Terms to Remember

A chronotrope is a substance that affects heart rate.
- Positive chronotrope = ↑ heart rate
- Negative chronotrope = ↓ heart rate

An inotrope is a substance that affects myocardial contractility.
- Positive inotrope = ↑ force of contraction
- Negative inotrope = ↓ force of contraction

A dromotrope is a substance that affects atrioventricular (AV) conduction velocity.
- Positive dromotrope = ↑ AV conduction velocity
- Negative dromotrope = ↓ AV conduction velocity

Remember: β_1-receptors affect the heart (you have one heart); β_2-receptors affect the lungs (you have two lungs).

Volume Expansion

TABLE 7-3 *Volume Expansion: Summary*

Crystalloid Solutions

Description	Isotonic solutions that provide transient expansion of the intravascular volume.
Examples	Normal saline—contains sodium chloride in water. Ringer's lactate—contains sodium chloride, potassium chloride, calcium chloride, and sodium lactate in water.
Advantages	Inexpensive, readily available, free from allergic reactions.
Disadvantages	Effectively expand the interstitial space and correct sodium deficits but do not effectively expand the intravascular volume because approximately three fourths of the infused crystalloid solution will leave the vascular space in about 1 hour. If administered in large enough amounts, Ringer's lactate may increase lactic acidodis and may increase the release of cytokines, while normal saline may worse intracellular depletion of potassium and produce hyperchloremic acidosis.

TABLE 7-3, *cont'd*

Colloid Solutions

Description	Contain molecules (typically proteins) that are too large to pass out of the capillary membranes. As a result, they remain in the vascular compartment and draw fluid from the interstitial and intracellular compartments into the vascular compartment to expand the intravascular volume.
Examples	5% albumin, fresh frozen plasma; synthetic colloids include hetastarch and dextran
Advantages	More efficient than crystalloid solutions in rapidly expanding the intravascular compartment; remain in the intravascular space for hours.
Disadvantages	More expensive than crystalloids, short shelf-life, potential for adverse effects or acute allergic reactions; can produce dramatic fluid shifts

Blood

Indications	Correction of a deficiency or functional defect of a blood component that has caused a clinically significant problem; severe acute hemorrhage
Notes	Red blood cells are the most frequently transfused blood component. They are given to increase the oxygen-carrying capacity of the blood and to maintain satisfactory tissue oxygenation.
	If blood is administered, it should be warmed before transfusion; otherwise, rapid administration may result in significant hypothermia.

Medication Administration

Although the terms *drug* and *medication* are often used interchangeably, a **drug** is any chemical compound that produces an effect on a living organism. **Medication** refers to drugs used in the practice of medicine as a remedy.

Administering medications to the pediatric patient is challenging because of changes that occur from birth through adolescence in body size, physiology, and general health. These changes affect the way in which the drug is absorbed, distributed, metabolized, and eliminated; where and how much of the drug is deposited in the body; and the therapeutic effects and side effects of the drug.

In the pediatric patient, medications may be administered via the oral, transmucosal, intranasal, rectal, pulmonary, subcutaneous (SubQ), intramuscular (IM), intravenous (IV), intraosseous (IO), or tracheal route. The route by which a drug is administered affects the rapidity with which the drug's onset of action occurs and may affect the therapeutic response that results.

TABLE 7-4 *Oral Medication Administration*

Advantages	Readily available route of administration Patient acceptance; painless Convenient, noninvasive Does not generally require special equipment for administration No risk of fluid overload, infection, or embolism as with IV medications
Disadvantages	Requires functioning GI tract and sufficient GI tract for absorption to occur Slow or erratic absorption following ingestion Limited value in an emergent situation Requires a responsive, cooperative patient with an intact gag reflex May cause gagging or aspiration if administered too rapidly
Examples	Activated charcoal, antibiotics, steroids
Notes	Do not administer oral medications in solid form (i.e., pills, capsules, tablets) to young children because of the danger of aspiration. A tuberculin syringe (needle removed) is ideal for administering liquid medications of 1 mL or less. A medicine cup can be used for older infants who are able to drink from a cup. Place an infant in a semireclining position or a child in a sitting or semireclining position. Position the infant or child securely. Place the syringe (or plastic dropper) along the side of the child's tongue, toward the back of the mouth. Administer the medication slowly and in small amounts, allowing the child sufficient time to swallow (Figure 7-1). If available, follow the medication with water, juice, or a frozen juice bar.

GI, gastrointestinal; IV, intravenous.

- When possible, use a length-based resuscitation tape to determine the correct dosage for medication administration or fluid resuscitation in children.
- Check each medication at least three times before administering it.
  - Check the medication when removing it from its storage container (i.e., drug box, code cart).
  - Check the medication again when preparing it for administration.
  - Check it once more at the patient's side before administering it.
- Question any medication dosage that is outside the normal range.
- Using age-appropriate language, explain to the child (and caregiver) why a medication is necessary.
- Children should always be praised for cooperating in taking their medications.
- If the child is uncooperative, restrain the child as necessary.

Considerations in Pediatric Medication Administration

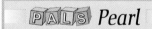 *Pearl*

Medication errors are common and preventable. Make it a habit to have a co-worker double-check your medication and dosage before administering it to an infant or child. This is particularly important for controlled substances (e.g., narcotics, sedatives), antiarrhythmics, heparin, insulin, and medications used during resuscitation.

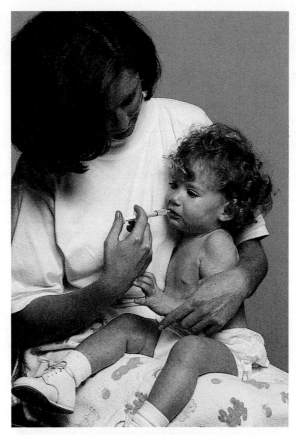

Figure 7-1 This child is partially restrained to ensure easy and comfortable administration of an oral medication using a tuberculin syringe.

TABLE 7-5 *Oral Transmucosal (Sublingual, Buccal) Medication Administration*

Advantages	Readily available route of administration Ease of administration Painless Rapid onset of action
Disadvantages	Requires a responsive, cooperative patient with an intact gag reflex Unsuitable for very young patients who may not understand your instructions Limited number of medications that can be administered via this route Variable absorption
Examples	Sedatives
Notes	Mucosal surfaces typically have a rich blood supply, allowing rapid drug transport to the systemic circulation

TABLE 7-6 *Intranasal Medication Administration*

Advantages	Easy to administer Rapid, reliable onset of action Relatively painless Obviates need for painful injections
Disadvantages	Some medications (e.g., midazolam) are associated with a burning sensation and lacrimation when administered intranasally Limited number of medications that can be administered via this route May cause gagging or aspiration if administered too rapidly
Examples	Fentanyl, midazolam, lorazepam, steroids
Notes	Intranasal medications are administered via spray, drops, or aerosol into the nasal cavity. The child should be placed in a supine position with the head tilted back so that the opening to the nares is almost horizontal (Figure 7-2). The child should remain in this position for approximately 1 minute after the medication has been instilled to ensure the medication reaches the nasal mucosa. The medication is being given too quickly if the child sputters, coughs, or swallows during administration. Do not administer medications via this route if the child has respiratory distress, copious nasal secretions, or nasal bleeding because of the increased risk of airway obstruction and aspiration.

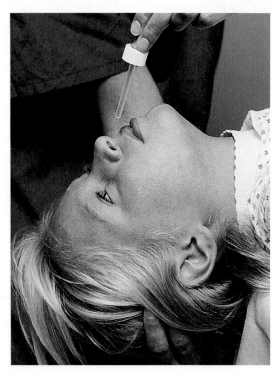

Figure 7-2 Patient positioning for intranasal medication administration.

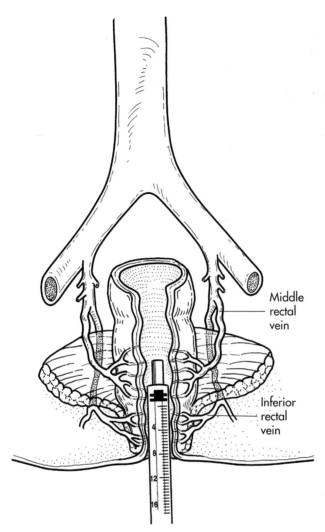

Figure 7-3   Venous drainage of the middle and inferior rectum and syringe insertion.

Middle rectal vein

Inferior rectal vein

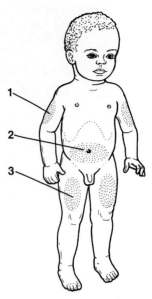

Figure 7-4   The most common sites used for subcutaneous injection are 1) the lateral aspect of the upper arms, 2) the abdomen from the costal margins to the iliac crests, and 3) the anterior thighs.

TABLE 7-7 *Rectal Medication Administration*

Advantages	Route is always available More easily accessible route during active seizures than intravenous route Rapid absorption Relatively painless
Disadvantages	Limited number of medications that can be administered via this route If the rectum is not empty when the medication is inserted, drug absorption may be delayed, diminished, or prevented Most children dislike this route of administration
Examples	Anticonvulsants, antipyretics, antiemetics, analgesics, sedatives
Notes	Rectal medication administration should be avoided in patients with rectal trauma and immunosuppressed patients in whom even minimal trauma could lead to formation of an abscess. To administer, draw up the appropriate drug dose into a lubricated 1-mL disposable tuberculin syringe. Insert the syringe (without the needle) into the rectum to the end of the syringe and inject the medication (Figure 7-3). Remove the syringe.

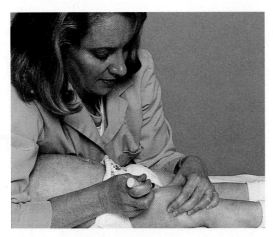

Figure 7-5 When administering an intramuscular (IM) injection, grasp the muscle between your thumb and index finger to isolate and stabilize the muscle and ensure IM delivery of the medication.

TABLE 7-8 *Pulmonary (Inhaled) Medication Administration*

Advantages	Painless Ease of administration Rapid onset of action
Disadvantages	Limited use with respiratory failure Medications used are limited to those with actions on or absorption through the respiratory tract
Examples	Oxygen, bronchodilators, nitrous oxide, steroids, antibiotics, antivirals
Notes	Administration may be difficult if the child is uncooperative; however, crying may improve medication delivery because of the child's deeper and more rapid ventilatory rate. Medication delivery is affected by airway size and the degree of obstruction within the airways due to mucous plugs, bronchoconstriction, and inflammation.

TABLE 7-9 *Subcutaneous Medication Administration*

Advantages	Readily available route Allows delivery of a variety of medications Less painful than intramuscular injection
Disadvantages	Painful; creates fear and anxiety in children and may cause a child to deny pain in order to avoid further injections of analgesics Inconvenient, time consuming Requires technical expertise to perform Volume of medication that can be delivered is limited to 0.5 to 1.0 mL (maximum of 1 mL in all age groups) Slower onset and lower peak effects than intravenous administration Can cause local tissue injury and nerve damage if improper technique used
Examples	Heparin, morphine, insulin, some vaccines, epinephrine, allergy desensitization, hormone replacement
Notes	Inappropriate route for medications that are irritating and are not water-soluble. Absorption may be rapid or slow depending on the water solubility of the drug and blood flow to the injection site. The most common sites used for SubQ injection are the lateral aspect of the upper arms, the abdomen from the costal margins to the iliac crests, and the anterior thighs (Figure 7-4). Use a 25-gauge, 1/2-inch needle for infant or thin child; 25-gauge, 5/8-inch needle for larger child. Insert the needle at a 90-degree angle, using a quick, dartlike motion. Some clinicians insert the needle at a 45-degree angle if the child has little SubQ tissue.

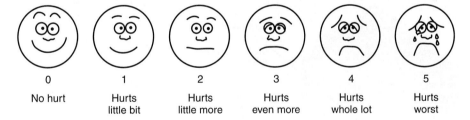

0	1	2	3	4	5
No hurt	Hurts little bit	Hurts little more	Hurts even more	Hurts whole lot	Hurts worst

Figure 7-6 Wong-Baker FACES Pain Rating Scale. To use this scale, point to each face using the words to describe the pain intensity. Ask the child to choose the face that best describes his or her own pain and record the appropriate number.

TABLE 7-10 *Intramuscular Medication Administration*

Advantages	Readily available route Allows delivery of a variety of medications
Disadvantages	Painful; creates fear and anxiety in children and may cause a child to deny pain in order to avoid further injections of analgesics Erratic absorption may cause discontinuous levels of analgesia Requires technical expertise to perform Volume of medication that can be delivered is limited by the site chosen and child's size More painful than SubQ injection Medication is given more slowly than SubQ injection Can cause local tissue injury and nerve damage if improper technique used Chronic injections may damage tissue (fibrosis, abscesses)
Examples	Antibiotics, some vaccines, sedatives, analgesics
Notes	Absorption may be rapid or slow depending on the water solubility of the drug and blood flow to the injection site. When administering an IM injection, grasp the muscle between your thumb and index finger to isolate and stabilize the muscle and ensure IM delivery of the medication (Figure 7-5). If the child is obese, spread the skin with your thumb and index finger to displace SubQ tissue and then grasp the muscle on each side.

IM, intramuscular; SubQ, subcutaneous.

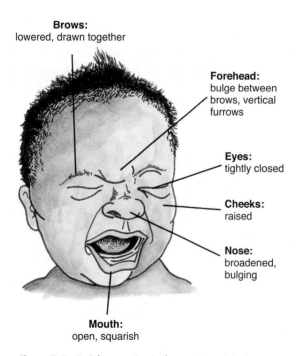

Brows:
lowered, drawn together

Forehead:
bulge between brows, vertical furrows

Eyes:
tightly closed

Cheeks:
raised

Nose:
broadened, bulging

Mouth:
open, squarish

Figure 7-7 Facial expression is the most consistent behavioral indicator of pain in infants.

TABLE 7-11 *Intravenous Medication Administration*

Advantages	Rapid onset of action for medications administered via this route Route is easily accessible Control over the level of the drug in the blood Useful for resuscitation medications and fluids
Disadvantages	Painful Limits patient mobility Time consuming Requires technical expertise to perform
Examples	Antiarrhythmics, sedatives, analgesics, antibiotics
Notes	No barriers to absorption since the drug is administered directly into the circulatory system Do not attempt intravenous access in a child experiencing respiratory distress unless the procedure is necessary for immediate lifesaving interventions.

TABLE 7-12 *Intraosseous Medication Administration*

Advantages	Rapid onset Control over the level of the drug in the blood Effective route when venous access is difficult or time consuming Useful for resuscitation medications and fluids
Disadvantages	Painful Limits patient mobility Requires technical expertise to perform
Examples	Antiarrhythmics
Notes	No barriers to absorption

TABLE 7-13 *Tracheal Medication Administration*

Advantages	Permits delivery of lipid-soluble medications into the pulmonary alveoli and systemic circulation via lung capillaries
Disadvantages	Limited number of medications that can be administered via this route Medication absorption may be negatively affected by the presence of blood, emesis, or secretions in the trachea or tracheal tube No fluid resuscitation possible via this medication route
Notes	Use the tracheal route for medication administration during resuscitation efforts if a tracheal tube is in place but intravenous or intraosseous access is not available. Tracheal medications should be diluted with approximately 5 mL of sterile normal saline When administering medications by means of a tracheal tube, temporarily stop chest compressions and instill the medication down the tracheal tube. Follow the medication with five positive-pressure ventilations to ensure adequate distribution of the drug, and then resume cardiopulmonary resuscitation.

Pain Management and Sedation

Pain is a subjective experience that is underestimated and inadequately treated by many healthcare professionals despite the availability of effective medications and other therapies. The safe and effective relief of pain should be a priority in the management of a patient of **any** age.

Barriers to Pain Assessment and Management

Pain Assessment in Infants and Children

The American Pain Society created the phrase "Pain: the fifth vital sign" to increase awareness of the importance of pain assessment.[1] The rationale for this initiative is that healthcare professionals should assess (and treat) pain with the same diligence and seriousness as evaluation of a patient's pulse, ventilatory rate, temperature, and blood pressure.

Pain should be assessed in *all* patients; however, the methods for assessing pain in the pediatric patient will vary according to the age of the child. Adequate pain management requires reassessment of the presence and severity of pain and the child's response to treatment. If pain is unrelieved, determine whether the cause is related to a new cause of pain, the progression of disease, procedure-related pain, or treatment-related pain.

Methods for assessing pain in the pediatric patient vary according to the age of the child. One approach to pain assessment is QUESTT[4]:

*Q*uestion the child

*U*se pain-rating scales

*E*valuate behavior and physiologic changes

*S*ecure parents' involvement

*T*ake cause of pain into account

*T*ake action

- Obtain a pain history from the child and his or her caregivers.
  - The answers a patient provides in response to questions about his or her pain is called a "self-report."
    - The patient's self-report is considered the most reliable method for assessing pain (in patients who can communicate verbally) because it is the *child's* verbal statement and description of pain.
    - Self-reporting is appropriate for most children 3 years and older.
    - Ascertain information related to the
      - Characteristics of the pain (e.g., duration, location, intensity, quality, exacerbating/alleviating factors)
      - Type of previous painful experiences

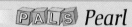 *Pearl*

Because no individual can feel another's pain, "Pain is whatever the experiencing person says it is, existing whenever s/he says it does."[2] The *patient*, not the healthcare professional, is the authority regarding his or her pain.

The most common reason for the undertreatment of pain in U.S. hospitals is the failure of clinicians to assess pain and pain relief.[3]

TABLE 7-14 *Fallacies and Facts about Children and Pain*

Fallacy	Fact
Infants do not feel pain.	Infants demonstrate behavioral (especially facial), and physiologic (including hormonal), indicators of pain. Fetuses have the neural mechanisms to transmit noxious stimuli by 20 weeks of gestation.
Children tolerate pain better than adults do.	A child's tolerance for pain increases with age. Younger children tend to rate procedure-related pain higher than older children do.
Children cannot tell you where they are hurt.	By 4 years of age, children can accurately point to the body area or mark the painful site on a drawing. Children as young as 3 years old can use pain scales, such as FACES.
Children always tell the truth about pain.	Children may not admit having pain to avoid an injection. Because of constant pain, they may not realize how much they are hurting. Children may believe that others know how they are feeling and not ask for analgesia.
Children become accustomed to pain or painful procedures.	Children often demonstrate *increased* behavioral signs of discomfort with repeated painful procedures.
Behavioral manifestations reflect pain intensity.	A child's developmental level, coping abilities, and temperament (e.g., activity level and intensity of reaction to pain) influence pain behavior. Children with more active, resisting behaviors may rate pain lower than children with passive, accepting behaviors.
Narcotics are more dangerous for children than they are for adults.	Narcotics (opioids) are no more dangerous for children than they are for adults. Addiction to opioids used to treat pain is extremely rare in children. Reports of respiratory depression in children are also uncommon. By 3 to 6 mo, healthy infants can metabolize opioids like other children.

Adapted from Hockenberry MJ, Wilson D, Winkelstein ML, et al. *Wong's nursing care of infants and children,* 7th ed. St. Louis: Mosby, 2003:1049.

- Present and past pain management strategies and their outcomes
  - Analgesic use
  - Nonpharmacologic comfort measures
- Past and present medical problems that may influence the pain and/or its management
- Medication allergies and side effects
- Relevant family history
- Current and past psychosocial issues or factors that may influence the pain and its management

Use physiologic or behavioral measures to assess pain if self-report is not available.

- Children may have difficulty verbally reporting their pain due to the following:
  - Immaturity (infants and children younger than 3 years)
  - Nonverbal or critically ill child
  - Cognitive impairment, severely emotionally disturbed, or sensory or motor impairment
  - Language of the child differs from that of the healthcare provider

- Use an age-appropriate pain rating scale (Figure 7-6). Many assessment tools are available. The same scale should be used consistently by all providers caring for the child.
- Observe the behavior and physiologic responses of the infant or child for cues regarding the intensity of pain (Figure 7-7).
  - Behavioral observations should be used for pain assessment of preverbal and nonverbal children and as an adjunct to the self-report of an older verbal child.
  - Specific behaviors associated with pain in young children include crying, facial grimaces, body posture, rigidity, changes in sleep, and consolability. Physiologic parameters evaluated in pain assessment include heart rate, ventilatory rate, oxygen saturation, restlessness, and diaphoresis.
- Because heart rate, ventilatory rate, blood pressure, and diaphoresis alter with a variety of stress-arousal events, they should not be used as measures of pain in the absence of other pain assessment methods or clinical indicators.[5]
  - Reassess behavior and vital signs after administration of an analgesic. Decreased irritability, cessation of crying, and decreased pulse, ventilations, and blood pressure are important parameters to assess when evaluating the effectiveness of pain management.
- Secure the caregiver's involvement.
  - Encourage the child's caregiver to take an active role in the assessment and management of the child's pain. The caregiver is often adept at noticing subtle changes in his or her child that could indicate pain, particularly in the preverbal or nonverbal child.
  - Studies have shown that although caregivers may be able to identify the presence of pain, they often underestimate the pain severity of others. Underestimation of pain may contribute to inadequate pain control.
- Take the cause of the pain or emotional distress into account.
  - Identify sources of anxiety or discomfort. Anxiety can increase the severity and intensity of pain and cause physical tension, which can generate pain.
  - Possible causes include the following:
    ◦ Pathology (e.g., sickle cell disease, sore throat)
    ◦ Absence of the child's caregiver, familiar toy, or blanket
    ◦ An overstimulating environment
- Take action and evaluate results.
  - Select appropriate therapeutic interventions on the basis of the initial pain assessment. The treatment goal should be complete relief of pain.

Some pain scales are difficult to use because of the length of time required for their use and their scoring complexity.

Remember that a child often regresses when stressed.

Physiologic and behavioral measures must be used with caution because discrepancies often exist between these measures and the child's self-report of pain.

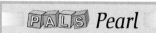

Analgesics used to manage severe pain usually cause sedation, but most sedatives do not provide analgesia.

- Therapeutic interventions may include child-parent teaching, analgesics, and nonpharmacologic techniques (e.g., coping strategies, guided visual imagery, distraction).

Sedation

Terminology

- Anxiolysis: relief of apprehension and uneasiness without alteration of awareness
- Amnesia: lack of memory about events occurring during a particular period
- Analgesia: absence of pain in response to stimulation that would normally be painful
- Anesthesia: a state of unconsciousness
- Sedation: depression of an individual's awareness of the environment and reduction of his or her responsiveness to external stimulation

Sedation: Indications

- Sedation may be used for the following[6]:
  - Help control anxiety or fear
  - Combat effects of toxic ingestions or withdrawal syndromes
  - Promote sleep
  - Decrease physical activity, metabolism, or oxygen consumption
  - Provide amnesia during procedures and neuromuscular paralysis
  - Facilitate management of mechanical ventilation
- If a procedure is not painful, a sedative is typically used. If pain is expected, analgesics are used, usually with a sedative. When selecting medications, consider the duration of action of the sedatives/analgesics and the duration of procedure.

Levels of Sedation/Analgesia

Sedation is a dose-dependent continuum from minimal sedation to general anesthesia (Table 7-15). Individual patient responses to a given dosage of a drug vary and the potential for serious adverse effects exists regardless of the medications selected or the route of administration. Because of this variation in patient response, the American Society of Anesthesiologists prefers the term *sedation-analgesia*[7] and the American College of Emergency Physicians (ACEP) uses the term *procedural sedation* instead of *conscious sedation*.

With each level of sedation/analgesia, the risk of the patient slipping into the next deeper level of sedation exists. The practitioner responsible for the procedure must have the skills and equipment necessary to safely manage patients who are sedated.

Nonpharmacologic techniques used to reduce pain and anxiety depend on the child's age, pain intensity, and abilities. Examples of nonpharmacologic techniques are listed in Table 7-16.

TABLE 7-15 *Levels of Sedation/Analgesia*

Level of Sedation/ Analgesia	Description	Comments
Minimal sedation/ analgesia	Anxiety reduction; cognitive function and coordination may be impaired Protective reflexes present Able to maintain patent airway independently and continuously Able to respond appropriately to verbal command (e.g., "Open your eyes") Ventilatory and cardiovascular functions intact	Equivalent to anxiolysis Examples of minimal sedation/analgesia include peripheral nerve blocks, local or topical anesthesia or a single, oral sedative or analgesic medication administered in doses appropriate for the unsupervised treatment of insomnia, anxiety, or pain
Moderate sedation/ analgesia	Minimally depressed level of consciousness Protective reflexes present; able to maintain patent airway independently and continuously Spontaneous ventilation is adequate Able to respond purposefully to verbal command (e.g., "Open your eyes"), either alone or accompanied by light tactile stimulation; reflex withdrawal from a painful stimulus is NOT considered a purposeful response Cardiovascular function is usually maintained	Moderate sedation/analgesia is equivalent to the term *conscious sedation* Risk of potential loss of protective reflexes exists
Deep sedation/ analgesia	Drug-induced state of depressed consciousness Cannot be easily aroused but responds purposefully following repeated or painful stimulation; reflex withdrawal from a painful stimulus is NOT considered a purposeful response Ability to maintain ventilatory function independently may be impaired Spontaneous ventilation may be inadequate Cardiovascular function is usually maintained	May be accompanied by loss of protective reflexes and ventilatory drive Assistance may be required to maintain a patent airway Positive-pressure ventilation may be required
General anesthesia	Drug-induced state of unconsciousness Unable to maintain patent airway independently Not arousable, even by painful stimulation Ability to maintain ventilatory function independently is often impaired Cardiovascular function may be impaired	Assistance often required to maintain a patent airway Positive-pressure ventilation may be required

Procedural Guidelines for Sedation and Analgesia

The following steps should be completed before beginning a procedure necessitating sedation/analgesia.

Pre-procedure Assessment

The pre-procedure assessment focuses on evaluation of the respiratory and cardiovascular systems and is performed to determine how the patient's condition might alter his or her response to sedation/analgesia.

Pharmacologic Methods of Pain Management and Sedation

TABLE 7-16 *Nonpharmacologic Methods of Pain Management*

Age	Nonpharmacologic Technique
Infant (1 to 12 mo)	Allow caregiver to remain with the child Promote relaxation with rocking, holding, light massage Allow the infant to suck on a pacifier Distract the infant with finger puppets, a rattle, plastic keys, music box, singing Cover injuries or deformities
Toddler (1 to 3 y)	Allow caregiver to remain with the child Promote relaxation with rocking, holding, light massage Distract the child with singing, listening to music, making funny faces, playing with a favorite toy, finger puppets, telling a story, using pop-up books or books with sound effects Cover injuries or deformities
Preschooler (4 to 5 y)	Allow caregiver to remain with the child Promote relaxation with rocking, holding, light massage Deep breathing exercises Cover injuries or deformities Distract the child with singing, listening to music, making funny faces, playing with a favorite toy, finger puppets, telling a story, using pop-up books or books with sound effects
School-age (6 to 12 y)	Allow caregiver to remain with the child Have the child visualize himself in a "safe" or beautiful place Deep breathing exercises Cover injuries or deformities Progressive muscle relaxation Distract the child with humor, telling stories, watching cartoons, playing games, or listening to familiar music on a tape or compact disk
Adolescent (13 to 18 y)	Allow caregiver to remain with the child, if child and caregiver desire Have the child visualize himself in a tranquil place Deep breathing exercises, rhythmic breathing Progressive muscle relaxation Distract the child with humor, watching a favorite movie, playing games, or listening to familiar music on a tape or compact disk Cover injuries or deformities

The clinician performing the procedure must obtain a history and physical examination that includes the following:

- Patient age, weight, and mental status
- AMPLE history
  - *A*llergies to food, medications, or latex
  - *M*edications (e.g., anticonvulsant medications [barbiturates, benzodiazepines], cardiac medications [digoxin, β-blockers, calcium channel blockers])

Allergies and medications may affect the choice of medications used during the procedure.

- *P*ast medical history
  - Airway abnormalities (e.g., snoring, sleep apnea)
  - History of adverse reaction to sedation/analgesia, as well as regional and general anesthesia

- History of tobacco, alcohol, or substance use or abuse
- Pregnancy status
- *L*ast oral intake (Table 7-17)
- *E*vents leading to the need for the procedure
- A focused physical examination
  - Obtain vital signs including pulse, blood pressure, ventilatory rate, and oxygen saturation.
  - Auscultate the heart and lungs.
  - Perform a general assessment of the patient's airway. Identify characteristics that suggest the possibility of a difficult tracheal intubation and/or increased risk of airway obstruction during the procedure.
  - Identify risk factors.
    - Upper respiratory infection (increased risk of upper airway obstruction due to secretions, laryngospasm)
    - Altered mental status (increased risk of tongue displacement into posterior pharynx)
    - Respiratory problems such as asthma with active wheezing (increased risk of apnea, hypoxemia, respiratory depression)
    - Cardiac disease with poor cardiac output (increased risk of hypotension, poor perfusion)

> A focused physical examination is performed to determine the patient's physiologic status and identify factors that may increase the risk of complications during the procedure.

TABLE 7-17 *American Society of Anesthesiologists Fasting Recommendations Before Elective Procedures*[a]

Ingested Material	Minimum Fasting Period
Clear liquids Examples of clear liquids: water, fruit juices without pulp, carbonated beverages, clear tea, black coffee	2 hours
Breast milk	4 hours
Infant formula	6 hours
Nonhuman milk Because nonhuman milk is similar to solids in gastric emptying time, the amount ingested must be considered when determining an appropriate fasting period.	6 hours
Light meal A light meal typically consists of toast and clear liquids. Meals that include fried or fatty foods or meat may prolong gastric emptying time. Both the amount and type of foods ingested must be considered when determining an appropriate fasting period.	6 hours

[a]These recommendations apply to healthy patients who are undergoing elective procedures. Following these recommendations does not guarantee complete gastric emptying has occurred.

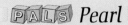
Age-appropriate and size-appropriate emergency equipment should be immediately available whenever medications capable of causing cardiorespiratory depression are administered.

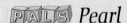
Oxygen is usually administered to patients receiving sedation/analgesia to reduce the incidence of hypoxia associated with some sedatives.

○ Seizure disorders (increased risk of depressed mental status with resultant airway and ventilation problems)

○ Newly born or young infant (increased risk of respiratory depression, apnea)

• Preprocedure laboratory testing should be guided by the patient's underlying medical condition and the likelihood that the results will affect the management of sedation/analgesia.

• Obtained informed consent.

Equipment and Personnel

Before administering a sedative or analgesic, ensure that age-appropriate and size-appropriate equipment is **immediately** available.

• Equipment
  • Visor or protective eyewear, disposable mask, and gloves
  • Length-based resuscitation tape or emergency medication sheet listing appropriate dosages for resuscitation
  • Airway equipment including oxygen and an oxygen source with regulator/flowmeter, oropharyngeal and nasopharyngeal airways, suction catheters (soft and Yankauer types), suction tubing, and a vacuum source; bag-mask with oxygen attachments and face masks of appropriate sizes; intubation equipment including laryngoscope, blades, tubes, and stylets; and pediatric laryngeal mask airways
  • IV equipment including gloves, tourniquet, alcohol wipes, gauze pads, IV catheters, tubing, and fluids; needles, syringes, and tape; intraosseous needles
  • Resuscitation medications (e.g., atropine, epinephrine) and reversal agents (e.g., naloxone, flumazenil)
  • Pulse oximeter, electrocardiogram (ECG) monitor/defibrillator capnometer
  • Noninvasive blood pressure monitor

• Personnel
  • The individual performing the procedure must have an understanding of the pharmacologic agents administered, the ability to monitor the patient's response to the medications given, and the skills necessary to intervene in managing all potential complications.
  • In addition to the individual performing the procedure, it is imperative to designate a qualified individual whose sole responsibility is to monitor the child during the procedure.
    ○ This individual must be capable of providing pediatric basic life support and be skilled in airway management and cardiopulmonary resuscitation; training in pediatric advanced life support is strongly encouraged.[8]

- ○ This individual
  - ▪ Is responsible for monitoring the child's airway patency, work of breathing, vital signs including oxygen saturation levels, mental status, circulatory status, and ECG.
  - ▪ Must be able to recognize signs of airway compromise and be able to open the child's airway, administer oxygen, and begin positive-pressure ventilation if required.
  - ▪ Should have an understanding of the pharmacologic agents administered including the role and actions of antagonists, and possible adverse effects of these agents.
  - ○ If available, another qualified individual should be designated to assist with the procedure.

Patient Monitoring and Documentation

Patient monitoring should begin before medications are administered and continue until the patient returns to his or her presedation level and recovery is complete (discharge criteria are met).

The following must be monitored and documented:

- Vital signs (pulse, blood pressure, ventilatory rate, oxygen saturation)
  - Document preprocedure (baseline) vital signs.
  - Monitor and document every 5 to 10 minutes during minimal and moderate sedation/analgesia.
  - Monitor and document at least every 5 minutes during deep sedation/analgesia.
  - Continue until the patient returns to his or her presedation level.
- Medication names, dosages, route, time, and effects of administration
- Sedation level and level of consciousness
- Airway patency, work of breathing, ventilatory pattern
- Any adverse effects including apnea, hypoxia, tachycardia or bradycardia, hypotension, and emesis
- Any necessary interventions and resolutions

Postsedation Monitoring and Discharge

Monitoring the patient in the immediate postprocedure period is imperative because the patient is at risk of complications from the medications used. Some patients may become more deeply sedated after the stimulus of the procedure is discontinued. Others may experience prolonged sedative effects because of the medications used. Children who received medications with a long half-life may require extended observation.

The patient can be discharged to a less intensely monitored level of care:

- When the patient has returned to his or her pre-procedure/pre-

TABLE 7-18 *Medications Used for Sedation/Analgesia*

Barbiturates	Sedation	Amnesia	Analgesia
	☺ ☺ ☺	–	–
Methohexital (Brevital)	Administered rectally Faster onset of action and recovery time than thiopental and twice as potent May precipitate seizures Use with extreme caution in patients in status asthmaticus Onset 5 to15 min; duration 30 to 90 min		
Pentobarbital (Nembutal)	Can increase pain perception; not useful as a sedative during painful procedures Onset IV 1 to 5 min, duration 15 to 60 min; onset IM 5 to 15 min, duration 2 to 4 h; onset PO 15 to 60 min, duration 2 to 4 h		
Thiopental (Pentothal)	Administered rectally Onset 5 to15 min; duration 60 to 90 min		

Benzodiazepines	Sedation	Amnesia	Analgesia
	☺ ☺ ☺	☺ ☺ ☺	–
Diazepam (Valium)	Sedative effects reversible with flumazenil Fat soluble Respiratory depressant effects are potentiated when administered in conjunction with opioids Slow administration decreases incidence of respiratory side effects and venous irritation Onset IV 2 to 3 min, duration 30 to 90 min; half-life about 30 h Onset per rectum 5 to 15 min, duration 2 to 4 h		
Lorazepam (Ativan)	Sedative effects reversible with flumazenil Respiratory depressant effects are potentiated when administered in conjunction with opioids IV administration can cause venous irritation Onset IV 3 to 5 min, duration 2 to 6 h Onset IM 10 to 20 min, duration 2 to 6 h Onset PO 60 min, duration 2 to 6 h		

Midazolam (Versed)	Sedative effects reversible with flumazenil
	Water soluble
	Two to four times more potent than diazepam and provides deeper sedation and more
	   amnesia than diazepam
	Respiratory depressant effects are potentiated when administered in conjunction with
	   opioids; respiratory depression is related to dosage given and rate of administration—
	   the faster the drug is given, the more likely apnea will result
	Compatible with many IV solutions and other medications; IV administration does not
	   result in venous irritation
	Onset IV 1 to 2 min, duration 30 to 60 min; onset IM 5 to 15 min, duration 30 to 60 min;
	   onset per rectum 5 to 10 min, duration 30 to 60 min; onset PO 10 min, duration 1 to 2 h		

CNS, central nervous system; IM, intramuscular; IV, intravenous; MRI, magnetic resonance imaging; NSAID, nonsteroidal antiinflammatory drug; ☺ ☺ ☺, heavy; ☺ ☺ moderate; ☺, minimal.

Continued

TABLE 7-18 *cont'd*

Opioids (Narcotics)	Sedation ☺ ☺	Amnesia –	Analgesia ☺ ☺ ☺
Fentanyl (Sublimaze)	Respiratory depression reversible with naloxone Synthetic opioid used for pain or anxiety associated with short procedures 50 to 100 times more powerful than morphine—recheck dosage carefully before administering Causes minimal or no release of histamine Infants younger than 3 mo may be more sensitive to respiratory depressant effects Respiratory depressant effects are potentiated when administered with benzodiazepines Chest wall rigidity may occur with large doses given rapidly Onset IV 2 min, duration IV 20 to 60 min; half-life about 20 min		
Morphine	Respiratory depression reversible with naloxone Used as a standard of comparison for all opioids Can stimulate histamine release Respiratory depressant effects are potentiated when administered in conjunction with benzodiazepines Hypovolemia makes the occurrence of hemodynamic side effects more common Onset IV 5 to 10 min, duration IV 2 to 4 h		

Other Agents

Chloral hydrate	Sedation ☺ ☺	Amnesia –	Analgesia –
	Sedative/hypnotic used for pediatric sedation for more than 100 y Used primarily for sedation for painless diagnostic procedures (e.g., MRI scan) Has CNS, respiratory, and cardiovascular depressant effects Increased risk of respiratory depression when administered concurrently with opioids or benzodiazepines Paradoxic agitation may occur; more likely in children with underlying developmental delays or neurologic disorders Onset PO or per rectum 15 to 30 min, duration 2 to 3 h		

Ketamine (Ketalar) *Sedation*	Sedation ☺ ☺ ☺	Amnesia ☺	Analgesia ☺ ☺ ☺
	Used for sedation during painful procedures Derivative of phencyclidine Child may appear awake with eyes open despite deep sedation May cause hypertension, hypotension, emergence reactions, tachycardia, laryngospasm, respiratory depression, and stimulation of salivary secretions Onset IV 1 to 2 min, duration 15 to 60 min; onset IM 3 to 10 min, duration 15 to 60 min		

Ketorolac (Toradol)	Sedation –	Amnesia –	Analgesia ☺ ☺ ☺
	NSAID used for moderate-to-severe pain IV route of administration in children is not yet recommended by the manufacturer, although it is well supported in the literature and in clinical practice Onset IV 10 to 15 min, duration 3 to 6 h		

CNS, central nervous system; IM, intramuscular; IV, intravenous; MRI, magnetic resonance imaging; NSAID, nonsteroidal antiinflammatory drug; ☺ ☺ ☺, heavy; ☺ ☺, moderate; ☺, minimal.

Continued

TABLE 7-18 *cont'd*

Propofol (Diprivan)	Sedation	Amnesia	Analgesia
	☺☺☺	☺	=

Used for sedation during procedures not associated with pain
Potent vasodilator, cardiac depressant, and respiratory depressant
Short duration of action necessitates administration by continuous IV infusion
Insoluble in water
Onset IV 1 to 2 min, duration 3 to 5 min

CNS, central nervous system; IM, intramuscular; IV, intravenous; MRI, magnetic resonance imaging; NSAID, nonsteroidal antiinflammatory drug; ☺☺☺, heavy; ☺☺, moderate; ☺, minimal.

sedation state with regard to his or her airway, breathing, circulation, and mental status:

- The patient is conscious and responds appropriately.
- Vital signs are stable and within acceptable limits for that patient.
- The patient's ventilatory status is not compromised.
- When the patient's pain and discomfort have been addressed
- If there are no new signs, symptoms, or problems
- If there is minimal nausea
- When hydration status is adequate
- When sufficient time (up to 2 hours) has elapsed following the last administration of reversal agents (naloxone, flumazenil) to ensure that the child does not become resedated after reversal effects have worn off.

TABLE 7-19 *Pharmacologic Antagonists (Reversal Agents)*

Agent	Remarks
Naloxone (opioid antagonist)	Effective for all opioids (narcotics). Effects of narcotics are usually longer than naloxone; thus, respiratory depression may return when naloxone has worn off. Monitor the patient closely and observe continuously for resedation for at least 2 h after the last dose of naloxone.
Flumazenil (benzodiazepine antagonist)	Effective for all benzodiazepines. Observe continuously for resedation for at least 2 h after the last dose of flumazenil. Administer as a series of small injections (not as a single bolus injection) to control the reversal of sedation to the approximate endpoint desired and minimize the possibility of adverse effects. Safety and efficacy in reversal of moderate sedation/analgesia in pediatric patients below the age of 1 y has not been established.

Common Medications used in Pediatric Emergency Care

Medication	Indication(s)	Dosage	Precautions	Special Considerations
Adenosine (Adenocard)	SVT	IV/IO: Initial dose 0.1 mg/kg (up to 6 mg) as rapidly as possible IV push followed by NS flush Second dose 0.2 mg/kg rapid IV push (maximum single dose 12 mg)	Dysrhythmias at time of rhythm conversion Use with caution in patients with asthma; severe bronchospasm has been reported in several asthmatic patients following adenosine administration Discontinue in any patient who develops severe respiratory difficulty Do not use in second-degree or third-degree heart block or sick sinus syndrome	Constant ECG monitoring is essential. Onset of action 10 to 40 sec; duration 1 to 2 min. Higher doses may be needed when a patient is taking methylxanthine preparations.
Albuterol (Proventil, Ventolin)	Bronchospasm, status asthmaticus	Nebulized albuterol (0.5% solution) 0.15 mg/kg/dose up to 5 mg diluted in 2 to 3 mL of NS Severe airflow obstruction may benefit from continuous albuterol nebulization (0.6 to 1 mg/kg/h) The patient in severe distress may require albuterol nebulizations every 20 min for up to 1 h. Repeated dosing produces incremental bronchodilation.	Watch for tachycardia, nausea, vomiting, tremor	The onset of action of inhaled bronchodilators is within 5 min. Their duration of action in severe asthma is unknown and may vary with the severity of the disease. Evaluate the patient's response to the initial inhaled albuterol treatments. Assess clinical signs of respiratory distress including pulse and ventilatory rate, oxygen saturation, and PEFR. Any deterioration may require prompt intervention.
Amiodarone (Cordarone)	Pulseless VT/VF Perfusing tachycardias—particularly ectopic atrial tachycardia, junctional ectopic tachycardia, and VT	IV/IO pulseless VT/VF: 5 mg/kg; may repeat twice up to 15 mg/kg; maximum single dose 300 mg IV/IO perfusing tachycardias: IV/IO 5 mg/kg loading dose over 20 to 60 min. Repeat as needed to max dose of 15 mg/kg/d.	Like all antiarrhythmic agents, amiodarone may cause a worsening of existing arrhythmias or precipitate a new arrhythmia. Common adverse effects include hypotension (most common), bradycardia, and AV block. Slow infusion rate or discontinue if seen. Forms a precipitate when mixed with sodium bicarbonate or heparin	The manufacturer has not established safety and efficacy in children and infants and therefore does not recommend its use in pediatric patients. Seek expert consultation before use for a patient who has a perfusing rhythm.

Medication	Indication(s)	Dosage	Precautions	Special Considerations
Atropine sulfate	Symptomatic bradycardia Anticholinesterase poisoning To reduce secretions during RSI or block reflex bradycardia induced by succinylcholine and laryngoscopy during RSI	Symptomatic bradycardia IV/IO: 0.02 mg/kg may repeat in 5 min Minimum single dose 0.1 mg. Maximum single dose 0.5 mg Tracheal: 0.04 to 0.06 mg/kg	Do not administer in less than minimum recommended dose—may cause paradoxic bradycardia (particularly in infants) with lower doses Monitor for tachycardia	Anticholinesterase poisonings may require large doses of atropine. Symptomatic bradycardia should first be treated with oxygenation and ventilation. Epinephrine is the drug of choice if bradycardia is due to hypoxia and oxygenation and ventilation do not correct the bradycardia. Give atropine before epinephrine if the bradycardia is due to increased vagal tone or if AV block is present.
Calcium chloride (10%)	Ionized hypocalcemia Hyperkalemia Hypermagnesemia Calcium channel blocker toxicity	IV/IO: 20 mg/kg (0.2 mL/kg) slowly, maximum single dose 2 g	Bradycardia with rapid IV injection. Stop administration if symptomatic bradycardia occurs. Precipitates with sodium bicarbonate. Do not administer IM or SubQ—can cause severe tissue necrosis, sloughing or abscess formation. Administration may be accompanied by peripheral vasodilation, with a moderate fall in blood pressure.	Ensure patency of IV line before administering. Monitor IV site closely. Routine administration is not recommended during cardiac arrest. Patient may experience pain, burning at the IV site, severe venous thrombosis, and severe tissue necrosis if solution extravasates. Incompatible with all medications. Flush line before and after administration.
Charcoal, activated	Acute ingestion of selected toxic substances	PO or via nasogastric tube: Children up to 1 year of age: 1 g/kg; Children 1 to 12 years: 25 to 50 g; Adolescents and adults: 25 to 100 g	Fatal hypernatremic dehydration has been reported after repeated doses of charcoal with sorbitol (a cathartic). Use products that do not contain sorbitol if repeated doses are necessary.	Iron, lithium, alcohols, ethylene glycol, alkalis, fluoride, mineral acids, and potassium do not bind to activated charcoal.

Medication	Indication(s)	Dosage	Precautions	Special Considerations
Chloral hydrate	Sedation	PO or rectally: 25 to 100 mg/kg; maximum 2 g	Avoid in liver or kidney failure Use with caution in patients with large tonsils/adenoids or other abnormalities of the upper airway Toxicity worsens when used concurrently with benzodiazepines, ethanol, or barbiturates; overdose can be fatal	Possesses CNS, respiratory, and cardiovascular depressant effects Gastric irritant Primary reason for failure of successful sedation is inadequate initial dose
Dexamethasone (Decadron)	Moderate to severe croup	IV/IM/PO: 0.6 mg/kg as a single dose (maximum dose 8 mg).	Use of corticosteroids is controversial. Some data show early treatment with dexamethasone may shorten the course and prevent the progression of croup to complete obstruction.	Further dosing and route of administration determined by clinical course.
Diazepam (Valium)	Status epilepticus Extreme anxiety or agitation	IV: 0.1 mg/kg every 2 min; maximum dose 0.3 mg/kg (maximum 10 mg/dose); administer at a rate no faster than 2 mg/min Rectal: 0.5 mg/kg up to 20 mg Onset after rectal administration is 5 to 10 min.	Do NOT give IM. Do not dilute with solutions or mix with other drugs in syringe, tubing, or IV container—incompatible. May cause local irritation when given rectally.	Does not provide analgesia Monitor oxygen saturation. Monitor IV site frequently for phlebitis, which may occur rapidly.
Digoxin (Lanoxin)	Heart failure due to poor left-sided ventricular contractility	IV digitalizing dose based on weight and age	Common adverse effects of chronic digoxin toxicity are visual disturbances and fatigue followed by weakness, nausea, loss of appetite, abdominal discomfort, psychological complaints, dizziness, abnormal dreams, headache, diarrhea, and vomiting. Visual disturbances include distorted yellow, red, and green color perception; blurred vision, and halos around solid objects.	Toxic-to-therapeutic ratio is narrow May result in toxicity in patients with hypokalemia or hypomagnesemia, because potassium or magnesium depletion sensitizes the myocardium to digoxin

Medication	Indication(s)	Dosage	Precautions	Special Considerations
Diphenhydramine (Benadryl)	Anaphylaxis Dystonic reactions	IM/IV: 1 mg/kg deep IM or slow IV push over 1 to 4 min; maximum dosage 50 mg	Should not be used in newborn or premature infants May cause hypotension. Do not give SubQ due to irritating effects.	May cause paradoxic CNS excitation, palpitations, and seizures in young children
Dobutamine (Dobutrex) infusion	Impaired cardiac contractility Cardiogenic shock	IV/IO: 2 to 20 mcg/kg/min; titrate to desired effect. For the child in shock, consider a starting dosage of 5 to 10 mcg/kg/min.	Tachycardia may occur with high doses. Other side effects include nausea, vomiting, hypertension, and hypotension. Extravasation may cause tissue ischemia and necrosis. Should only be infused via an infusion pump.	Correct hypovolemia before treatment with dobutamine. Patient response varies widely—continuously monitor ECG and blood pressure.
Dopamine (Intropin, Dopastat) infusion	Persistent hypotension or shock after volume resuscitation and stable cardiac rhythm Inadequate cardiac output Cardiogenic shock, septic shock	IV/IO: 2 to 20 mcg/kg/min; titrate to desired effect. For the child in shock, consider a starting dosage of 10 mcg/kg/min.	Gradually taper drug before discontinuing the infusion. Tachycardia, palpitations, dysrhythmias (due to increased myocardial oxygen demand) Extravasation may cause necrosis and sloughing. Should only be infused via an infusion pump.	Monitor blood pressure, ECG, and drip rate closely. Dose-related effects: **Low dose** (0.5 to 5 mcg/kg/min), mesenteric, renal, and coronary vessel vasodilation. **Moderate dose** (5 to 10 mcg/kg/min), increases myocardial contractility, and stroke volume, increasing cardiac output. **High dose** (10 to 20 mcg/kg/min), systemic vasoconstriction

Medication	Indication(s)	Dosage	Precautions	Special Considerations
Epinephrine for bronchospasm	Asthma/reactive airway disease Anaphylaxis	SVN: 0.5 mL/kg of 1:1000 (1 mg/mL) in 3 mL NS (maximum dose is 2.5 mL for 4 y or younger, 5 mL for older than 4 y) *Racemic* epinephrine 2.25% inhalation solution 0–20 kg: 0.25 mL in 2 mL with NS via nebulizer 20–40 kg: 0.50 mL in 2 mL with NS via nebulizer Above 40 kg: 0.75 mL in 2 mL with NS via nebulizer	Adverse effects include transient, moderate anxiety, apprehensiveness, restlessness, tremor, weakness, dizziness, sweating, palpitations, pallor, nausea and vomiting, headache	After inhalation, the patient's sputum may be pink in color due to a chemical reaction between mucous secretions and the epinephrine solution. Large doses of epinephrine may be required in the treatment of some anaphylactic reactions (e.g, latex allergy). A continuous epinephrine infusion may be necessary.
Epinephrine for symptomatic bradycardia and cardic arrest	Symptomatic bradycardia Cardiac arrest	IV/IO: 0.01 mg/kg (0.1 mL/kg) of 1:10,000 solution. May repeat every 3 to 5 min. Tracheal: 0.1 mg/kg (0.1 mL/kg) of 1:1000 solution Max IV/IO dose = 1 mg; max tracheal dose 2.5 mg	Should not be administered in the same IV line as alkaline solutions—inactivates epinephrine.	Tracheal absorption is unpredictable.
Epinephrine infusion	Continued shock after volume resuscitation	IV/IO: Start at 0.1 mcg/kg/min. Titrate according to patient response up to 1 mcg/kg/min.	Increases myocardial oxygen demand Check IV site frequently for evidence of tissue sloughing Extravasation may cause necrosis and sloughing. Should only be infused via an infusion pump.	Low-dose infusions (less than 0.3 mcg/kg/min) primarily produce β-adrenergic effects. Infusions above 0.3 mcg/kg/min produce a mix of β-adrenergic and α-adrenergic effects.

Medication	Indication(s)	Dosage	Precautions	Special Considerations
Etomidate (Amidate)	Sedative used in RSI	0.2 to 0.6 mg/kg (child older than 10 yrs)	Use with caution in asthmatics. Myoclonus (jerky, muscular contractions) may be seen after administration. Monitor oxygen saturation.	Possesses no analgesic or amnestic properties May cause minor pain during administration Produces little alteration in hemodynamics, cerebral blood flow, respiratory function, or coronary oxygenation Rapid onset with a very short duration of action
Fentanyl (Sublimaze)	Pain Sedative used in RSI	Pain IV: 0.5 to 2 mcg/kg Administer slowly over several minutes. Repeat dose as necessary for clinical effect. Sedation in RSI: IV: 2 to 3 mcg/kg slowly over several minutes; give 1 to 3 min before intubation	Respiratory depression is common and dose dependent; reversible with naloxone Chest wall rigidity with large doses given rapidly Do not use with MAO inhibitors Increased incidence of apnea when combined with other sedative agents, particularly benzodiazepines	Fentanyl is an opiate. 50 to 100 times more powerful than morphine but causes minimal or no release of histamine No significant cardiovascular effects at usual therapeutic doses Provide respiratory support as necessary
Flumazenil (Romazicon)	Benzodiazepine intoxication	IV: Initial dose: 0.01 mg/kg (max. dose: 0.2 mg), then 0.005–0.01 mg/kg (max. dose: 0.2 mg) given Q 1 min to a max. total cumulative dose of 1 mg. Doses may be repeated in 20 min up to a maximum of 3 mg in 1 hr.	Seizure activity after flumazenil administration has occurred in patients physically dependent on benzodiazepines and those receiving benzodiazepines for control of seizures. May precipitate acute withdrawal in dependent patients. Safety and efficacy in reversal of moderate sedation/analgesia in pediatric patients younger than 1 y have not been established.	Observe continuously for resedation for at least 2 h after the last dose of flumazenil. Administer as a series of small injections (not as a single bolus injection) to control the reversal of sedation to the approximate endpoint desired and minimize the possibility of adverse effects.
Furosemide (Lasix)	Congestive heart failure Fluid overload	IV/IO/IM: 1 mg/kg; if given IV/IO, give slowly	Potassium depletion, low blood pressure, dehydration, hyponatremia Because furosemide is a sulfonamide derivative, it may induce allergic reactions in patients with sensitivity to sulfonamides (sulfa drugs).	Monitor intake and output, daily weight, and serum electrolytes regularly. Ototoxicity and transient deafness can occur with rapid administration.

Medication	Indication(s)	Dosage	Precautions	Special Considerations
Glucose	Hypoglycemia	IV/IO: 0.5 to 1 g/kg Newborn: 5–10 mL/kg $D_{10}W$ Infants and Children: 2–4 mL/kg $D_{25}W$ Adolescents: 1–2 mL/kg $D_{50}W$	Administer through a large vein. Determine glucose levels before and during administration. Extravasation can cause severe local tissue damage.	If large volumes of dextrose are administered, include electrolytes to prevent hyponatremia and hypokalemia. Diluting a 50% dextrose solution 1:1 with sterile water or NS = $D_{25}W$. Diluting 50% dextrose solution 1:4 with sterile water or NS = $D_{10}W$.
Ipratropium bromide (Atrovent)	May be beneficial for moderate to severe exacerbations of asthma	Administered via nebulizer	Side effects include nervousness, dizziness, drowsiness, headache, upset stomach, constipation, cough, dry mouth or throat irritation, skin rash, and blurred vision.	Anticholinergic. Anticholinergics produce preferential dilation of the larger central airways, in contrast to β-agonists, which affect the peripheral airways. Onset 30 to 60 min to maximum effect.
Ketamine (Ketalar)	Sedation/analgesia Adjunct to RSI	Sedation/analgesia IM: 1 to 2 mg/kg IV: 0.5 to 1 mg/kg Adjunct to RSI IV: 1 to 2 mg/kg Rate of IV infusion should not exceed 0.5 mg/kg/min and should not be administered in less than 60 sec.	May increase blood pressure, heart rate, and oral secretions Contraindicated in eye injuries, increased intracranial pressure Emergence reactions (hallucinations, nightmares) common in children older than 11 y Higher doses and rapid IV administration can result in apnea	A PCP derivative that is rapid acting in producing a "dissociative" anesthesia Provides amnesia, analgesia, and sedation Often used for RSI in children with respiratory failure caused by asthma because this drug causes bronchodilation Monitor oxygen saturation. Be prepared to provide respiratory support.

Medication	Indication(s)	Dosage	Precautions	Special Considerations
Ketorolac (Toradol)	Moderate to severe pain	Children 2-16 years of age should receive only a single dose of Toradol injection, as follows: IM dosing: One dose of 1 mg/kg up to a maximum of 30 mg. IV: One dose of 0.5 mg/kg up to a maximum of 15 mg.	Anaphylactoid reactions may occur in patients without a known previous exposure or hypersensitivity to aspirin, ketorolac, or other NSAIDs, or in individuals with a history of angioedema, asthma, and nasal polyps.	NSAID Possesses no amnesic or sedative properties
Lidocaine	Stable ventricular tachycardia Adjunctive agent in RSI	Ventricular dysrhythmias IV/IO/: 1 mg/kg (give over 1 to 2 min), maximum dose 100 mg Adjunctive agent in RSI IV/IO/ET: 1 to 2 mg/kg Maximum IV bolus dose is 3 mg/kg.	Signs and symptoms of lidocaine toxicity are primarily CNS related (e.g., drowsiness, disorientation, muscle twitching, seizures)	Diminishes the cough and gag reflexes, and may diminish the rise in ICP associated with intubation. If indicated, administer 2 to 5 min before RSI procedure.
Lidocaine infusion	Stable ventricular tachycardia	IV/IO: 20 to 50 mcg/kg/min	Metabolized (90%) in the liver; decrease infusion rate in congestive heart failure or liver impairment (infusion rate should not exceed 20 mcg/kg/min)	If there is a delay of more than 15 min between the initial dose of lidocaine and the start of the infusion, consider giving a second bolus of 0.5 to 1 mg/kg to reestablish a therapeutic level.
Lorazepam (Ativan)	Status epilepticus Adjunct for intubation	IV/IM: 0.05 to 0.1 mg/kg Repeat doses every 10 to 15 min for clinical effect. Maximum single dose 4 mg. Onset of action IV is about 15 to 30 min, IM is 30 to 60 min	Increased incidence of apnea when combined with other sedative agents	Does not provide analgesia. Monitor oxygen saturation. Be prepared to provide ventilatory support.
Magnesium sulfate	TdP Severe asthma Documented hypomagnesemia	IV/IO: 25 to 50 mg/kg slow bolus over 10 to 20 min.; may be given faster when rhythm is TdP. Maximum dose 2 g.	Rapid administration may result in hypotension, bradycardia, and decreased cardiac contractility	While treating TdP, search for possible reversible causes of the dysrhythmia, such as an electrolyte disturbance. Monitor magnesium levels.

Medication	Indication(s)	Dosage	Precautions	Special Considerations
Methyl-prednisolone (Solu–Medrol)	Reactive airway disease Anaphylaxis Croup	Reactive airway disease/anaphylaxis IV: 1 to 2 mg/kg every 6 h Croup IV: 1 to 2 mg/kg then 0.5 mg/kg every 6 to 8 h	Rapid administration of large doses may result in hypotension and cardiovascular collapse	Contraindicated in premature infants because the Act-O-Vial system and the accompanying diluent contain benzyl alcohol. Benzyl alcohol is reportedly associated with a fatal "gasping syndrome" in premature infants.
Midazolam (Versed)	Sedative used in RSI Sedation/anxiolysis	6 mo to 5 yrs: 0.05–0.1 mg/kg; total dose up to 0.6 mg/kg 6–12 yrs: 0.025–0.05 mg/kg; total dose up to 0.4 mg/kg 12–16 yrs: 0.3–0.35 mg/kg; total dose up to 0.6 mg/kg	May cause decreased blood pressure, heart rate, respiratory depression Monitor oxygen saturation.	Midazolam is a benzodiazepine reversible with flumazenil. Possesses antianxiety, amnesic, anticonvulsant and sedating properties but possesses no analgesic properties.
Morphine sulfate	Pain "Tet spell"	IV (slowly) or IM: 0.05 to 0.1 mg/kg. Repeat dose as necessary until desired effect is achieved.	Watch closely for bradycardia, CNS depression, nausea/vomiting, respiratory depression, hypotension. Histamine release can cause bronchospasm, hypotension, and facial itching. Hypovolemia makes the occurrence of hemodynamic side effects more common.	Monitor the patient's vital signs and oxygen saturation. Be prepared to provide ventilatory support. Ensure naloxone and airway equipment is readily available before administration. Respiratory depressant effects are potentiated when administered in conjunction with benzodiazepines

Medication	Indication(s)	Dosage	Precautions	Special Considerations
Naloxone (Narcan)	Coma of unknown etiology to rule out (or reverse) opioid-induced coma Opiate-induced respiratory depression	Acute opiate intoxication IV/IO/IM/ET: If 5 y or younger or 20 kg or less: 0.1 mg/kg. If older than 5 y or more than 20 kg: 2 mg. Lower doses should be used to reverse respiratory depression that is associated with therapeutic opioid use.	May induce acute withdrawal in opioid dependency resulting in nausea, vomiting, sweating, tachycardia, increased blood pressure, tremor, seizures, or cardiac arrest. IM absorption may be erratic in the hypoperfused patient.	Effects of narcotics are usually longer than naloxone; thus, respiratory depression may return when naloxone has worn off. Monitor the patient closely and observe for at least 2 h after the last dose of naloxone.
Nitrous oxide	Moderate to severe pain	Self-administered and self-regulated by the patient who must hold the mask to the face to create an airtight seal until the pain is significantly relieved or the patient drops the mask. The child must be old enough to follow the instructions for use and large enough so that the mask creates an airtight seal. Give oxygen during intervals that nitrous oxide is not being used.	Contraindications: Unresponsive patient Inability to comply with instructions Head injury with altered mental status Abdominal pain, unless intestinal bowel obstruction has been completely ruled out Possible drug overdose Respiratory compromise or distress (pulmonary edema, pneumothorax) Otitis, air embolism, decompression sickness (expands air pockets and can exacerbate these problems) Administration by a healthcare provider or anyone other than the patient	Produces CNS depression and decreases sensitivity to all types of pain. Effects dissipate within 2 to 5 min after cessation of administration. Produces sedation and some amnesia.
Nitroprusside (Nipride) infusion	Immediate reduction of blood pressure in a hypertensive emergency or hypertensive urgency	IV: 0.5 to 8 mcg/kg/min Begin infusion at 0.1 mcg/kg/min and titrate slowly upward to desired clinical response (up to 8 mcg/kg/min).	Cover the bottle, burette, or syringe pump (but not the IV tubing) with protective foil to avoid breakdown by light. Can cause precipitous decreases in blood pressure—monitor continuously. Cyanide toxicity can result from large doses and/or prolonged infusions.	Do not mix with NS. Onset of action is 1 to 2 min. Effects stop quickly upon discontinuation of infusion. Administer via an infusion pump.

Medication	Indication(s)	Dosage	Precautions	Special Considerations
Norepinephrine (Levophed) infusion	Inadequate cardiac output Septic shock, neurogenic shock, anaphylaxis, drug overdose with significant α-adrenergic blocking effects (e.g, tricyclic antidepressants)	IV/IO: 0.1 to 2 mcg/kg/min Begin infusion at 0.1 mcg/kg/min and titrate slowly upward to desired clinical response (up to 2 mcg/kg/min).	Extravasation into surrounding tissue may cause necrosis and sloughing.	Correct volume depletion with appropriate fluid and electrolyte replacement therapy before administration of norepinephrine. Should be administered via an infusion pump into a central vein or a large peripheral vein to reduce the risk of necrosis of the overlying skin from prolonged vasoconstriction.
Oxygen	All arrest situations Hypoxemia and/or respiratory distress Carbon monoxide poisoning Shock	During cardiac or respiratory arrest, deliver positive-pressure ventilations with supplemental oxygen For the patient who has a perfusing rhythm, administer supplemental oxygen as needed to maintain an oxygen saturation level of 94% or higher	With prolonged administration of high-concentration oxygen, concern regarding toxic effects on the lungs and, in premature infants, on the eyes	Do NOT withhold oxygen if signs of hypoxemia are present.
Pancuronium (Pavulon)	Nondepolarizing agent used during RSI	IV: 0.06 to 0.1 mg/kg; 0.02 mg/kg in neonates Conditions satisfactory for intubation are usually present within 2 to 3 min of administration.	Tachycardia Contraindicated in renal failure, tricyclic antidepressant use Does not alter the level of responsiveness, provide analgesia or amnesia Monitor oxygen saturation.	Long-acting neuromuscular blocker that requires ventilatory assistance for at least 1 hour. For neonates, it is recommended that a test dose of 0.02 mg/kg be given first to measure responsiveness. Can be used when succinylcholine is contraindicated.
Pentobarbital (Nembutal)	Sedation	IV: 1 to 3 mg/kg; may repeat up to 6 mg/kg; administer at a rate no faster than 50 mg/min IM: 2 to 5 mg/kg PO: 2 to 3 mg/kg Maximum dose: 150 mg	Avoid in hypotensive or hypovolemic patients Respiratory depression is dose related	Barbiturate with an intermediate duration of action; no analgesic effects When given IV, may rapidly induce general anesthesia No advantage over phenobarbital for seizure control

Medication	Indication(s)	Dosage	Precautions	Special Considerations
Procainamide (Pronestyl)	Wide range of atrial and ventricular dysrhythmias, including SVT and VT	IV/IO: 15 mg/kg slow infusion over 30 to 60 min	Contraindicated in complete AV block in the absence of an artificial pacemaker, patients sensitive to procaine or other ester-type local anesthetics, patients with a prolonged QRS duration or QT interval because of the potential for heart block; preexisting QT prolongation/TdP; digitalis toxicity (procainamide may further depress conduction)	During administration, carefully monitor the patient's ECG and blood pressure. Observe ECG closely for increasing PR and QT intervals, widening of the QRS complex, heart block, and/or onset of TdP. If the QRS widens to more than 50% of its original width or hypotension occurs, stop the infusion.
Propofol (Diprivan)	Sedation Sedative/hypnotic used in RSI	Sedation dosage: IV: 0.5 to 1 mg/kg; may repeat in 0.5 mg/kg boluses; may give as a titrated continuous infusion of 25 to 100 mcg/kg/min RSI dosage: 2.5–3.5 mg/kg (3 to 16 years of age)	Has been associated with laryngospasm and bronchospasm Hypotension may occur, particularly in hypovolemic patients The FDA recommends propofol not be used to sedate critically ill or injured children. Contraindicated in patients with soybean or egg allergies	Lowers intracranial pressure but also decreases intracranial blood flow Potent vasodilator, cardiac depressant, and respiratory depressant A white, milky, alcohol emulsion that consists of 1% propofol, 10% soybean oil, 2.25% glycerol, and 1.25% egg lecithin—contaminates easily. Use quickly after opening.
Rocuronium (Zemuron)	Nondepolarizing agent used during RSI	IV: 0.6 to 1.2 mg/kg Satisfactory conditions for intubation usually occur 45 to 60 sec after administration.	The use of rocuronium bromide injection in pediatric patients younger than 3 mo and older than 14 y has not been studied. Ventilatory support is necessary. Monitor oxygen saturation.	Minimal effect on heart rate or blood pressure Precipitates when in contact with other medications so flush IV line before and after use Does not alter level of responsiveness or provide analgesia or amnesia
Sodium bicarbonate	Severe metabolic acidosis Tricyclic antidepressant overdose Hyperkalemia	IV/IO: 1 mEq/kg per dose slowly–administer only after ensuring ventilation is adequate.	Extravasation may lead to tissue inflammation and necrosis Do not mix with parenteral drugs because of the possibility of drug inactivation or precipitation.	Administer slowly. The solution is hyperosmotic. Routine administration is not recommended during cardiac arrest.

Medication	Indication(s)	Dosage	Precautions	Special Considerations
Succinylcholine (Anectine)	Depolarizing agent used during RSI	IV: 2 mg/kg infants/small children; 1 mg/kg older children/adolescents IM: Double the IV dose Satisfactory conditions for tracheal intubation generally occur 30 to 45 sec after IV administration and 3 to 5 min after IM administration.	Muscle fasciculations Hypertension, life–threatening hyperkalemia Increased intracranial, intraocular, intragastric pressure Contraindications for use include known or suspected hyperkalemia, penetrating eye injuries, burns or crush injuries several hours old, history of malignant hyperthermia, rhabdomyolysis.	Monitor oxygen saturation Atropine administration should be standard for all children younger than 1 year, children who are bradycardic, children younger than 5 y who are to receive succinylcholine, and adolescents who receive a second dose of succinylcholine.
Thiopental (Pentothal)	Sedative used in RSI Sedation	Dosage in RSI: IV: 2 to 4 mg/kg Dosage for sedation: 25 mg/kg rectally; maximum 1 g/dose	May cause respiratory depression, histamine release, hypotension; monitor oxygen saturation. Decreases ICP and cerebral blood flow May increase oral secretions, cause bronchospasm and laryngospasm; contraindicated in status asthmaticus	Thiopental is a short-acting barbiturate that possesses no analgesic properties. Rapid onset; short duration Cerebroprotective effect During RSI, avoid or use reduced dose (1 to 2 mg/kg) in patients with known or suspected shock or hypovolemia.
Vasopressin	Cardiac arrest	Current resuscitation guidelines do not make a recommendation for or against the routine use of vasopressin in cardiac arrest.	Tissue necrosis if extravasation occurs	Causes constriction of peripheral, coronary, and renal vessels
Verapamil (Isoptin, Calan)	SVT	IV/IO: 0.1 to 0.3 mg/kg in older children	Contraindicated in patients younger than 1 y or with ventricular dysfunction, sick sinus syndrome, second–degree or third-degree heart block, atrial fibrillation or flutter Monitor blood pressure and heart rate closely	Administer slowly and in small doses; continuous ECG monitoring is essential Extreme bradycardia and hypotension may occur if used in infants younger than 1 y; avoid use

AV, atrioventricular; ECG, electrocardiogram; ET, endotracheal; FDA, Food and Drug Administration; ICP, intracranial pressure; IM, intramuscular; IO, intraosseous; IV, intravenous; MAO, monoamine oxidase; NS, normal saline; NSAID, nonsteroidal antiinflammatory drug; PCP, phencyclidine; PEFR, peak expiratory flow rate; RSI, rapid sequence intubation; SubQ, subcutaneous; SVN, small volume nebulizer; SVT, supraventricular tachycardia; TdP, torsades de points; VF, ventricular fibrillation; VT, ventricular tachycardia.

Case Study Resolution

Pain should be assessed in *all* patients; however, the methods for assessing pain in the pediatric patient will vary according to the age of the child. In this situation, ask the child to rate his degree of discomfort using a tool such as the Wong-Baker FACES Pain Rating Scale. Observe the child's behavior and physiologic responses (e.g., heart rate, ventilatory rate, blood pressure) as adjuncts to his or her verbal statement and description of pain.

References

1. Campbell J. Pain. The Fifth Vital Sign [Presidential Address], American Pain Society, Los Angeles, CA, November 11, 1995.
2. McCaffery M, Pasero CL. When the physician prescribes a placebo. *Am J Nurs* 1998;98:52–53.
3. Max MB, Payne R, Edwards WT. *Principles of analgesic use in the treatment of acute pain and cancer pain.* 4th ed. Glenview, IL: American Pain Society; 1999.
4. Wong DL, Hess CS. *Wong and Whaley's clinical manual of pediatric nursing,* 5th ed. St. Louis: Mosby, 2000.
5. McGrath PA, de Veber LL, Hearn MT. Multidimensional pain assessment in children. In: Fields HL, Dubner R, Cervero F, eds. *Proceedings of the Fourth World Congress on pain: advances in pain research and therapy.* New York: Raven Press, 1985:387–393.
6. Sherif M, Mokhtar MS, Carlson RW. Sedation monitoring. In: Kruse JA, Fink MP, Carlson RW, eds. *Saunders manual of critical care.* Philadelphia: Elsevier, 2003, pp. 800-802.
7. Task Force on Sedation and Analgesia by Non-Anesthesiologists. Practice guidelines for sedation and analgesia by non-anesthesiologists: a report by the American Society of Anesthesiologists task force on sedation and analgesia by non-anesthesiologists. *Anesthesiology* 2002;96:1004–1017.
8. American Academy of Pediatrics Committee on Drugs. Guidelines for monitoring and management of pediatric patients during and after sedation for diagnostic and therapeutic procedures: addendum. *Pediatrics* 2002;110:836 –838.

Chapter Quiz

1. When administering medications by means of a tracheal tube you should:
   A) Continue chest compressions throughout administration of the medication.
   B) Insert a needle through the wall of the tracheal tube to administer the medication.
   C) Temporarily stop chest compressions, instill the medication down the tracheal tube, ventilate 5 times with a bag-mask device, then resume CPR.
   D) Temporarily stop chest compressions, instill the medication down the tracheal tube, ventilate the patient for a minimum of 5 minutes with a bag-mask device to ensure the drug is dispersed through the alveoli, and then resume CPR.

2. Anxiolysis is:
   A) Relief of apprehension and uneasiness without alteration of awareness.
   B) Lack of memory about events occurring during a particular period.
   C) Absence of pain in response to stimulation that would normally be painful.
   D) A state of unconsciousness.

3. The drug of choice for a stable but symptomatic child in supraventricular tachycardia is:
   A) Atropine.
   B) Amiodarone.
   C) Adenosine.
   D) Procainamide.

4. Medications used to maintain cardiac output include:
   A) Midazolam, epinephrine, and naloxone.
   B) Lorazepam, midazolam, and naloxone.
   C) Diazepam, dopamine, and dobutamine.
   D) Dopamine, epinephrine, and dobutamine.

5. The term "conscious sedation" is equivalent to:
   A) Minimal sedation/analgesia.
   B) Moderate sedation/analgesia.
   C) Deep sedation/analgesia.
   D) General anesthesia.

6. Bronchodilation and vasodilation are effects that occur with stimulation of:
   A) β-1 receptors.
   B) β-2 receptors.
   C) α-1 receptors.
   D) Dopaminergic receptors.

7. Select the **incorrect** statement regarding benzodiazepines.
   A) The respiratory depression associated with benzodiazepines may be reversed with naloxone.
   B) Benzodiazepines have potent amnestic effects.
   C) Diazepam, lorazepam, and midazolam are examples of benzodiazepines.
   D) Benzodiazepines decrease patient anxiety.

8. Activation of the parasympathetic division of the autonomic nervous system:
   A) Prepares the body for emergencies (i.e., the "fight-or-flight" response).
   B) Results in an increase in blood pressure.
   C) Results in a decrease in heart rate.
   D) Results in bronchodilation and peripheral vasoconstriction.

9. Which of the following medications should be administered first to an infant or child with severe symptomatic bradycardia that persists despite effective oxygenation and ventilation?
   A) Epinephrine.
   B) Atropine.
   C) Dopamine.
   D) Amiodarone.

10. Which of the following is **NOT** a common site used for subcutaneous injections in the pediatric patient?
    A) The lateral aspect of the upper arms.
    B) The abdomen from the costal margins to the iliac crests.
    C) The anterior thighs.
    D) The buttocks.

11. Medications used for moderate sedation/analgesia most often include:
    A) Paralytics, barbiturates, and benzodiazepines.
    B) Benzodiazepines, opioids, and barbiturates.
    C) Paralytics, barbiturates, and opioids.
    D) Paralytics, opioids, and benzodiazepines.

12. Indications for the use of amiodarone include:
    A) Asystole.
    B) Severe bradycardia.
    C) Ventricular fibrillation.
    D) Sinus tachycardia.

13. The minimum recommended single dose of atropine in the pediatric patient is:
    A) 0.03 mg/kg.
    B) 0.04 mg/kg.
    C) 0.1 mg.
    D) 1 mg.

14. What is the recommended dose of naloxone for infants and children from birth to 5 years of age (or up to 20 kg of body weight)?

A) 0.1 mg.

B) 0.1 mg/kg.

C) 2 mg.

D) 3 mg/kg.

Chapter Quiz Answers

1. C. When administering medications by means of a tracheal tube, temporarily stop chest compressions, instill the medication down the tube, ventilate several times with a bag-valve device, then resume CPR.

2. A. Anxiolysis is relief of apprehension and uneasiness without alteration of awareness. Amnesia is a lack of memory about events occurring during a particular period. Analgesia is the absence of pain in response to stimulation that would normally be painful. Anesthesia is a state of unconsciousness.

3. C. In stable patients with SVT, adenosine is the drug of choice because of its rapid onset of action and minimal effects on cardiac contractility.

4. D. Dopamine, epinephrine, and dobutamine are medications used to maintain cardiac output. Midazolam (Versed), lorazepam (Ativan), and diazepam (Valium) are benzodiazepines used for sedation. Naloxone (Narcan) is an opioid (narcotic) antagonist.

5. B. Sedation is dose-dependent continuum from minimal sedation to general anesthesia. Individual patient responses to a given dosage of a drug vary. Because of this variation in patient response, the American Society of Anesthesiologists (ASA) prefers the term "sedation-analgesia" and the American College of Emergency Physicians (ACEP) uses the term "procedural sedation" instead of "conscious sedation."

6. B. Bronchodilation and vasodilation are effects of β-2 adrenergic receptor stimulation.

7. A. The respiratory depression associated with benzodiazepines may be reversed with flumazenil. Benzodiazepines such as diazepam, lorazepam, and midazolam are sedative-hypnotic agents with potent amnestic effects that decrease patient anxiety.

8. C. Activation of the parasympathetic division of the autonomic nervous system (ANS) prepares the body for the ingestion and digestion of food, resulting in a decrease in heart rate and the strength of myocardial contractions, a decrease in blood pressure, and an increase in blood flow to the stomach and intestines. Activation of the *sympathetic* division of the ANS prepares the body for emergencies (i.e., the "fight-or-flight" response).

9. A. After oxygen, epinephrine is the first medication that should be administered to an infant or child with severe symptomatic bradycardia that persists despite effective oxygenation and ventilation.

10. D. In the pediatric patient, the most common sites used for a subcutaneous injection are the lateral aspect of the upper arms, the abdomen from the costal margins to the iliac crests, and the anterior thighs.

11. B. Medications used for moderate sedation/analgesia most often include benzodiazepines, opioids, and barbiturates. Paralytics are not routinely used for moderate sedation/analgesia.

12. C. Amiodarone may be used in the treatment of pulseless VT/VF and perfusing tachycardias – particularly ectopic atrial tachycardia, junctional ectopic tachycardia, and ventricular tachycardia.

13. C. The minimum recommended single dose of atropine in the pediatric patient is 0.1 mg.

14. B. For total reversal of narcotic effects, the recommended dose of naloxone for infants and children from birth to 5 years of age (or up to 20 kg of body weight) is 0.1 mg/kg. Smaller doses may be used if complete reversal is not required.

Trauma and Burns

8

Case Study

A 12-year-old girl has fallen from a third-story window in an apartment complex. At the scene, the child was found lying on her side on a sidewalk. Neighbors placed pillows under her head and instructed her not to move. Witnesses said she landed on her feet and then fell over, striking the concrete sidewalk.

Emergency Medical Technicians (EMTs) stabilized the child on a long backboard. She has arrived at your facility by ambulance. The child is awake. She knows her name and where she is, but does not remember the fall or events immediately preceding it. She says nothing hurts. There is an abrasion over the child's left eye, blood oozing from her left ear, and an open fracture of her left tibia/fibula.

What would you do next?

Objectives

1. Identify common mechanisms and types of injury in infants and children.
2. Explain the difference between primary and secondary brain injury.
3. Compare and contrast an epidural hematoma and subdural hematoma.
4. Explain the initial management of the patient with a head injury.
5. Explain mechanisms of injury that indicate spinal stabilization may be required.
6. Differentiate the clinical presentation of neurogenic shock from hypovolemic shock.
7. Explain the pathophysiology and initial management of a flail chest, open pneumothorax, tension pneumothorax, pulmonary contusion, and traumatic asphyxia.
8. State the immediately life-threatening and potentially life-threatening thoracic injuries.
9. Predict abdominal injuries based on blunt and penetrating mechanisms of injury.
10. Discuss mechanisms of burn injuries.
11. Identify and describe the depth classifications of burn injuries.

12. Describe how to determine the body surface area percentage of a burn injury by using the "rule of nines" and the "rule of palms."
13. Describe the initial management of a thermal burn injury.

Mechanism of Injury/Anatomic and Physiologic Considerations

Blunt trauma is the most common mechanism of serious injury in the pediatric patient.

Kinematics is the process of predicting injury patterns.

- Acute injury occurs when there is a transfer of energy from an external source to the human body that exceeds the ability of one or more body tissues to absorb that energy without loss of cellular or structural integrity.[1]
- The extent of injury is determined by the type of energy applied, how quickly it is applied, and to what part of the body it is applied.
- Recognizing the anatomic differences and injury patterns in children and the child's response to injury can assist healthcare professionals in the delivery of appropriate emergency care.
- Common childhood injuries by age group are shown in Table 8-1.
- The most common factor in acute traumatic injuries is kinetic energy (the energy of motion) and the dissipation of that energy. A child's small size and shape permits distribution of intense force over a smaller area.
- "Children are small, with less fat and elastic connective tissue, and have multiple organs in close proximity to a very pliable skeleton. Because of the smaller body mass, the transmitted injury from whatever mechanism is distributed over a smaller body that is ill-equipped to withstand this intense force, resulting in transmission of injury throughout the body and multi-system injuries in almost 50% of children with serious trauma."[2]

TABLE 8-1 *Common Childhood Injuries by Age Group*

Age Group	Common Childhood Injuries
Infant	Child abuse, burns, falls, drowning
Toddler	Burns, drowning, falls, poisonings
School-age	Pedestrian injuries, bicycle-related injuries (the most serious usually involve motor vehicles), motor vehicle occupant injuries, burns, drowning
Adolescent	Motor vehicle occupant trauma, drowning, burns, intentional trauma, work-related injuries

With the exception of burns, poisonings, and foreign bodies, trauma may be divided into two broad categories: blunt and penetrating. Because the extent and seriousness of a child's injuries may not be readily apparent on initial evaluation, knowledge of specific mechanisms of trauma is important to predict resultant injury.

- **Penetrating trauma** is any mechanism of injury that causes a cut or piercing of the skin. A penetrating injury typically results from a gunshot, stab wound, or blast injury, but may also result from a child's toy or foreign body. Penetrating trauma usually affects organs and tissues in the direct path of the wounding object.
- **Blunt trauma** is any mechanism of injury that occurs without actual penetration of the body and typically results from motor vehicle crashes (MVCs), falls, sports injuries, or assaults with a blunt object. Blunt trauma produces injury first to the body surface, and then to the body's contents resulting in compression and/or stretching of the tissue beneath the skin. The amount of injury depends on the length of time of compression, the force of compression, and the area compressed.

Motor Vehicle Crashes

MVCs include those involving automobiles, motorcycles, all-terrain vehicles, and tractors. An MVC may be classified by the type of impact. These include head on (frontal), lateral, rear end, rotational, and rollover. In an MVC, three separate impacts occur as kinetic energy is transferred

- The vehicle strikes an object.
- The occupant collides with the interior of the vehicle. This includes a seatbelt, airbag, or the dashboard.
- Internal organs collide with other organs, muscle, bone, or other supporting structures inside the body. The lungs, brain, liver, and spleen are particularly vulnerable to this trauma.
- A fourth impact may occur if loose objects in the vehicle become projectiles.

The injuries that result depend on

- The type of collision.
- The position of the occupant inside the vehicle.
- The use or nonuse of active or passive restraint systems.

Child safety seats are available in several shapes and sizes to adapt to the different stages of physical development including infant carriers, toddler seats, and booster seats. Safety seats use a combination of lap belts, shoulder belts, full body harnesses, and harness and shield apparatus to protect the child during vehicle crashes. When used properly, the restraints transfer the force of the impact from the patient's body to the restraint belts and restraint system.

An improperly worn restraint may not protect against injury in the event of a crash and may even cause injury. For example, if an infant is properly restrained in a car seat but the car seat is not properly secured to the vehicle, the infant may be ejected from the vehicle or strike various parts of the vehicle during a crash.

Predictable injuries that may occur even with proper use of a child safety seat include blunt abdominal trauma, change of speed injuries from deceleration forces, and neck and spinal injury.

Motor Vehicle/Pedestrian Crashes

Adults will typically turn away if they are about to be struck by an oncoming vehicle, resulting in lateral or posterior injuries. In contrast, a child will usually face an oncoming vehicle, resulting in anterior injuries. Factors affecting the severity of injury include

- The speed of the vehicle.
- The point of initial impact.
- Additional points of impact.
- The height and weight of the child.
- The surface on which the child lands.

Pedestrian versus MVCs have three separate phases, each with its own injury pattern.

- Initial impact (Figure 8-1)
  - Because a child is usually shorter, the initial impact of the automobile occurs higher on the body than in adults.
  - The bumper typically strikes the child's pelvis or legs (above the knees) and the fender strikes the abdomen.
  - Predictable injuries from the initial impact include injuries to the chest, abdomen, pelvis, or femur.
- Second impact (Figure 8-2)
  - The second impact occurs as the front of the vehicle's hood continues forward and strikes the child's thorax. The child is thrown backward, forcing the head and neck to flex forward.
  - Depending on the position of the child in relation to the vehicle, the child's head and face may strike the front or top of the vehicle's hood. An impression from the child's head may be left on the hood or windshield. Primary and contrecoup injuries to the head are common in this situation.
  - Predictable injuries from the second impact include facial, abdominopelvic, and thoracic trauma and head and neck injury.
- Third impact (Figure 8-3)
  - The third impact occurs as the child is thrown to the ground.
  - Because of the child's smaller size and weight, the child may:

In the United States, left-sided injuries are more common because automobiles are driven on the right side of the road.

The injury pattern experienced by a child involved in a pedestrian injury is referred to as Waddell triad because the child experiences (a) extremity trauma, (b) thoracic and abdominal trauma, and (c) head trauma.

The velocity of a motor vehicle need be only 40 miles per hour for the force of the impact to knock a child out of his shoes.[1]

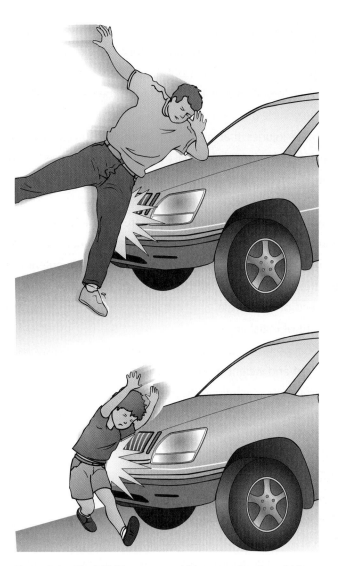

Figure 8-1   The initial impact on a child occurs when the vehicle strikes the child's upper leg or pelvis.

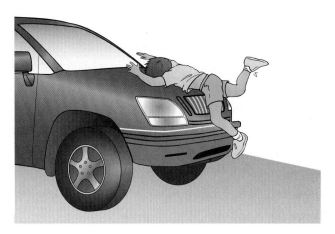

Figure 8-2   The second impact occurs when the child's head and face strike the top of the vehicle's hood.

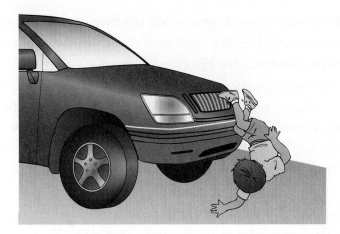

Figure 8-3   The third impact occurs as the child is thrown to ground. The child may fall under vehicle and be trapped and dragged for some distance, fall to side of vehicle and the child's lower limbs run over by a front wheel, or fall backward and end up completely under the vehicle.

- Fall under the vehicle and be trapped and dragged for some distance.
- Fall to the side of the vehicle and the child's lower limbs are run over by a front wheel.
- Fall backward and end up completely under the vehicle. In this situation, almost any injury can occur (e.g., run over by a wheel, being dragged).

Falls

- Falls are the single most common cause of injury in children. Factors to consider in a fall include the following:
  - The height from which the child fell.
  - The mass of the child.
  - The surface the child landed on.
  - The part of the child's body that struck first.
- In general, the greater the height from which the child falls, the more severe the injury. However the type of surface onto which the child falls (concrete and trash are the most common) and the degree to which the fall is broken on the way down affect the type and severity of injuries.
- The average age of patients injured in falls from heights is approximately 5 years. Infants fall from low objects such as changing tables, high chairs, countertops, and beds. Preschool children usually fall from windows. Older boys fall from dangerous play areas, such as rooftops and fire escapes.[3]
- Children younger than 3 years are much less likely to have serious injuries than are older children who fall the same distance. It is thought that younger children may better dissipate the energy transferred by the fall because they have more fat and cartilage and less muscle mass than older children.[4]

- Fatalities occur primarily when a child falls from a height of more than two stories or 22 feet (e.g., a fall from a roof, window, or balcony), or when the head of a child hits a hard surface (e.g., concrete).

- Because witnessed falls of two stories or less usually do not result in serious injury, consider the possibility of child abuse in a child with serious injuries from a fall that was reportedly from a low height, particularly if the fall was unwitnessed.[3] Some children jump to avoid beatings or fires, and some are pushed by siblings or parents.[5]

Falls from greater heights tend to occur in warm weather, probably because windows are more likely to be open.

- Most severe and fatal bicycle injuries involve head trauma. Other injuries associated with bicycle crashes include facial and extremity trauma and abdominal injuries (from striking the handle bars).

- The use of helmets can reduce the risk of head injury. A helmet absorbs some of the energy and dissipates the blow over a larger area for a slightly longer time. The skull provides another layer of protection and absorbs additional energy.[6]

- Studies indicate that helmets are very effective, reducing the risk of head injury by 85% and serious brain injury by 88%.[7] Helmets also protect against injuries to the mid and upper face.

- All young children should wear a bicycle helmet, whether they are riding a bicycle, tricycle, or are a passenger on a parent's bicycle. Bicycle helmets for children ages 1 to 5 cover a larger portion of the head than helmets for older individuals.

Bicycle Injuries

Assessment of the Pediatric Trauma Patient

Detailed information regarding patient assessment has been discussed in a previous chapter. Specific points to consider during assessment of the pediatric trauma patient are presented here.

On arrival, assess the scene for safety, mechanism of injury, and other victims. Ensure the scene is safe before proceeding with your assessment of the patient.

Scene Safety

From a distance, use the Pediatric Assessment Triangle (PAT) to the child's appearance, work of breathing, circulation, and the presence of obvious injuries to determine the severity of the child's injury and assist you in determining the urgency for care. If the child's condition is urgent, proceed immediately with rapid assessment of airway, breathing, and circulation. Treat problems as you find them.

The Pediatric Assessment Triangle

Primary Survey

Airway and Cervical Spine Protection

- Assume spinal injury if the child is unresponsive or has an altered mental status, has experienced blunt trauma above the nipple line, has a significant mechanism of injury, complains of neck or back pain, numbness or tingling, loss of movement or weakness, or if the child has multiple injuries of any cause.

- If cervical spine injury is suspected (by examination, history, or mechanism of injury), manually stabilize the head and neck in a neutral in-line position or maintain spinal stabilization if already completed.

  - If the patient is not already stabilized, do not take the time to apply a cervical collar until the primary survey is finished. Maintain manual in-line cervical spine stabilization throughout the assessment and management of the patient until cervical spine injury has been ruled out or until the patient has been properly secured to a backboard.

  - Do NOT apply traction to the neck. In a child with possible cervical spine trauma, the application of traction can exacerbate an existing injury or convert a stable cervical fracture to an unstable fracture. If an attempt to move the head and neck into a neutral in-line position results in any of the following, STOP any movement and stabilize the head in that position.
    - Compromise of the airway or ventilation.
    - Neck muscle spasm.
    - Increased pain.
    - Onset or increase of a neurologic deficit such as numbness, tingling, or loss of motor ability.

- The prominent occiput of infants and young children often causes passive flexion of the neck when the child is placed in a supine position on a flat surface (Figure 8-4). Flexion of the neck may compromise air exchange or aggravate an existing spinal cord injury.

- To maintain the cervical spine in a neutral position, it is often necessary to place padding under the child's torso. The padding should be firm, evenly shaped, and extend from the shoulders to the pelvis (Figure 8-5). Use of irregularly shaped or insufficient padding or placing padding only under the shoulders can result in movement and misalignment of the spine.

- If the child is unresponsive and trauma is suspected, use the jaw-thrust without head tilt maneuver to open the airway. If the airway is open, move on to evaluation of the patient's breathing. If the airway is not open, assess for sounds of airway compromise (snoring, gurgling, or stridor). Look in the mouth for blood, broken teeth, gastric contents, and foreign objects (e.g., loose teeth, gum). Suction as needed.

For an infant or small child, the padding should be of appropriate thickness so that the child's shoulders are in horizontal alignment with the ear canal.

If blood, vomitus, or other secretions are visible, suction the oropharynx with a rigid (tonsil tip) suction catheter before manually opening the airway.

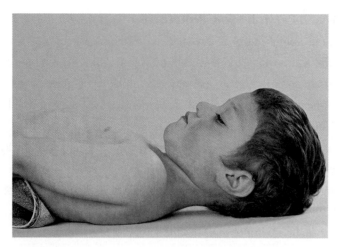

Figure 8-4   The prominent occiput of an infant or young child often causes passive flexion of the neck when the child is placed in a supine position on a flat surface.

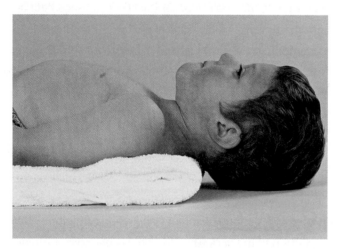

Figure 8-5   To maintain the cervical spine in a neutral position, it is often necessary to place padding under the torso of an infant or young child. The padding should be of appropriate thickness so that the child's shoulders are in horizontal alignment with the ear canal.

- Insert an oropharyngeal airway (OPA) as needed to maintain an open airway.
  - Use of a nasopharyngeal airway (NPA) is not recommended if trauma to the mid-face is present or in cases of a known or suspected basilar skull fracture. If a basilar or cribriform plate fracture is present, the NPA may enter the cranial vault during insertion.
- Perform tracheal intubation if airway patency cannot be maintained by other means.
  - Rapid sequence intubation (RSI) should be considered for those

patients in whom intubation may otherwise be difficult due to combativeness, seizures, clenched teeth, or posturing.

- RSI provides a controlled method of achieving airway access while limiting the risk of complications, such as aspiration of stomach contents.

Intubation can be performed with simultaneous in-line stabilization of the cervical spine.

- Indications for tracheal intubation in the injured child include the following:[8]
  - Inability to ventilate the child by bag-mask methods.
  - The need for prolonged control of the airway.
  - Prevention of aspiration in a comatose child.
  - The need for controlled hyperventilation in patients with serious head injuries.
  - Flail chest with pulmonary contusion.
  - Shock unresponsive to fluid volume replacement.
- After intubation, remember to confirm placement of the tracheal tube with both assessment methods and at least one mechanical method (e.g., end-tidal carbon dioxide [ETCO$_2$], chest radiograph).
- Although rarely necessary in the pediatric patient, cricothyroidotomy may be necessary if less invasive airway methods have been unsuccessful. Needle cricothyroidotomy is preferred over surgical cricothyroidotomy in a child younger than 10 years.

Breathing

Gastric distention is a cause of ventilatory compromise that is frequently overlooked.

Expose the child's chest and abdomen. Look for surface trauma, penetrating wounds, paradoxic motion, and retractions. If the patient is breathing, determine if breathing is adequate or inadequate.

Look at the rate and depth of breathing.

- Assess the chest and abdomen for ventilatory movement.
- Evaluate the depth (tidal volume) and symmetry of movement with each breath.
- Determine if the patient's ventilatory rate is within normal limits for the child's age.

Listen for the presence and quality of bilateral breath sounds and briefly listen to heart sounds.

- To minimize the possibility of sound transmission from one side of the chest to the other, listen along the midaxillary line (under each armpit) and in the midclavicular line under each clavicle. Alternate from side to side and compare your findings.
- Briefly listen to heart sounds to establish a baseline from which to compare (e.g., development of muffled heart sounds).

Feel for air movement from the nose or mouth against your chin, face, or palm. Palpate the chest for tenderness, instability, and crepitation. Assess for the presence of respiratory distress/failure. Note signs of increased work of breathing (ventilatory effort).

If breathing is adequate, provide supplemental oxygen and move on to assessment of circulation. If breathing is inadequate:

- Ensure the airway is clear of blood, vomitus, and foreign material.
- Provide supplemental oxygen and, if necessary, positive-pressure ventilation.
- Ensure the patient's chest wall rises with each ventilation. Continue the primary survey.

If breathing is absent but a pulse is present:

- Insert an airway adjunct (if not previously done and not contraindicated) and ventilate with a pocket mask or bag-mask with supplemental oxygen.
- Ensure the patient's chest wall rises with each ventilation. Continue the primary survey.

If an open pneumothorax is present (i.e., sucking chest wound), cover the wound with a sterile occlusive dressing taped on three sides (Figure 8-6). If signs of a tension pneumothorax are present, needle decompression is indicated.

All injured children should receive supplemental oxygen when indicated. Attempt to keep the SpO_2 at 94% or higher.

Circulation and Bleeding Control

Rapidly assess the child for signs of shock.

- Look for visible external hemorrhage.
  - Control major bleeding, if present. Apply direct pressure over the bleeding site with sterile dressings.
- Consider possible areas of major internal hemorrhage.
  - Significant internal hemorrhage may occur in the chest, abdomen, pelvis, retroperitoneum, and femoral areas. Pain or swelling in any of these areas may signal possible internal hemorrhage.

Heart rate, capillary refill (in children younger than 6 years), and mental status are signs that are particularly helpful in detecting shock.

Internal bleeding should be suspected if the child shows signs of shock but there is no evidence of external volume loss.

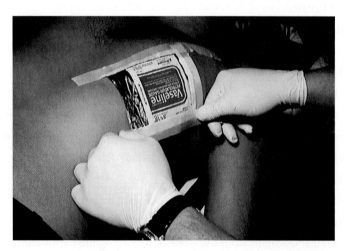

Figure 8-6   If an open pneumothorax is present (i.e., sucking chest wound), cover the wound with a sterile occlusive dressing taped on three sides.

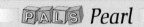 Pearl

In an injured patient, tachycardia may be a compensatory response to hypovolemia, but may also be a response to fear, pain, anxiety, or stress. Prolonged capillary refill and cool extremities may indicate poor perfusion, but may also occur as a result of fright or cold weather. Be sure to correlate your patient's vital signs with your assessment findings when considering your treatment plan.

PALS Pearl

Thoracic Injuries
Immediately life-threatening injuries that must be identified and managed in the primary survey include the following:
• Airway obstruction
• Open pneumothorax
• Tension pneumothorax
• Massive hemothorax
• Flail chest
• Cardiac tamponade

Before applying the cervical collar, assess the neck veins and palpate the position of the trachea to determine if it is in a midline position.

• Compare the strength and quality of central and peripheral pulses.
  • If a pulse is absent, begin chest compressions immediately and consider possible causes of the arrest (e.g., hypovolemia, tension pneumothorax, cardiac tamponade). Begin appropriate interventions.
  • If a pulse is present, determine if the patient's heart rate is within normal limits for the child's age. Note the quality of the pulse (thready, bounding, weak, or irregular).
• Evaluate skin color, temperature, moisture, and capillary refill.

If signs of shock are present, establish vascular access. If decompensated shock is present, establish access in two sites using large-bore catheters. In the field, the presence of shock in an infant or child indicates rapid stabilization and transport are needed immediately. Obtain intravenous (IV) or intraosseous (IO) access quickly or on the way to an appropriate receiving facility. Transport must not be delayed for multiple vascular access attempts at the scene. Begin fluid resuscitation with 20 mL/kg of an isotonic crystalloid solution (e.g., normal saline or Ringer's lactate).

Disability (Mental Status)

Use the Glasgow Coma Scale (GCS) modified for pediatric use (see Chapter 2) to assess the patient's neurologic status and document the patient's progress over time.

Avoid vague terms such as "lethargic" or "obtunded" when describing a patient's level of responsiveness. Use descriptive phrases that describe the child's awareness of his or her environment and the appropriateness of his or her response. For example, "cries vigorously and fights attempts at venipuncture."

Expose/Environment

Undress the patient. Preserve body heat and maintain appropriate temperature. Respect the child's modesty. Keep the child covered if possible and replace clothing promptly after examining each body area.

Cervical Spine stabilization

• After completing the primary survey, apply a rigid cervical collar if a device of appropriate size is available. Maintain the neck in a neutral position before and during application of the collar. A rigid cervical collar should be applied *only if it fits properly*. Estimate the distance between the angle of the jaw and the top of the shoulder and use a collar of that width. The collar should be measured in width from the top of the shoulder to the chin when the head is in a neutral position.
• A collar that is too tight may cause airway compromise or compress the veins of the neck, causing circulatory compromise. A collar that is too loose may accidentally cover the anterior chin, mouth, and nose, resulting in an airway obstruction. A collar that is too short will permit

significant flexion, ineffectively limiting motion. A collar that is too large may cause hyperextension or full motion if the chin is inside of it, or push the jaw posteriorly, occluding the airway.

- If a properly fitting device is not available, use towels, washcloths, or blanket rolls (depending on the child's size) and adhesive tape across the forehead to stabilize the head as best as possible. Avoid the use of IV bags or sand bags; their weight may push the cervical spine out of alignment.

Possible contraindications for spinal stabilization include the following:[9]

- Combative child
  - Efforts to forcefully stabilize a combative child with a possible head or spinal injury may result in further manipulation of the spine and exacerbate the injury.
  - If the risks of agitation and increased spinal movement from full spinal stabilization are greater than the benefits, defer the stabilization procedure and consider other stabilization options. For example, enlist the assistance of the child's parent or caregiver to hold the child in a position the child can tolerate that has a neutral effect on the spine and minimizes movement.
- Penetrating foreign body to the neck with hemorrhage.
- Massive cervical swelling.
- Presence of a tracheal stoma that is integral to the management of the patient's airway.
- Requirement for any maneuver to ensure adequate oxygenation and ventilation.

> If full spinal stabilization is indicated but not performed, be sure to clearly document the circumstances in the patient's medical record.

> Manual stabilization is better in these situations.

Transfer/Transport Decision

At the end of the primary survey, you should have sufficient information to make important decisions about your patient's care.

- In the field, it is important to remember that definitive care for a trauma patient requires physician evaluation of the patient at an appropriate facility. With this in mind, limit scene time to 10 minutes or less if the patient's condition is critical. The patient should be rapidly packaged after initiating essential field interventions and transported to the closest appropriate facility.
- In an urgent care or hospital setting, the physician evaluating the patient should determine if the patient requires transfer to another facility for definitive care. If this decision is made, additional patient care and evaluation can be performed while preparations are made for the patient's transfer. Communication between the referring physician and receiving physician is essential.

PALS Pearl

When used alone, a rigid cervical collar does not stabilize. A rigid collar is used to
- Temporarily splint the head and neck in a neutral position
- Limit movement of the cervical spine
- Support the weight of the head while the patient is in a sitting position
- Help maintain alignment of the cervical spine when

the patient is in a supine position
- Remind the patient and healthcare professionals that the integrity of the patient's cervical spine is questionable because of the mechanism of injury

For effective stabilization, a rigid collar must be used with manual stabilization or mechanical stabilization provided by a suitable spine stabilization device.

PALS Pearl

Spinal Stabilization: Indications
- Mechanisms of injury involving blunt or penetrating trauma directly to the spine or forces applied to the spine involving flexion, extension, or rotation of the head and neck (e.g., sports injuries, falls from heights)
- If the mechanism of injury may have resulted in rapid, forceful head movement
- Consider in any child with an altered mental status

and no history available, found in setting of possible trauma, or near drowning with history or probability of diving
- Neurologic deficit in the arms or legs
- Significant helmet damage
- Local tenderness or deformity in the cervical, thoracic, or lumbar region

Pediatric Trauma Score

The Pediatric Trauma Score (PTS) is a scoring tool used to evaluate the severity of injury in the pediatric patient and assist in pediatric triage decisions. The PTS consists of six parameters that are evaluated during the initial assessment of an injured child. Each parameter is assessed and given a numeric score based on three variables: +2 (no injury or non–life threatening), +1 (minor injury or potentially life-threatening), or –1 (life-threatening). The scores are then added together. Children with a PTS less than 8 should be treated in a designated trauma center.

Secondary Survey

In the prehospital setting, perform the secondary survey en route to an appropriate facility if you have a priority (critical) patient. If the patient is stable, the secondary survey can be performed on the scene; however, factors such as time of day, traffic and weather conditions, and distance from an appropriate receiving facility may affect your decision to do so.

Potentially life-threatening injuries that must be identified and for which treatment must begin in the secondary survey include pulmonary contusion, myocardial contusion, aortic disruption, traumatic diaphragmatic rupture, tracheobronchial disruption, and esophageal disruption.

TABLE 8-2 *Pediatric Trauma Score*

Clinical Category	Score		
	+2	+1	−1
Size	Child/adolescent Above 20 kg (44 lb)	Toddler 10-20 kg (22–44 lb)	Infant Less than 10 kg (22 lb)
Airway	Patent; no assistance required	Maintainable by patient but observation needed to ensure adequate airway (e.g., positioning, suctioning)	Unmaintainable; airway devices needed to maintain airway (e.g., oral airway, tracheal tube, cricothyroidotomy)
Mental status (AVPU)	Awake; no loss of consciousness	Obtunded; responds to Verbal or Painful stimulus; any loss of consciousness	Coma, Unresponsive, decerebrate
Systolic blood pressure (or central pulse)	Above 90 mm Hg Good peripheral pulses	50-90 mm Hg Weak carotid/femoral pulse palpable	Below 50 mm Hg Very weak or no pulses
Skeletal (fractures)	None seen or suspected	Single closed fracture anywhere or suspected	Open or multiple fractures
Open wounds	No visible injury	Minor contusion, abrasion, laceration smaller than 7 cm not through fascia, burns less than 10% and not involving hands, face, feet, or genitalia	Major/penetrating; tissue loss, any gunshot wound or stab through fascia; burns more than 10% or involving hands, face, feet, or genitalia

Scoring: 9-12 minor trauma; 6-8, potentially life-threatening; 0-5 life-threatening; below 0, usually fatal.
Adapted from Tepas JJ III, Mollitt DL, Talbert JL. The pediatric trauma score as a predictor of injury severity in the injured child. *J Pediatr Surg* 1987; 22; 14–18.

Focused History

In addition to the SAMPLE history, consider the following questions when obtaining a focused history for a pediatric trauma patient. This list will require modification based on the patient's age, mechanism of injury, and patient's chief complaint.

Remember to use age-appropriate language when asking questions of the patient.

Mechanism of injury

• How did the injury occur? When?

• Circumstances of the incident: Does the explanation for how the trauma occurred fit the injury and the child's abilities?

Fall injury

• Height of the fall?

• What type of surface did the child land on?

Motor vehicle crash

- Site of impact (e.g., lateral, frontal)? Estimated speed? What was struck (e.g., moving or stationary object)? Amount of damage to the vehicle?
- Where was the child located in the vehicle? Was the child restrained? Was the child's safety seat properly secured?
- Was the vehicle equipped with an air bag? If so, did the air bag deploy (open)?
- Ejected from the vehicle? Prolonged extrication required? Scene fatalities?

Pedestrian injury

- If the child was struck by a car and thrown while walking, roller-skating, or bicycling, was a helmet worn? If so, is it still in place or was it knocked off the head on impact? Is there damage to the helmet?
- How fast was the car traveling?
- Where was the child struck?
- How far was the child thrown?
- What type of surface did the child land on?

Bicycle injury

- If struck by a motor vehicle, was the vehicle moving or stationary? If moving, estimated speed?
- Was the child wearing a helmet? If so, is it still in place or was it knocked off the head on impact? Is there damage to the helmet?

Burns

- Location of the burn?
- What caused the burn (e.g., fire, scalding, electrical shock, chemicals)?
- How long ago did the injury occur?
- What treatment has been given?

Penetrating trauma

- Location of the wound(s)?
- Type/caliber/velocity of the weapon.
- Distance from which the child was shot (close range or long range) or stabbed?
- Presence of powder burns surrounding the wounds?
- Number of shots or stab wounds?
- Estimated blood loss at the scene?

Chronology

- Initial Glasgow Coma Scale score?
- Behavior immediately after the incident (e.g., crying, stunned, seizure, unconscious)?
- Loss of consciousness immediately or shortly after the incident? Duration?
- Any breathing problems following the injury?

Physical Examination

A detailed physical examination is presented here; however, a focused physical examination may be more appropriate, based on your patient's presentation and chief complaint.

- Obtain vital signs, attach a pulse oximeter, electrocardiogram (ECG) monitor, and blood pressure (BP) monitor. Evaluate the information obtained and determine if it is within normal range for the patient's age.
- Inspect and palpate each of the major body areas for DCAP-BLS-TIC (**D**eformities, **C**ontusions, **A**brasions, **P**enetrations/punctures, **B**urns, **L**acerations, **S**welling/edema, **T**enderness, **I**nstability, **C**repitus).

Head and Face

- Inspect the scalp and skull for DCAP-BLS. Palpate for DCAP-BLS-TIC, depressions, or protrusions.
  - In a child younger than 14 months, gently palpate the anterior and posterior fontanelles. Feel for any bulging beyond the level of the skull. A bulging fontanelle in a quiet infant may indicate increased intracranial pressure (ICP).
  - Assess for other signs of a head injury. If brain tissue is visible, cover it with a saline-moistened sterile dressing.
- Inspect the ears for DCAP-BLS, postauricular ecchymosis (Battle sign), and blood or clear fluid in the ears. Palpate for tenderness or pain.
- Inspect the face for DCAP-BLS, singed facial hair, and symmetry of facial expression. Palpate the orbital rims, zygoma, maxilla, and mandible for DCAP-BLS-TIC, neurovascular impairment, muscle spasm, false motion, or motor impairment.
- Inspect the eyes for DCAP-BLS, foreign body, blood in the anterior chamber of the eye (hyphema), presence of eyeglasses or contact lenses, periorbital ecchymosis (raccoon eyes), color of sclera and conjunctiva, periorbital edema, pupils (size, shape, equality, reactivity to light), and eye movement (dysconjugate gaze, ocular muscle function).
- Inspect the nose for DCAP-BLS, blood or fluid from the nose, singed nasal hairs, and nares for flaring. Palpate the nasal bones.
- Inspect the mouth for DCAP-BLS, blood, absent or broken teeth, gastric contents, foreign objects (e.g., loose teeth, gum, small toys); injured or swollen tongue; color of the mucous membranes of the mouth; note presence and character of fluids and vomitus; and note sputum color, amount, and consistency (Figure 8-7). Listen for hoarseness and inability to talk. Note unusual odors (e.g., alcohol, acetone, almonds).

Neck

- Inspect the neck for DCAP-BLS, neck veins (flat or distended), use of accessory muscles, presence of a hematoma, presence of a stoma, and presence of a medical identification device.

A scalp laceration can result in significant blood loss in an infant or child. If present, control bleeding as quickly as possible.

In a trauma patient, unequal or fixed and dilated pupils suggest severe brain injury.

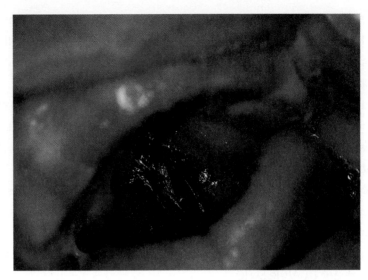

Figure 8-7   This infant's soft palate was shredded by repeated stabs with a sharp object. He presented with a report of spitting up blood and no history of trauma.

- Palpate for DCAP-BLS-TIC, subcutaneous emphysema, and tracheal position. Subcutaneous emphysema feels like "Rice Krispies" or bubble wrap.

Chest

- Inspect the chest. Assess work of breathing, symmetry of movement, use of accessory muscles, and presence of retractions. Note abnormal breathing patterns, DCAP-BLS, and presence of vascular access devices.
- Auscultate the chest. Assess the equality of breath sounds and presence of adventitious breath sounds (e.g., crackles, wheezes). Evaluate heart sounds for rate, rhythm, murmurs, bruits, gallops, friction rub, and muffled heart tones.
- Palpate for DCAP-BLS-TIC, chest wall tenderness, symmetry of chest wall expansion, and subcutaneous emphysema.

Abdomen, Pelvis, and Genitalia

Intraabdominal bleeding is a common cause of reversible shock.

- Inspect the abdomen for DCAP-BLS, distention, scars from healed surgical incisions or penetrating wounds, feeding tubes, use of abdominal muscles during respiration, signs of injury, discoloration, tire marks, and signs of seatbelt injury.
- Auscultate the presence or absence of bowel sounds in all quadrants.
- Palpate all four quadrants for DCAP-BLS, guarding or distention, rigidity, and masses.
- In the hospital setting, examine the perineum for lacerations, hematomas, or active bleeding and examine the rectum for integrity of the wall, muscle tone, prostatic injury, and occult gastrointestinal bleeding.
- Assess the integrity of the pelvis.
  - First, gently palpate for point tenderness.

- Next, place your hands on each iliac crest and press gently inward. If pain, crepitation, or instability is elicited, suspect a fracture of the pelvic ring. No further assessment is necessary if this assessment reveals positive findings.
- If this assessment is negative, simultaneously push down on both iliac crests. Then place one hand on the pubic bone (over the symphysis pubis) and apply gentle pressure.

Extremities

Examine each extremity for the five P's: pain, pallor, paralysis, paresthesia, and pulses. Compare an injured extremity to an uninjured extremity and document your findings.

Assess and document pulses, motor function, and sensory function before and after splinting.

- Inspect each extremity for DCAP-BLS and abnormal extremity position.
- Palpate for DCAP-BLS-TIC.
  - Assess skin temperature, moisture, and capillary refill in each extremity.
  - Assess the strength and quality of pulses, motor function, and sensory function (PMS) in each extremity.
  - If the child is alert, assess sensation by lightly touching the extremity and asking, "Do you feel me brushing your skin? Where?"
  - Assess motor function in an upper extremity in an alert patient by instructing the child to "Squeeze my fingers in your hand." To assess motor function in a lower extremity, instruct the child to "Push down on my fingers with your toes."
  - When assessing a child's sensory function, carefully consider the method you will use. A pinch in a child may result in more distress, distrust, and/or a lack of cooperation. Consider a less distressing method such as, "Can you feel my hand touching your toes?"

Posterior Body

Ensure manual in-line stabilization of the head and spine during examination of the posterior body.

- Inspect the posterior body for DCAP-BLS, purpura, petechiae, rashes, and edema.
- Auscultate the posterior thorax.
- Palpate the posterior trunk for DCAP-BLS.

Head Trauma

The head of the pediatric patient is vulnerable to injury because of the following:

- The skull of an infant and child is thin and pliable and is more likely to transfer force to the brain beneath it instead of fracturing and absorbing some of the force along the fracture line.
- The disproportionately large size and weight of the head adds to the momentum of acceleration-deceleration forces and accounts for the fact that infants and children tend to "lead with their head" when falling or when thrown (whether bodily or ejected from a motor vehicle).
- Underdeveloped cervical ligaments, relatively weak neck muscles, and anteriorly wedged cervical vertebrae make an infant susceptible to extreme hyperflexion and hyperextension of the neck and greater head motion when subjected to acceleration-deceleration forces.[10]

Brain Perfusion

CPP = MAP − ICP

Edema, hypotension, and bleeding can interfere with CPP.

Maintenance of an adequate blood volume and BP is critical for brain perfusion. If the BP is reduced, so is cerebral perfusion pressure (CPP).

- CPP is determined by the difference between mean arterial blood pressure (MAP) and ICP.
- A mechanism called autoregulation regulates the body's BP to maintain CPP. It is generally believed that attempts to maintain the CPP above 70 mm Hg improves outcome; however, there are no systematic scientific studies to validate this.[11]
- The brain can compensate for changes in ICP by manipulating one of three major components of the skull (a decrease in any one of these will lower ICP):
  - Brain tissue (occupies 78% of the skull).
  - Blood volume (occupies 12%).
  - Cerebrospinal fluid (CSF) (occupies 10%).
- Increases in ICP cause characteristic changes in vital signs including hypertension, bradycardia, and an irregular breathing pattern (Cushing triad). Cushing's triad is a LATE sign of increased ICP; however, the absence of Cushing's triad does not rule out the presence of increased ICP.

General Categories of Injury

- Coup injuries: injury directly below point of impact.
- Contrecoup injuries: injury at another site, usually opposite the impact.
- Diffuse axonal injury (DAI): shearing, tearing, stretching force of nerve fibers with axonal damage.
- Focal injury: an identifiable site of injury limited to a particular area or region of the brain.

Primary (direct) injury

- Refers to the direct damage incurred during the actual injury/impact to the head.
- Damage resulting in dysfunction occurs to the scalp and skull, neurons, axons, and blood vessels.
- Examples of primary injuries include skull fractures, concussions, contusions, lacerations, axon-shearing injuries, and neuronal and vascular damage.

Secondary or tertiary (indirect) injury

- Secondary injury: The result of metabolic events precipitated by the trauma that produce damage to the brain minutes, hours, or days after the initial event.
  - Examples of secondary injuries include cerebral ischemia and brain edema, which may result from systemic hypotension, hypercapnia, and hypoxemia.
  - Vasospasm, seizures, meningitis, and hydrocephalus may also produce secondary injury.
- Tertiary injury: Caused by apnea, hypotension, pulmonary resistance, and change in ECG.

Concussion (Mild Diffuse Axonal Injury)

- A brain insult with transient impairment of consciousness followed by rapid recovery to baseline neurologic activity.
- Most common result of blunt trauma to the head.
- Infrequently associated with structural brain injury and rarely leads to significant long-term sequelae.
- Concussion grades
  - Grade 1 definition: Transient confusion, no loss of consciousness, and duration of mental status abnormalities less than 15 minutes.
  - Grade 2 definition: Transient confusion, no loss of consciousness, and duration of mental status abnormalities of more than 15 minutes.
  - Grade 3 definition: Concussion involving loss of consciousness.
- Assessment: Confusion, disorientation, amnesia of the event; anorexia, vomiting, or pallor common soon after the insult.

Moderate Diffuse Axonal Injury

- Shearing, stretching, or tearing results in minute petechial bruising of brain tissue.
- Brainstem and reticular activating system may be involved, leading to unresponsiveness.
- Commonly associated with basilar skull fracture, most survive but neurologic impairment common.

Causes of Brain Injury

If left untreated, secondary injuries can exacerbate the primary injury.

Diffuse Axonal Injury

- Assessment
  - May result in immediate unresponsiveness or persistent confusion, disorientation, and amnesia of the event extending to amnesia of moment-to-moment events.
  - May have focal deficit.
  - Residual cognitive (inability to concentrate), psychologic (frequent periods of anxiety, uncharacteristic mood swings), and sensori-motor deficits (sense of smell altered) may persist.

Severe Diffuse Axonal Injury

- Formerly called brainstem injury.
- Involves severe mechanical disruption of many axons in both cerebral hemispheres and extending to the brainstem.
- Assessment: Unresponsiveness for prolonged period, posturing is common, other signs of increased ICP occur depending on various degrees of damage.

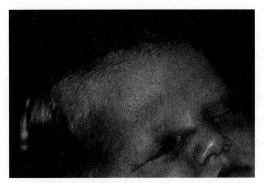

Figure 8-8   Bilateral black eyes are seen in this 12-day-old. His father reported that he had fallen on the stairs while holding the baby in a football hold and that, in the fall, the baby hit the steps face first with the father landing on top of him. The absence of an associated forehead hematoma or frontal fracture and the presence of an occipital fracture consistent with impact against a hard surface (not the father's chest) belied this story. Nevertheless, abuse was not suspected and the baby was sent home. He returned 3 months later in extremis with massive intracranial injury and died. On this occasion, the father said he had found the infant choking and gasping for breath and that he picked him up and shook him to revive him.

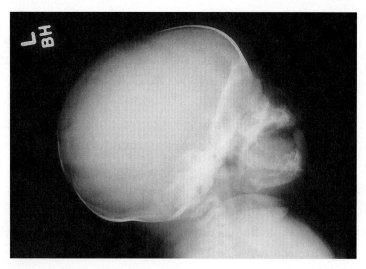

Figure 8-9   This linear skull fracture was found in the infant shown in
Figure 8-7.

Skull Fractures

Types

- Linear
  - Line crack in the skull (Figures 8-8 and 8-9).
  - Most common type of skull fracture; makes up approximately 60% to 90% of skull fractures in children.
  - Most linear fractures have an overlying hematoma or soft tissue swelling, although the swelling may not be detectable if the child is evaluated within a short period of the trauma or if the swelling is underlying the patient's hair.
  - Larger hematomas or hematomas in the temporal or parietal regions are more likely to indicate fracture.
  - Rarely require therapy and are often associated with good outcomes; uncomplicated linear skull fractures heal spontaneously within 6 months without surgical treatment.
  - Linear fractures that may be associated with a less favorable outcome include those that overlie a vascular channel, a fracture that extends through a suture line, or a fracture that extends over the area of the middle meningeal artery.
- Depressed
  - Pieces of bone are pushed inward pressing on, and sometimes causing tearing of brain tissue.
  - Most commonly seen in the parietal area. A fracture in this area causes concern because the underlying brain may have been bruised or lacerated and there is a higher likelihood of intracranial hemorrhage.
  - In some cases, the fracture is open (a compound fracture) or comminuted, and requires neurosurgical débridement and inspection.

Focal Injuries

Significance is in the amount of force involved.

○ A neurosurgeon may consider surgical elevation of the bony edges if the depression is greater than either the thickness of the skull or 5 mm.

- Neurologic signs and symptoms are evident.
- Cover the depressed area with a sterile dressing moistened with sterile saline.
- Monitor closely for signs of increased ICP.
- Basilar
  - Extension of linear fracture to floor of skull, may not be seen on radiograph or computed tomography (CT) scan.
  - Frequently involve the temporal bone with resultant bleeding into the middle ear, but may occur anywhere along the base of the skull
  - Fracture may cause a dural tear, which can lead to CSF leak and exposure to microorganisms of the upper airway (with potential for meningitis).
  - Signs and symptoms depend on amount of damage.
  - Clinical signs and symptoms.
    ○ CSF/blood from ear(s) or nose (frequency of occurrence is approximately 15% to 30%).
    ○ Bilateral black eyes (raccoon eyes).
    ○ Bruising behind ear(s): Battle sign; usually presents 12 to 24 hours after the injury.
    ○ Hemotympanum.
    ○ Hearing loss occurs in up to half of patients and may be permanent in a small number of patients.
    ○ May have seizures due to irritation of blood on brain tissue.
  - Most heal spontaneously within 7 to 10 days.
- Open skull fractures.
  - Severe force involved, brain tissue may be exposed.
  - Neurologic signs and symptoms evident.

Assessment

- Linear fractures may be missed.
  - Depressed and open skull fractures usually found on palpation of head.
  - Use balls of fingers to palpate.
- Airway patency and breathing adequacy are a priority; vomiting and inadequate respirations are common.
- Assess for signs and symptoms of increased ICP.
  - Infant
    ○ Full fontanelle, altered mental status, paradoxic irritability, persistent vomiting, and inability to fully open the eyes (referred to as the "setting sun" sign).

Children are particularly prone to basilar skull fractures.

Leakage of CSF from the ear (otorrhea) or nose (rhinorrhea) is evidence that a basilar fracture communicates with the subarachnoid space and indicates the presence of a pathway for infection from the exterior to the subarachnoid space.

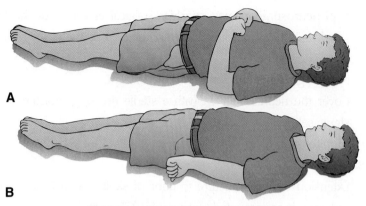

Figure 8-10 **Decorticate and decerebrate posturing. A,** In decorticate posturing, the legs are extended and the arms are flexed. **B,** In decerebrate posturing, all extremities are extended and rotated inward.

- Child
  - ◦ Headache, stiff neck, photophobia, altered mental status, persistent vomiting, cranial nerve involvement, Cushing triad, and decorticate or decerebrate posturing.
  - ◦ In decorticate posturing, the legs are extended and the arms are flexed (Figure 8-10). In decerebrate posturing, all extremities are extended and rotated inward. Progression from decorticate to decerebrate posturing is an ominous sign.
- Current data do not indicate that prophylactic antibiotic therapy significantly reduces the incidence of meningitis in a child with a basilar skull fracture.

Cerebral Contusion

- A focal brain injury in which brain tissue is bruised and damaged in a local area. It may occur at both the area of direct impact (coup) and/or on the side opposite (contrecoup) the impact.
- Assessment
  - Airway patency and breathing adequacy a priority.
  - Alteration in level of responsiveness.
  - Confusion or unusual behavior common.
  - May complain of progressive headache and/or photophobia.
  - May be unable to lay down memory; repetitive phrases common.
  - Assess for signs and symptoms of increased ICP.

Intracranial Hemorrhage

Epidural Hematoma

- An epidural hematoma is a rapidly accumulating hematoma between the dura and the cranium (Figure 8-11). Eighty five percent are associated with an overlying skull fracture; the most serious lacerate the middle meningeal artery.

TYPES OF HEMATOMAS AND THE MENINGES

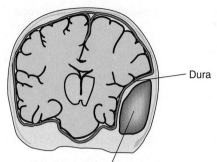

A. EXTRADURAL OR EPIDURAL HEMATOMA
Blood fills space between
dura and bone

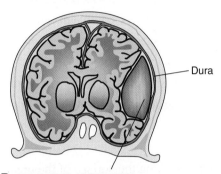

B. SUBDURAL HEMATOMA
Blood fills space between dura
and arachnoid

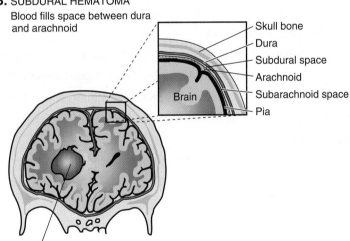

C. INTRACEREBRAL HEMATOMA

Figure 8-11   **Types of cerebral hematomas and the meninges. A,** Epidural
hematoma. **B,** Subdural hematoma. **C,** Intracerebral hematoma.

- In adults, an epidural hematoma is usually from an arterial tear, usually of the middle meningeal artery.
- Occasionally, a pediatric epidural hematoma may be the result of *venous* bleeding, which predisposes the infant or child to a subtle and more subacute presentation over days.[12]
- Most patients experience a loss of consciousness followed by a lucid, awake interval often associated with a severe headache. If untreated, this abruptly evolves to deterioration and death within 15 to 60 minutes.

- Other signs and symptoms include headache, vomiting, and altered mental status, early dilation of the ipsilateral pupil, and contralateral hemiparesis.

- Early diagnosis and treatment results in a good prognosis; delayed treatment results in a poor prognosis and possible death. Emergent surgical evacuation is usually necessary.

The hallmark sign is a dilated and fixed pupil on the same side as the impact.

Subdural Hematoma

- Usually results from tearing of the bridging veins between the cerebral cortex and dura; blood fills the space between the dura and the arachnoid.

- A subdural hematoma may be acute or chronic.

- A newborn or infant often presents with focal seizures, decreased level of consciousness, bulging fontanelle, weak cry, pallor, and vomiting. Retinal hemorrhages, which may occur as a result of the primary injury, are common.

Subdural hematomas most commonly occur in patients younger than 2 years, with 93% of cases involving children younger than 1 year.[12]

- In children older than 2 to 3 years, signs and symptoms often include pupillary changes, hemiparesis, restlessness, focal neurologic signs, and altered mental status.

Subarachnoid Hematoma

- Usually confined to the CSF space along the surface of the brain.
- Results in bloody CSF and meningeal irritation.

Intracerebral Hematoma

- Occurs within the brain substance; many small, deep intracerebral hemorrhages are associated with other brain injuries (especially DAI).
- Neurologic deficits depend on the associated injuries and the region involved, the size of the hemorrhage, and whether bleeding continues.

Assessment

- May be impossible to tell which type of hematoma is present.
  - History is important: What were they doing? What happened? What is wrong now? What doesn't seem right?
  - More important to recognize the presence of brain injury.
- Signs/symptoms of increasing ICP
  - Headache that becomes increasingly severe
  - Vomiting
  - Lethargy
  - Confusion
  - Changes in consciousness
  - Comatose
  - Pupil changes
  - Pulse slows or becomes irregular
  - Ventilations become irregular
  - Posturing
  - Seizures

- Signs/symptoms of neurologic deficit: early signs and symptoms of alterations in level of consciousness.
- Signs of brain irritation: change in personality, irritability, lethargy, confusion, repeating words or phrases, changes in consciousness, paralysis of one side of the body, seizures.
- GCS.

General Management of Head/Brain Injuries

- Suspect cervical spine injury; cervical spine precautions.
- Maintain airway and adequate ventilation.
  - Hypoxia must be prevented to prevent secondary injury to brain tissue.
  - Tracheal intubation is often necessary for the child with a severe head injury. Consider RSI and the use of lidocaine before the procedure to reduce ICP.
  - Ensure the availability of suction. Spontaneous emesis in the first 30 to 60 minutes following head injury is common in children. Consider placement of an orogastric tube.
- Elevate the head of the backboard 30 degrees.
- Establish vascular access
  - Start IV of isotonic fluid (normal saline [NS] or lactated Ringer's [LR]) and titrate to BP.
  - Prevent hypotension to preserve CPP.
  - If hypotension present, look for internal bleeding.
  - Stop external bleeding.
- Pharmacologic treatment
  - Possible use of diuretics.
  - Paralytics/sedation.
  - Avoid glucose unless hypoglycemia confirmed.
- Nonpharmacologic treatment
  - Position: Elevate the head of the backboard 30 degrees.
  - Decrease central nervous system stimulation: quiet, calm atmosphere; avoid bright lights due to photophobia.
- Perform serial neurologic checks including vital signs, arousability, size, and reactivity of the pupils to light, and extent and symmetry of motor responses.
  - Every 15 to 30 minutes until the child is alert.
  - Then every 1 to 2 hours for 12 hours.
  - Then every 2 to 4 hours thereafter.
  - Use the GCS for serial comparisons. A GCS score that falls two points suggests significant deterioration; urgent patient reassessment is required.

PALS Pearl

If a penetrating object is present, do not remove it. The only indications for nonsurgical removal of an impaled object are the following:
- It is not possible to ventilate the child without removing the foreign body (e.g., the object is impaled in the patient's cheek).
- The presence of the object would interfere with chest compressions.

Manually secure the object, expose the wound area, control bleeding if present, and use a bulky dressing to help stabilize the object in place.

- Treat seizures if present.
- Consider CT scan. Do not send for CT without adequate stabilization. Minimum requirements include heart rate and pulse oximetry monitoring.
- Psychological support for patient and family.

Reassessment is crucial to detecting signs of increasing ICP.

Spinal Trauma

- Children can have spinal nerve injury without damage to the vertebrae, a condition called spinal cord injury without radiographic abnormality (SCIWORA). SCIWORA is thought to be attributable to the increased mobility of a child's spine due to the relatively large size of the child's head, weakness of the soft tissues of the neck, incomplete development of the bony spine, and frequency with which ligamentous injuries occur without cervical spine injury.
- Although spinal cord and spinal column injuries are uncommon in the pediatric patient, children younger than 8 years tend to sustain injury to the upper (C1 and C2) cervical spine region. Adults and older children tend to have cervical spine injuries in the lower cervical spine area (between C5-C6 and C6-C7). As a child approaches 8 to 10 years of age, the spinal anatomy and injury pattern more closely approximate those of adult injuries.
- Since the high cervical region is the most likely area of spinal injury in a pediatric patient, it is particularly dangerous to have a child's neck in a flexed position. Proper stabilization requires either a special board with a recess for the back of the head, allowing the head to rest in line with the body, or placement of padding under the shoulders to elevate the neck in line with the head.
- It is possible to have a spinal **column** injury (i.e., bony injury) with or without spinal **cord** injury. It is also possible to have spinal **cord** injury with or without spinal **column** injury.

- Primary injury
  - Occurs at time of impact/injury.
  - Causes include cord compression, direct cord injury (sharp or unstable bony structures), interruption in the cord's blood supply.
- Secondary injury
  - Occurs after initial injury.
  - Causes include swelling, ischemia, movement of bony fragments.
  - Cord concussion results from temporary disruption of cord-mediated functions.

Hypotension can contribute to secondary injury after acute spinal cord injury by further reducing spinal cord blood flow and perfusion.

Nearly 80% of injuries in children younger than 2 years affect the upper cervical spine region.

Types of Spinal Cord Injuries

- Cord contusion
  - Bruising of the cord's tissues.
  - Temporary loss of cord-mediated function.
- Cord compression
  - Pressure on the cord.
  - Causes tissue ischemia.
  - Must be decompressed to avoid permanent loss/damage to cord.
- Laceration
  - Tearing of the cord tissue.
  - May be reversed if only slight damage.
  - May result in permanent loss if spinal tracts are disrupted.
- Hemorrhage
  - Bleeding into the cord's tissue due to injured blood vessels.
  - Injury related to amount of hemorrhage.
  - Damage or obstruction to spinal blood supply results in local ischemia.
- Cord transection
  - Complete
    - All tracts of the spinal cord completely disrupted.
    - Cord-mediated functions below transection are permanently lost.
    - Accurately determined after at least 24 hours after injury.
    - Results in
      - Quadriplegia
        - Injury at the cervical level.
        - Loss of all function below injury site.
      - Paraplegia
        - Injury at the thoracic or lumbar level.
        - Loss of lower trunk only.
  - Incomplete
    - Some tracts of the spinal cord remain intact.
    - Some cord-mediated functions intact.
    - Potential for recovery; function may only be temporarily lost.
- Neurogenic shock
  - Occurs secondary to spinal cord injury.

Differentiate neurogenic shock (↓ BP, ↓ heart rate) from hypovolemic shock (↓ BP, ↑ heart rate).

  - Injury disrupts the body's sympathetic compensatory mechanism.
    - Loss of sympathetic tone to the vessels.
      - Arteries and arterioles dilate, enlarging the size of the vascular container and producing a relative hypovolemia.
      - Skin will be warm and dry due to cutaneous vasodilation.
    - Relative hypotension.
    - Relative bradycardia.

- Shock presentation is usually the result of hidden volume loss (e.g., chest injuries, abdominal injuries).
- Treatment focus is primarily on volume replacement.

Signs and symptoms of possible spinal trauma include the following:

Signs and Symptoms of Spinal Trauma

- Pain to the neck or back.
- Pain on movement of the neck or back.
- Pain on palpation of the posterior neck or midline of the back.
- Deformity of the spinal column.
- Guarding or splinting of the muscles of the neck or back.
- Priapism.
- Signs and symptoms of neurogenic shock (peripheral vasodilation, bradycardia, and hypotension).
- Paralysis, paresis, numbness, or tingling in the arms or legs at any time after the incident.
- Diaphragmatic breathing.

- The use and effectiveness of steroids in spinal cord injuries is controversial.

General Management of Spinal Injuries

- Principles of spinal stabilization
  - Primary goal is to prevent further injury.
  - Treat the spine as a long bone with a joint at either end. Stabilize the joint above (head) and the joint below (pelvis) the injury. Always use "complete" spine stabilization; impossible to isolate and splint specific injury site.
  - Stabilization of the spine begins in the primary survey and continues until the spine is completely stabilized on a long backboard or evidence of spinal injury has been definitively ruled out.
  - The head and neck should be placed in a neutral in-line position unless contraindicated.
  - Backboards
    ○ To stabilize a pediatric patient on a backboard:
      ▪ Manually stabilize the child's head and neck.
      ▪ Apply a properly sized rigid cervical collar (Figure 8-12A). If a properly sized device is not available, use towels, washcloths, or other material to stabilize the head as best as possible.
      ▪ Log roll the child onto a rigid board (Figure 8-12B).
        • To maintain the cervical spine in a neutral position, it is often necessary to place padding under the child's torso.
        • The padding should be firm, evenly shaped, and extend from the shoulders to the pelvis. For an infant or young child, the padding should be of appropriate thickness so

Do NOT pull on the child's head or neck. Slide the child out of the seat as a unit.

that the child's shoulders are in horizontal alignment with the ear canal.

◦ Secure the child to the board with straps around the chest, pelvis, and legs to restrict patient movement from side to side and to prevent the child from sliding up and down on the backboard. Secure the torso to the board first and the head to the board last (Figure 8–12C).

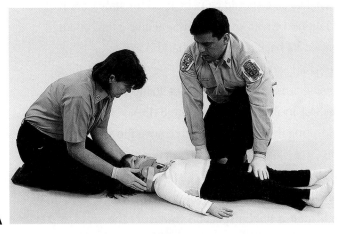

A

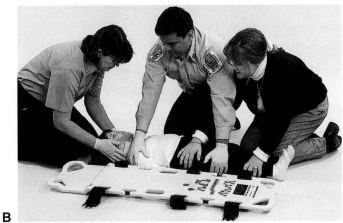

B

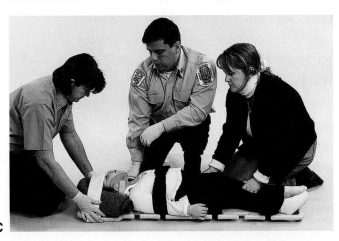

C

Figure 8-12 Stabilizing a pediatric patient on a backboard. A, Apply a properly sized rigid cervical collar. **B,** Log roll the child onto a rigid board. **C,** Secure the child to board with straps around the chest, pelvis, and legs. Secure the head to the board last.

- Manual stabilization can be discontinued after the head has been secured to the board.
- Additional padding may be necessary along the torso and between the legs.
    - Secure the board to the stretcher and reassess the patient.
- Child safety seats
    - If a child is critically injured or the child's condition has the potential to worsen, a safety seat should NOT be used for stabilization. Instead, the child should be removed from the seat onto a rigid board.
        - Place the seat on its back onto a long backboard.
        - Unstrap the child and slide him or her onto the long backboard using a padded board splint to keep the child's spine in a neutral, in-line position (Figure 8-13A).
        - Slide the child along the backboard and remove the safety seat (Figure 8-13B).
        - Stabilize the child to the backboard.
    - If the child's condition is stable, a child safety seat can be used for stabilization only after a brief inspection to ensure the seat has not sustained any major structural damage and only if the safety seat can be secured appropriately in the ambulance.
        - Manually stabilize the child's head and neck (Figure 8-14A).
        - If the seat includes a protection plate over the child's chest, remove it to enable easy visualization and assessment of the child's chest.
            - If a chest plate is not present, use the chest straps to secure the child in place whenever possible.
            - Additional padding and/or cravats between the straps and the child or tightening of the straps may be needed.
        - If a properly fitting rigid cervical collar is available, apply it and use towel rolls to limit movement. If a rigid cervical collar of appropriate size is not available, use towels, washcloths, or small blankets (depending on the child's size) and adhesive tape across the forehead to stabilize the head (Figure 8-14B). Use a cravat or similar material around the head to prevent forward movement (Figure 8-14C).
        - Use small blankets, towels, or similar materials to pad all open areas around the child's body so the child does not move.
        - Once adequately stabilized, the patient and seat should be transferred to the ambulance and carefully secured to the stretcher or captain's seat so that it is not mobile during transport (Figure 8-14D).

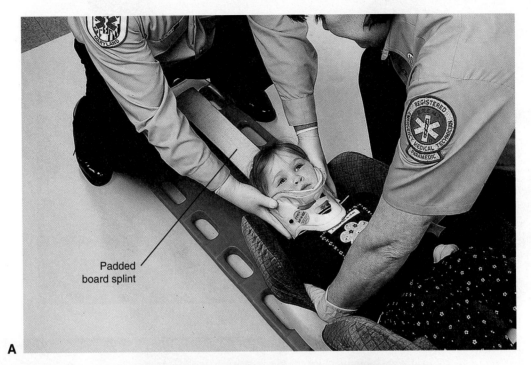

Padded
board splint

A

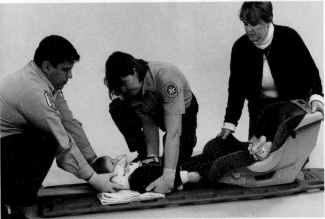

B

Figure 8-13   A, Place the seat on its back onto a long backboard. Unstrap the child and slide him or her onto the long backboard using a padded board splint to keep the child's spine in a neutral, in-line position. **B,** Slide the child along the board and remove the safety seat. Stabilize the child to the backboard.

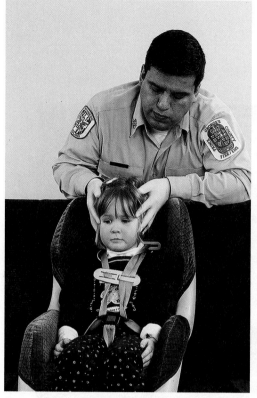

A

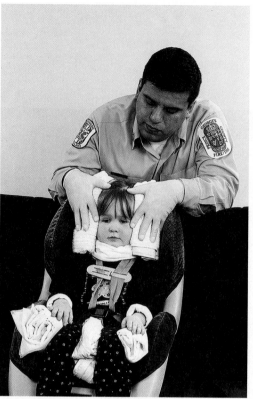

B

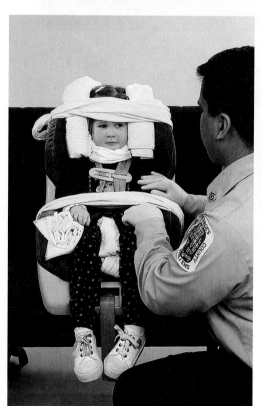

C

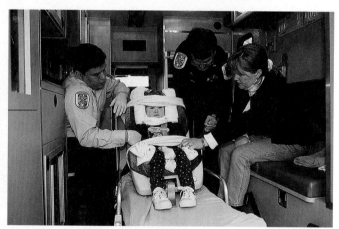

D

Figure 8-14 **A**, Manually stabilize the child's head and neck. Use the safety seat's chest straps to secure the child in place whenever possible. **B**, If a properly fitting rigid cervical collar is not available, use towels, washcloths, or small blankets (depending on the child's size) and adhesive tape across the forehead to stabilize the head. **C**, Use a cravat or similar material around the head to prevent forward movement. Use small blankets, towels, or similar materials to pad all open areas around the child's body so the child does not move. **D**, Secure the safety seat in place for transport.

- Helmeted patients
  - Special assessment needs for patients wearing helmets.
    - Airway and breathing.
    - Fit of helmet and movement within the helmet.
    - Ability to gain access to airway and breathing.
  - Indications for leaving the helmet in place.
    - Good fit with little or no head movement within helmet.
    - No impending airway or breathing problems.
    - Removal may cause further injury.
    - Proper spinal stabilization could be performed with helmet in place.
    - No interference with ability to assess and reassess airway.
  - Indications for helmet removal.
    - Inability to assess or reassess airway and breathing.
    - Restriction of adequate management of the airway or breathing.
    - Improperly fitted helmet with excessive head movement within helmet.
    - Proper spinal stabilization cannot be performed with helmet in place (Figure 8-15).
    - Cardiac arrest.

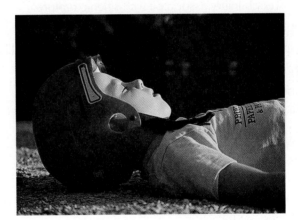

Figure 8-15 Neck flexion caused by a helmet on a child.

Thoracic Trauma

The most common thoracic injuries seen in children are pneumothorax, hemothorax, pulmonary contusion, fractures, damage to major blood vessels, the heart, and diaphragm.[13]

In children, thoracic trauma is associated with a high mortality rate. The greater elasticity and resilience of the chest wall in children makes rib and sternum fractures less common than in adults; however, force is more easily transmitted to the underlying lung tissues, resulting in pulmonary contusion, pneumothorax, or hemothorax.

Rib Fractures

Chest Wall Injuries

- Children are less likely to sustain rib fractures than adults are because a child's chest wall is more flexible than that of an adult. The presence of a rib fracture suggests significant force caused the injury.
- Most frequently caused by blunt trauma and may be associated with injury to the underlying lung (pulmonary contusion) or the heart (myocardial contusion). The seriousness of the injury increases with age, the number of fractures, and the location of the fractures.
  - Left lower rib injury associated with splenic rupture.
  - Right lower rib injury associated with hepatic injury.
  - Multiple rib fractures may result in inadequate ventilation and pneumonia.
- Signs and symptoms
  - Localized pain at the fracture site that worsens with deep breathing, coughing, or moving. Pain often causes the patient to "splint" the injury by holding his or her arm close to the chest.
  - Pain on inspiration.
  - Shallow breathing (to decrease the pain associated with breathing).
  - Tenderness on palpation.
  - Deformity of chest wall.
  - Crepitus (grating sound produced by bone fragments rubbing together).
  - Swelling and/or bruising at the fracture site.
  - Possible subcutaneous emphysema (a crackling sensation felt under the fingers during palpation). The presence of subcutaneous emphysema suggests laceration of a lung and the leakage of air into the pleural space.

- Management
  - Airway and ventilation.
    - Oxygen therapy.
    - Positive-pressure ventilation if needed.
    - Encourage coughing and deep breathing.
  - Pharmacologic: analgesics.
  - Nonpharmacologic.
    - Splint, but avoid circumferential splinting.
    - Do not apply tape or straps to the ribs or chest wall.
      - Limits chest wall motion.
      - Reduces effectiveness of ventilation.

Flail Chest

- Flail chest is a life-threatening injury.
- Most commonly occurs because of a vehicle crash but may also occur because of falls from a height, assault, and birth trauma.
  - Because a child's ribs are flexible, flail chest is uncommon in children.
- Pathophysiology
  - Flail chest results when two or more adjacent ribs are fractured at two points, allowing a freely moving segment of the chest wall to move in paradoxic motion.
    - The section of the chest wall between the fractured ribs becomes free-floating because it is no longer in continuity with the thorax. This free-floating section of the chest wall is called the "flail segment."
    - The injured portion of the chest wall (flail segment) does not move with the rest of the rib cage when the patient attempts to breathe (paradoxic movement). When the patient inhales, the flail segment is drawn inward instead of moving outward. When the patient exhales, the flail segment moves outward instead of moving inward.
  - Respiratory failure may be caused by the following:
    - Bruising of the underlying lung and associated hemorrhage of the alveoli, reducing the amount of lung tissue available for gas exchange.
    - Instability of the chest wall and pain associated with breathing, leading to decreased ventilation and hypoxia.
    - Interference with the normal "bellows" action of the chest, resulting in inadequate gas exchange.
    - Associated chest injuries.
  - Paradoxic movement of the chest (may be minimal because of muscle spasm).
  - Pain: reduces thoracic expansion, decreases ventilation.
  - Pulmonary contusion.

- Decreased ventilation.
- Impaired venous return with ventilation-perfusion mismatch.
- Hypercapnia, hypoxia.
- Signs and symptoms: chest wall contusion, respiratory distress, paradoxic chest wall movement, pleuritic chest pain, crepitus, pain and splinting of affected side, tachypnea, tachycardia.
- Management
  - Supplemental oxygen; positive-pressure ventilation may be needed.
  - Evaluate the need for tracheal intubation.
  - Positive end-expiratory pressure (PEEP).
  - Pharmacologic: analgesics.
  - Nonpharmacologic: positioning; tracheal intubation, and positive-pressure ventilation.

Pulmonary Contusion

Injury to the Lung

A pulmonary contusion is one of the most frequently observed chest injuries in children.

- Potentially life-threatening injury.
- Frequently missed due to presence of other associated injuries.
- Pathophysiology.
  - Alveoli fill with blood and fluid because of bruising of the lung tissue.
  - Area of the lung available for gas exchange is decreased.
  - Severity of signs and symptoms depends on the amount of lung tissue injured.
- Signs and symptoms
  - Evidence of blunt chest trauma, apprehension, anxiety, tachypnea, tachycardia, cough, hemoptysis, dyspnea, wheezes, crackles, and decreased breath sounds. Subcutaneous emphysema may or may not be present.

  The child may initially be asymptomatic but may develop symptoms a few hours later.

  - Arterial blood gas changes precede clinical symptoms; reflect increased $Paco_2$ level and decreased Pao_2 level.
- Management
  - Mild contusion: observation and supportive care.
  - More severe contusion: tracheal intubation and mechanical ventilation with PEEP.
  - Maintain normal blood volume.

A simple pneumothorax may occur as a result of blunt or penetrating chest trauma (i.e., rib fractures or central line placement).

Simple Pneumothorax
- Pathophysiology
  - Air enters the chest cavity causing a loss of negative pressure and a partial or total collapse of the lung. Air may enter the chest cavity through a hole in the chest wall (sucking chest wound) or a hole in the lung tissue, bronchus, or the trachea. As air enters and fills the pleural space, lung tissue is compressed, reducing the amount of lung tissue available for gas exchange.
  - Signs and symptoms will depend on the size of the pneumothorax
    - Small tears may self-seal, resolving by themselves; patient may not experience dyspnea or other signs of respiratory distress.
    - Larger tears may progress, resulting in signs and symptoms of respiratory distress.
  - If the child is sitting or standing, air will accumulate in the apices; check there first for diminished breath sounds; if the child is supine, air will accumulate in the anterior chest.
  - Trachea may tug toward the effected side.
  - Ventilation/perfusion mismatch.
- Signs and symptoms: tachypnea, tachycardia, respiratory distress, absent or decreased breath sounds on affected side, decreased chest wall movement, dyspnea, slight pleuritic chest pain.
- Management
  - Small pneumothorax (less than 15%) may not require treatment other than observation.
  - Positive-pressure ventilation if necessary.
  - Monitor for development of tension pneumothorax.

Open Pneumothorax
- Pathophysiology
  - Open defect in the chest wall
    - Allows communication between pleural space and atmosphere.
    - Prevents development of negative intrapleural pressure.
    - Produces collapse of ipsilateral lung.
    - Inability to ventilate affected lung.
    - Ventilation/perfusion mismatch.
  - Severity of an open pneumothorax depends on the size of the wound.
  - Direct lung injury may be present.
- Signs and symptoms: defect in the chest wall, penetrating injury to the chest that does not seal itself, sucking sound on inhalation, tachycardia, tachypnea, respiratory distress, subcutaneous emphysema, decreased breath sounds on affected side.

- Management
  - Positive-pressure ventilation if necessary.
  - Monitor for development of tension pneumothorax.
  - Nonpharmacologic.
    - Promptly close the chest wall defect with an occlusive (airtight) dressing (plastic wrap, petroleum gauze, or a defibrillation pad are examples of dressings that may be used).
      - Tape the dressing on three sides (flutter-valve effect—the dressing is sucked over the wound as the patient inhales, preventing air from entering; the open end of the dressing allows air to escape as the patient exhales)
    - Tube thoracostomy: in-hospital management

Tension Pneumothorax

- Life-threatening chest injury that can occur because of blunt or penetrating trauma or as a complication of treatment of an open pneumothorax

- Pathophysiology
  - May result from an opening through the chest wall and parietal pleura (open pneumothorax) or from a tear in the lung tissue and visceral pleura (closed pneumothorax).
  - Air enters the pleura during inspiration and progressively accumulates under pressure. The flap of injured lung acts as a one-way valve, allowing air to enter the pleural space during inspiration, but trapping it during expiration (Figure 8-16).

> Tension pneumothorax is common in children.
>
> Shifting of the trachea to the side opposite the injury is called **tracheal deviation**. Shifting of the heart and major blood vessels to the side opposite the injury is called **mediastinal shift**.

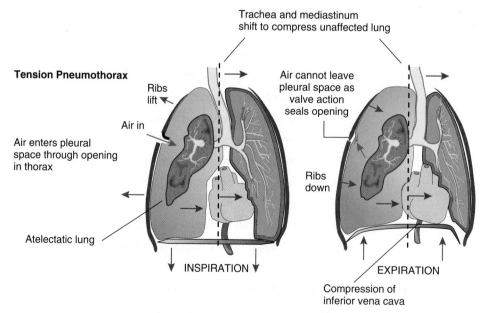

Tension Pneumothorax

Ribs lift

Air in

Air enters pleural space through opening in thorax

Atelectatic lung

INSPIRATION

Trachea and mediastinum shift to compress unaffected lung

Air cannot leave pleural space as valve action seals opening

Ribs down

EXPIRATION

Compression of inferior vena cava

Figure 8-16 Tension pneumothorax.

A tracheal shift is difficult to detect in young children. JVD may not be prominent if hypovolemia is present.

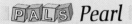

Pearl

Diagnosis of tension pneumothorax in children is complicated by false transmission of breath sounds. Uncertainty as to the side of the tension pneumothorax should not prohibit initiation of empirical treatment if the patient is deteriorating. Decompression of the other side should be performed if immediate improvement is not seen with the initial needle or tube thoracostomy.[14]

A hemothorax requires a minimum of 10 mL/kg of blood to be visualized on chest radiograph.[14]

- The injured lung collapses completely and pressure rises, forcing the trachea, heart, and major blood vessels to be pushed toward the opposite side. Shifting of the major blood vessels causes them to kink, resulting in a backup of blood into the venous system. The backup of blood into the venous system results in jugular venous distention (JVD), decreased blood return to the heart, and signs of shock.
- Signs and symptoms: cool, clammy skin; increased pulse rate, cyanosis (a late sign), JVD, hypotension, severe respiratory distress; agitation, restlessness, anxiety; bulging of intercostal muscles on the affected side, decreased or absent breath sounds on the affected side, tracheal deviation toward the unaffected side (late sign), and possible subcutaneous emphysema in the face, neck, or chest wall.
- Management
  - Positive-pressure ventilation if necessary.
  - Relieve tension pneumothorax to improve cardiac output.
  - Nonpharmacologic
    ○ If the patient has an open chest wound with signs of a tension pneumothorax.
      ■ Remove the dressing over the wound for a few seconds. If the wound in the chest wall has not sealed under the dressing, air will rush out of the wound.
      ■ Reseal the wound with the occlusive dressing once the pressure has been released. This procedure may need to be repeated periodically if pressure again builds up in the chest.
      ■ If this procedure does not relieve the signs of a tension pneumothorax, needle decompression should be performed.
    ○ Needle decompression.
    ○ Tube thoracostomy: in-hospital management.

Hemothorax
- Life-threatening injury that frequently requires urgent chest tube and/or surgery.
- Pathophysiology
  - Occurs as a result of blunt or penetrating trauma when large amounts of blood accumulate in the pleural space and compress the lung.
  - Massive hemothorax indicates great vessel or cardiac injury.
  - Respiratory insufficiency dependent on amount of blood.
  - Hypotension and inadequate perfusion may result from blood loss.

- Signs and symptoms: tachypnea, tachycardia, dyspnea, respiratory distress, hypotension, narrowed pulse pressure, flat neck veins, pleuritic chest pain; pale, cool, moist skin; decreased breath sounds and dullness to percussion on affected side with or without obvious respiratory distress.
- Management
  - Positive-pressure ventilation if necessary.
  - Tracheal intubation if necessary.
  - Treat hypovolemia and shock with IV fluids, blood administration as indicated.
  - Tube thoracostomy: in-hospital management (ensure IV fluid resuscitation is initiated before procedure).

Signs of shock are often the initial indicators of a large hemothorax.

Traumatic Asphyxia

- Pathophysiology
  - Sudden compression force to the chest or upper abdomen, with the lungs full of air and glottis closed, causes a sudden increase in intrapleural and intraabdominal pressure.
  - This raises the pressure in the superior vena cava, causing the blood in the veins of the thorax and neck to be forced into the chest, lungs, neck, head, and brain. Increased venous pressure causes rupture of capillaries, which results in violet color of skin in the head and neck area, bilateral subconjunctival hemorrhages, and facial edema.
- Signs and symptoms: cyanosis of the face and upper neck; JVD; swelling or hemorrhage of the conjunctiva; skin below area remains pink; tachypnea; disorientation; hemoptysis; epistaxis; signs of respiratory insufficiency.
- Management
  - Manage associated injuries (e.g., pulmonary contusion).
  - Supportive care.

Pericardial Tamponade

- Pathophysiology
  - Rapid accumulation of fluid in the pericardial sac over a period of minutes to hours leads to increases in intrapericardial pressure.
  - Compresses heart and decreases cardiac output due to restricted diastolic expansion and filling.
  - Hampers venous return.
- Signs and symptoms: tachycardia, respiratory distress, pulsus paradoxus, cyanosis of head, neck, upper extremities, Beck's triad (narrowing pulse

pressure, neck vein distention, muffled heart tones), dysrhythmias (e.g., bradycardia, pulseless electrical activity, asystole).

Beck's triad is not often evident in the pediatric patient. If profound hypovolemia is present, JVD will be absent. If bradycardia occurs, the patient is about to arrest.

- Management
  - Airway and ventilation.
  - IV fluid challenge (may transiently increase cardiac output by increasing the filling pressure of the heart).
  - Nonpharmacologic management (in-hospital).
  - Echocardiographically guided pericardiocentesis.
  - Percutaneous balloon pericardiotomy.
  - Emergency department thoracotomy.
  - Operative intervention.

Abdominal and Pelvic Trauma

Mechanism of Injury

Abdominal trauma is the third leading cause of traumatic death, after head and thoracic injuries, and is the most common cause of unrecognized fatal injury in children. The abdominal organs of an infant or child are susceptible to injury for several reasons.

- The abdominal wall is thin, so the organs are closer to the surface of the abdomen.
- Children have proportionally larger solid organs, less subcutaneous fat, and less protective abdominal musculature than adults do.
- The liver and spleen of a small child are lower in the abdomen and less protected by the rib cage.
- Blunt mechanisms (85% of cases)
  - Blunt abdominal trauma in an infant or child is primarily caused by motor vehicle collisions, motorcycle collisions, falls, sports-related injuries, pedestrian crashes, and child abuse.
  - Blunt trauma related to motor vehicle collisions causes more than 50% of the abdominal injuries in children and is the most lethal.
  - The effects of bicycle injuries may not be seen on initial presentation, with the mean elapsed time to onset of symptoms being nearly 24 hours.[12]
- Penetrating mechanisms (15% of cases)
  - Energy imparted to the body.
  - Low velocity: knife, ice pick, scissors.
  - Medium velocity: gunshot wounds, shotgun wounds.
  - High velocity: high-power hunting rifles, military weapons.

- Splenic injuries
  - Most frequently injured abdominal organ during blunt trauma (e.g., motor vehicle collisions, sudden deceleration injuries, and contact sports–related injuries).
  - Commonly associated with other intraabdominal injuries.
  - May present with left upper quadrant abdominal pain radiating to the left shoulder (Kehr sign; result of diaphragm irritation).
  - Patient presentation may range from stable to persistent hypotension to cardiovascular collapse. Stable patients may undergo CT for radiologic evaluation or bedside ultrasound.
  - Bleeding from a minor splenic injury often stops spontaneously without requiring operative intervention; however, spontaneous splenic rupture 3 to 5 days after the injury has been described.
  - Patients with splenic injury should be admitted to the hospital, with frequent repeated assessments.
- Liver injuries
  - The liver is vulnerable to injury because of its large size and fragility.
  - Second most commonly injured solid organ in the pediatric patient with blunt abdominal trauma but the most common cause of lethal hemorrhage.
  - Injuries may be the result of blunt or penetrating trauma; a firm blow to the right upper quadrant or right-sided rib fractures may cause liver injury.
  - Absence of localized bruises or abrasions does not rule out the possibility of serious laceration or rupture.
- Kidney injuries
  - Kidney injury is usually caused by blunt trauma (e.g., deceleration forces) and is rarely caused by penetrating trauma.
  - Often present with hematuria, back pain.
  - Most injuries are minor and can be managed without surgical intervention.
- Pancreas
  - Contusion most common type of injury to the pancreas.
  - Common mechanisms include falling from a bicycle with injury caused by the handlebars, pedestrian traffic collisions, motor vehicle collisions, and child abuse.
  - Lacerations cause hemorrhage and release of enzymatic contents toxic to surrounding tissues.
  - Penetrating trauma requires surgical evaluation.

Solid-Organ Injuries

All patients with suspected splenic injury should be evaluated by a surgeon.

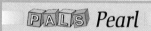 *Pearl*

A child who is wearing a seatbelt with no shoulder harness during a motor vehicle collision may sustain a Chance fracture and abdominal injuries involving the pancreas, duodenum, or intestines, with the potential for hematomas and bowel rupture. A Chance fracture (also called a seatbelt fracture) is a horizontal fracture of the thoracic or lumbar spine caused by a hyperflexion injury with little or no compression of the vertebral body.

Hollow-Organ Injuries

- Morbidity/mortality secondary to blood loss and content spillage.
- May result from blunt or penetrating injuries.
- Common mechanisms include seatbelt injuries, bicycle handlebar injuries, and child abuse.
- Small and large intestines
  - Most often injured as a result of penetrating injuries.
  - Can occur with deceleration injuries.
- Stomach
  - Most often injured as a result of blunt trauma.
  - Full stomach before incident increases risk of injury.
- Duodenum
  - Most often injured as a result of blunt trauma.
  - Recognition often delayed.
- Bladder
  - Most often injured as a result of blunt trauma due to automobile or automobile-pedestrian collisions.
  - Full bladder before incident or inappropriate use of seatbelts may increase risk of bladder injury.
  - Penetrating injuries may be caused by guns, knives, or fractured pelvic bones.

Abdominal Wall Injuries

Evisceration

- Do not touch or try to replace the exposed organ.
- Carefully remove clothing from around the wound.
- Cover exposed organs and wound.
  - Apply a large sterile dressing, moistened with sterile water or saline, over the organs and wound.
  - Secure the dressing in place with a large bandage to retain moisture and prevent heat loss.

Pelvic Fractures

Because the pelvis contains major blood vessels, the patient with a pelvic fracture is at significant risk for serious hemorrhage.

- Fractures of the pelvis in children are uncommon.
- Associated soft tissue injuries may be severe and require emergency treatment.
- Many pelvic fractures occur in children struck by moving vehicles.
- Treatment of a pelvic fracture depends on the type of fracture. Follow local protocol.

Extremity Trauma

- Fractures are among the most frequently missed injuries in children with multiple trauma.
- Bilateral femur fractures can cause significant blood loss, resulting in hypovolemic shock.
- Be alert for evidence of possible child abuse:
  - Fractures of differing ages.
  - Spiral fracture.
  - Discrepancy between history and injury.
  - Prolonged and/or unexplained delay in treatment.
  - Different stories at different times.
  - Poor health and hygiene.
- Extremity stabilization
  - Stabilize the joint above and below the fracture site.
  - Assess and document pulses, motor function, and sensation in the affected extremity before and after stabilization.
  - Do not attempt to realign a fracture or dislocation, or straighten any angulation, unless obvious vascular compromise necessitates a position change.
- Amputated part
  - If a complete amputation has occurred:
    - Apply a sterile dressing soaked in normal saline to the stump, then splint it.
      - If profuse bleeding is present, apply direct pressure with a soft dressing.
      - Stabilize the limb to prevent further injury.
    - Gently rinse dirt and debris from the amputated part with sterile saline or LR solution.
      - Do not scrub.
      - Clean water is an acceptable alternative if sterile isotonic solution is not available.
    - Put the amputated part in a plastic bag or waterproof container.
    - Place the plastic bag or waterproof container in water with a few ice cubes. Never place ice in direct contact with the amputated part.
    - Transport the amputated part with the patient.
  - Do not use dry ice.
  - Do not allow the part to freeze. Freezing renders tissues non-replantable.
  - Do not place the amputated part directly on ice or in water.
  - Do not complete partial amputations.

- Stabilize suspected fractures and dislocations and administer an analgesic before obtaining radiographs.
- Consult an orthopedic surgeon to evaluate a child with a compartment syndrome, other causes of neurovascular compromise, or an open fracture.

Thermal Burns

- Thermal burns are caused by exposure to some form of heat (e.g., flames, hot liquids, or hot solid objects).
- Depth classification of a burn injury
  - It is often days before depth can be determined accurately.
  - Superficial burn (first degree) (Figure 8-17)
    - Example: sunburn.
    - Only epidermis involved.
    - Dry, no blisters.
    - Minimal or no edema.
    - Painful and erythematous.
    - Heal in 2 to 5 days with no scarring.

Any blistering qualifies as a second-degree burn.

- Partial-thickness burn (second degree).
    - Often caused by scalds.
    - Epidermis and dermis involved, but dermal appendages spared.
    - Superficial second-degree burns are blistered and painful.

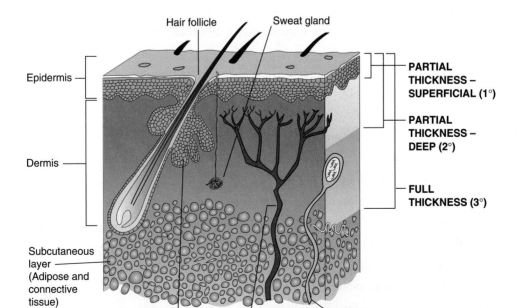

Figure 8-17   Depth classification of a burn injury.

- ○ Deep second-degree burns may be white and painless.
  - ○ Healing
    - ▪ Superficial: 5 to 21 days with no grafting.
    - ▪ Deep partial: 21 to 35 days with no infection. If infected, converts to full thickness.
- • Full-thickness burn (third degree).
  - ○ Typically result from flame or contact injuries.
  - ○ Epidermis and dermis involved; may include fat, subcutaneous tissue, fascia, muscle, and bone.
  - ○ Color may vary from yellow or pallid to black and charred, with a dry, waxy, or leathery appearance.
  - ○ Often insensate to pinprick because nerve endings have been destroyed.
  - ○ Large areas require grafting. Small areas may heal from the edges after weeks.
- • Methods for determining body surface area percentage of a burn injury.
  - • The extent of a burn is classified as a percentage of the total body surface area (BSA).
  - • "Rule of nines" (Figure 8-18)
    - ○ The adult body is divided into anatomic regions that have surface area percentages that are all multiples of 9%.
    - ○ Less accurate for children who tend to have proportionally larger heads and smaller legs: pediatric version developed.
    - ○ Calculations with the rule of nines tend to overestimate burn size.
  - • "Rule of palms"
    - ○ May be used to estimate burns encompassing 5% total BSA or less.
    - ○ The surface area of the patient's palm is estimated to be about 1% of the patient's total BSA.
  - • Lund and Browder Chart
    - ○ Adult and pediatric versions are widely used in burn care.
- • Initial treatment guidelines
  - • Remove all clothing and jewelry.
  - • Assess for associated injuries or shock; be sure to assess the posterior surface of the patient for burn injury.
  - • Keep burned extremities elevated above the level of the heart.
  - • Keep the burned patient warm.
  - • Monitor vital signs at least every 15 to 30 minutes.
  - • Establish vascular access with LR solution. Two commonly used burn resuscitation formulas are the Parkland burn formula (4 mL/kg

When determining the extent of a burn, include only partial-thickness and full-thickness burns in the estimate.

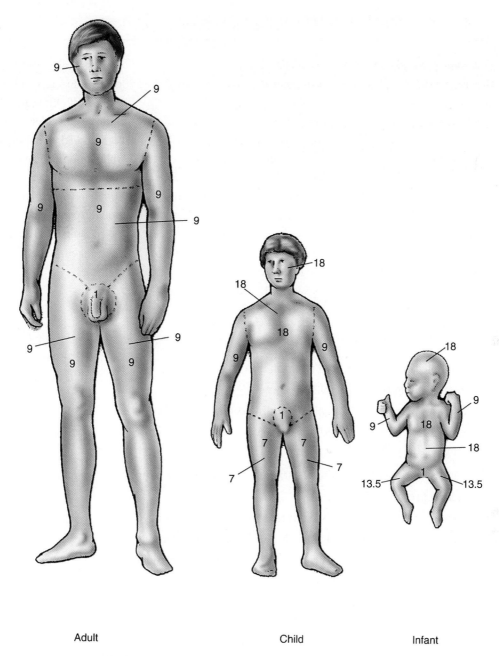

Adult   Child   Infant

Figure 8-18 The rule of nines for an adult, child, and infant.

divided by the percentage of total BSA burned) and the consensus formula (2 to 4 mL/kg divided by the percentage of total BSA burned). The resulting number is administered over the first 8 hours after a burn injury. A maintenance fluid containing dextrose is also used in very young children (younger than 2 years) because very young children have a low reserve of glycogen. Glycogen depletion causes hypoglycemia and subsequent brain damage in this age group.

Burns Best Treated in a Burn Center[15]

- Partial thickness burns greater than 10% TBSA
- Burns that involve the face, hands, feet, genitalia, perineum, or major joints
- Third-degree burns in any age group
- Electrical burns, including lightning injury
- Chemical burns
- Inhalation injury
- Burn injury in patients with preexisting medical disorders that could complicate management, prolong recovery, or affect mortality
- Any patients with burns or concomitant trauma (such as fractures) in which the burn injury poses the greatest risk of morbidity or mortality. In such cases, if the trauma poses the greater immediate risk, the patient initially may be stabilized in a trauma center before being transferred to a burn unit.
- Physician judgement is necessary in such situations and should be concert with the regional medical control plan and triage protocols
- Burned children in hospitals without qualified personnel or equipment for care of children
- Burn injury in patients who will require special, emotional, or long-term rehabilitative intervention

TBSA, total body surface area

- Urinary catheter insertion for fluid resuscitation or as indicated.
- Give patient nothing by mouth (NPO).
- Insert a nasogastric tube for all air transport patients, burns affecting more than 20% total BSA, or those who are intoxicated or intubated, or as indicated.
- Give intramuscular injection of tetanus toxoid if patient has not been immunized in preceding 5 years.
- Pain management: IV analgesia is often necessary to treat pain. Do not attribute combativeness or anxiety to pain until adequate perfusion, oxygenation, and ventilation are established. Consider narcotic therapy for pain management.
- Give pain medication IV in small increments, titrated to level of comfort.
- Provide emotional support to patient and family.

Case Study Resolution

After performing a primary survey to ensure there are no immediate life-threatening injuries, perform a thorough physical examination to determine the extent of known injuries and locate any other injuries. Try to obtain a thorough history. Administer oxygen, establish vascular access, and evaluate the patient's vital signs. The patient's ventilatory rate is 18 breaths per minute, heart rate is 96 beats per minute, BP is 140/80 mm Hg, and her skin is pink, warm, and dry. SpO$_2$ on room air is 98%. Clean and dress the abrasion over the left eye and cover the left ear with a sterile dressing. Place the patient on a cardiac monitor and obtain a beside glucose test. Obtain necessary radiographs and laboratory studies and perform additional interventions based on your assessment findings and test results.

References

1. Templeton JM. Jr. *Mechanism of injury: biomechanics in pediatric trauma: prevention, acute care, rehabilitation.* Eichelberger MR. St. Louis: Mosby–Year-Book, 1993.

2. Stafford PW, Blinman TA, Nance ML. Practical points in evaluation and resuscitation of the injured child. *Surg Clin North Am* 2002;82:273–301.

3. Committee on Injury and Poison Prevention. American Academy of Pediatrics. Falls from heights: windows, roofs, and balconies. *Pediatrics* 2001;107:1188–1191.

4. Meller JL, Shermeta DW. Falls in urban children: a problem revisited. *Am J Dis Child* 1987;141:1271–1275.

5. Barlow B, Niemirska M, Gandhi R, et al. Ten years of experience with falls from a height in children. *J Pediatr Surg* 1983;18:509–511.

6. Committee on Injury and Poison Prevention. American Academy of Pediatrics. Bicycle helmets. *Pediatrics* 2001;108:1030–1032.

7. Rivara FP, Grossman D. Injury control. In: Kliegman RM, Behrman RE, Jenson HB, eds. *Nelson textbook of pediatrics,* 18th ed. New York: WB Saunders, 2007.

8. Gerardi MJ. Evaluation and management of the multiple trauma patient. In: Strange GR, Ahrens WR, Lelyveld S, et al, eds. *Pediatric emergency medicine: a comprehensive study guide,* 2nd ed. New York: McGraw-Hill, 2002.

9. Carruthers GN. Spinal immobilization. In: Dieckmann RA, Fiser DH, Selbst SM, eds. *Illustrated textbook of pediatric emergency & critical care procedures,* St. Louis: Mosby–Year Book, 1997.

10. Davis HW, Carrasco MM. Child abuse and neglect. In: Zitelli BJ, Davis HW, eds. *Atlas of pediatric physical diagnosis,* 4th ed. St. Louis: Mosby, 2002.

11. Evans RW, Wilberger JE. Traumatic disorders. In: Goetz CM, ed. *Textbook of clinical neurology,* 2nd ed., New York: Elsevier, 2003.

12. Cantor RM, Leaming JM. Pediatric trauma. In: Marx JA, Hockberger RS, Walls RM, eds. *Rosen's emergency medicine: concepts and clinical practice,* 5th ed. St. Louis: Mosby, 2002.

13. Jarjosa JL. Blunt thoracic and abdominal traum. In: Custer JW, Rau RE, eds. The Harriet Lane handbook: a manual for pediatric house officers, 18th ed. Philadelphia: Mosby, 2009.

14. Lucid WA, Taylor TB. Thoracic trauma. In: Strange GR, Ahrens WR, Lelyveld S, et al., eds. *Pediatric emergency medicine: a comprehensive study guide,* 2nd ed. New York: McGraw-Hill, 2002.

15. Reprinted from Committee on Trauma. (2006). Guidelines for the operations of burn units: Resources for optimal care of the injured patient (pp 79-86). Chicago: American College of Surgeons.

Chapter Quiz

1. True or False: Penetrating trauma is the most common mechanism of serious injury in the pediatric patient.

2. The single most common cause of injury in children is:
   A) Motor vehicle crashes
   B) Falls
   C) Pedestrian injuries
   D) Firearm-related injuries

3. What is the earliest clinical manifestation of compensated shock in children?
   A) Restlessness
   B) Hypotension
   C) Tachycardia
   D) Diminished peripheral pulses

4. A 10-year-old child presents with a knife impaled in his skull. Your best course of action regarding the impaled object will be to:
   A) Secure the object in place.
   B) Apply an occlusive dressing over the object.
   C) Remove the object immediately and apply direct pressure to the wound to minimize bleeding.
   D) Complete the primary survey and then remove the object to assess the length of the blade.

5. Which of the following is a manifestation of Cushing's triad?
   A) Hypotension
   B) Tachycardia
   C) Hypoglycemia
   D) Bradycardia

6. With which type of injury is a Chance fracture most commonly associated?
   A) Gunshot wound
   B) Child abuse
   C) Lapbelt use
   D) Bicycle handlebars

7. Which of the following is the most common type of skull fracture in the pediatric patient?
   A) Basilar
   B) Linear
   C) Depressed
   D) Open

8. Which of the following is an immediately life-threatening chest injury that must be identified and treated during the primary survey?

   A) Tension pneumothorax

   B) Pulmonary contusion

   C) Myocardial contusion

   D) Aortic disruption

9. When performing spinal stabilization, which of the following body areas should be secured to the backboard last?

   A) Head

   B) Chest

   C) Pelvis

   D) Legs

10. Under what conditions can an infant or child found in a safety seat be used to transport the child to the hospital?

Chapter Answers

1. False. Blunt trauma is the most common mechanism of serious injury in the pediatric patient.

2. B. Falls are the single most common cause of injury in children.

3. C. Tachycardia is the earliest clinical manifestation of compensated shock in children. Hypotension is a late sign of shock.

4. A. Leave the impaled object in place. The only indications for nonsurgical removal of an impaled object are: 1) It is not possible to ventilate the child without removing the foreign body (e.g., the object is impaled in the patient's cheek), or 2) the presence of the object would interfere with chest compressions. Manually secure the object, expose the wound area, control bleeding if present, and use a bulky dressing to help stabilize the object in place.

5. D. Increases in intracranial pressure cause characteristic changes in vital signs including hypertension, bradycardia, and an irregular breathing pattern (Cushing's triad). Cushing's triad is a **LATE** sign of increased ICP.

6. C. A Chance fracture is a horizontal fracture of the thoracic or lumbar spine caused by hyperflexion injuries with little or no compression of the vertebral body. Chance fractures are also called seatbelt fractures, since they are commonly associated with the wearing of lap-type seatbelts.

7. B. Linear skull fractures make up approximately 60% to 90% of skull fractures in children.

8. A. Immediately life-threatening injuries that must be identified and managed in the primary survey include airway obstruction, open pneumothorax, tension pneumothorax, massive hemothorax, flail chest, and cardiac tamponade. Potentially life-threatening injuries that must be identified and for which treatment must begin in the secondary survey include pulmonary contusion, myocardial contusion, aortic disruption, traumatic diaphragmatic rupture, tracheobronchial disruption, and esophageal disruption.

9. A. When performing spinal stabilization, secure the child's torso to the board first, the legs next, and the head last.

10. If the child's condition is stable, a child safety seat can be used for stabilization only after a brief inspection to ensure the seat has not sustained any major structural damage and only if the safety seat can be secured appropriately in the ambulance. If a child is critically injured or the child's condition has the potential to worsen, a safety seat should **NOT** be used for stabilization. Instead, the child should be removed from the seat onto a rigid backboard and stabilized.

Toxicological Emergencies

9

Case Study

An 18-month-old boy was found holding a bottle of bleach. When his mother yelled, the child dropped the bottle and some bleach spilled onto the front of him. It is unknown if the child actually drank any of the bleach. You find the child crying. His color is pink and he does not show any obvious signs of respiratory distress.

What should you do next?

Objectives

1. Define poison.
2. Explain the role of a Poison Control Center (PCC).
3. Describe the routes of entry of toxic substances into the body.
4. Explain why children are at risk for toxic exposures.
5. Identify the pediatric age group at the greatest risk for unintentional poisoning.
6. Define toxidrome.
7 List five common toxidromes and typical signs and symptoms associated with each.
8. Describe the general management principles for a toxic exposure by ingestion.
9. List the principles of gastric decontamination.
10. Identify the types of ingestions for which activated charcoal should be used.
11. Describe the use of specific therapies for poisonings caused by acetaminophen, β-blockers, calcium channel blockers, iron, opiates, salicylates, and tricyclic antidepressants.

Introduction

A **poison** is a substance that, on ingestion, inhalation, absorption, application, injection, or development within the body in relatively small amounts, may cause structural damage or functional disturbance.

- Poisons can be found in four forms: solid, liquid, spray, or gas.
- Poisons may enter the body through ingestion, inhalation, injection, or absorption (Figure 9-1).

  Poisoning by ingestion is the focus of this chapter.

- Poisonings may be unintentional or intentional.
  - Most poisonings are unintentional (accidental) and may occur because of dosage errors, idiosyncratic reactions, environmental exposure, occupational exposure, or childhood poisoning.
  - Intentional poisonings may result from acts of terrorism, suicide (self-poisoning), or homicide (murder).

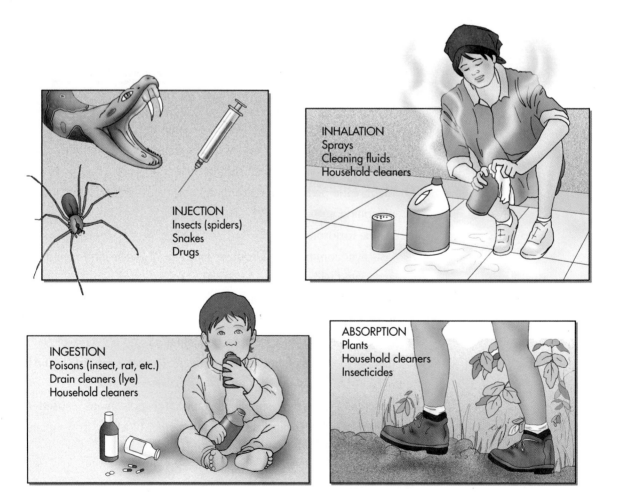

Figure 9-1   Poisons may enter the body through ingestion, inhalation, injection, and absorption.

Poison Control Centers

In the United States, poison centers are information sources and do not provide direct patient treatment.

- PCCs provide free, 24-hour emergency telephone service for the public and medical professionals. 1-800-222-1222 is the telephone number for every poison center in the United States. Call this number 24 hours a day, 7 days a week to talk to a poison expert.[1]

- The telephone is staffed by medical personnel highly trained in the recognition and assessment of poisonings, first-aid treatment, and drug information, reducing the time required to diagnose and establish definitive care for the poisoned patient.

- The PCC is often contacted from the scene by emergency medical services (EMS) personnel requesting information and advice regarding the management of a poisoned patient. The ability to accept treatment orders/instructions from a PCC is based on local medical direction and local protocols.

Toxic Exposure and the Pediatric Patient

Children younger than 6 years are at the greatest risk for unintentional poisoning.

- Children are at risk for toxic exposures because of their developmental and environmental characteristics.
  - Developmental
    - Curious by nature.
    - Mobile.
    - Explore their environment by putting most things in their mouths.
    - Imitate the behavior of others.
    - Inability to discriminate a toxic substance from a nontoxic one.
    - Drawn to attractive packaging and smell of many products found around the home.

Many poisonings take place during mealtime or when the family routine is disrupted.

  - Environmental
    - Toxic substances (e.g., household cleaning agents, gardening chemicals, plants) are often accessible to a child (Figure 9-2).
      - Improper storage.
      - Availability of substances in their immediate environment.
    - Inattentiveness of caregiver/inadequate supervision.

Poisonings in older children and adolescents usually represent manipulative behavior, chemical or drug abuse, or genuine suicide attempts.[2]

- Of the more than 2 million human poisoning exposures reported to the Toxic Exposure Surveillance System (TESS) of the American Association of Poison Control Centers (AAPCC) in 2002:
  - More than 50% (51.6%) occurred in children younger than 6 years.
  - More than 30% occurred in children younger than 3 years.
- Most pediatric toxic exposures.
  - Are unintentional.
  - Occur in the home.
  - Involve only a single substance.

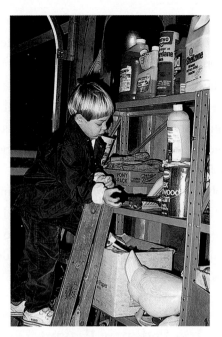

Figure 9-2   Toxic substances such as household cleaning agents and gardening chemicals are often within reach of a curious child.

Tox Fact

Substances Most Frequently Involved in Pediatric Exposures[3] (Children Younger than 6 Years)	
Substance	%*
Cosmetics and personal care products	13.3
Cleaning substances	10.3
Analgesics	7.4
Foreign bodies	7.1
Topicals	7.0
Plants	5.1
Cough and cold preparations	5.1
Pesticides	4.1
Vitamins	3.7
Gastrointestinal preparations	3.2
Antimicrobials	2.8
Antihistamines	2.6
Arts/crafts/office supplies	2.6
Hormones and hormone antagonists	2.3
Hydrocarbons	1.8

*Percentages are based on total number of exposures in children under 6 years (1,227,381) rather than the total number of substances.

Drug Pearl
Activated Charcoal

- Activated charcoal is a fine, black, tasteless powder produced from organic materials that effectively adsorbs (binds with) toxins and prevents their systemic absorption. Charcoal can only bind a drug that is *not yet absorbed* from the GI tract.
- Activated charcoal should *never* be administered to a patient who has a depressed gag reflex or altered mental status unless it is administered by nasogastric tube and the airway is protected by a tracheal tube. Aspiration of charcoal may cause a severe and potentially fatal pneumonitis.
- Activated charcoal looks like mud. The patient may be more willing to drink it if he or she cannot see it. Consider placing the medication in a covered opaque container and

have the child drink through a straw. Before administering activated charcoal, shake the container thoroughly. If it is too thick to shake well, remove the cap and stir it until well mixed.
- Be prepared for vomiting. (Charcoal stains any clothing it contacts.) Have suction readily available.
- Activated charcoal is contraindicated in poisonings involving ingestion of caustics (e.g., hydrochloric acid, bleach, ammonia) or hydrocarbons (e.g., gasoline, kerosene).
- Activated charcoal is ineffective for iron, lithium, heavy metals, and most solvents and is not recommended for poisonings involving these substances.

- Death due to unintentional poisoning in young children is uncommon because of increased product safety measures (e.g., child-resistant packaging), increased poison prevention education, early recognition of exposure, and improvements in medical management.

Assessment of the Child with a Possible Toxic Exposure

Scene Safety

Consider the possibility of a toxic exposure in any situation involving a patient with an altered mental status.

Upon arrival at a scene, perform a scene size-up to determine the nature of the incident and request additional support, if necessary. Ensure the scene is safe before proceeding with patient assessment.

If the caller identified the nature of the incident at the time of dispatch (e.g., ingestion of a relative's medication, swallowed bleach, or acetaminophen overdose), contact with your poison center may be advisable to determine the toxicity of the substance and identify an appropriate treatment plan. However, you may not be aware that the situation involves a toxic exposure until arrival at the scene. The environment may reveal fire, smoke, spilled liquids, open containers, or a chemical odor indicating a toxic exposure. In such situations, determine the need for special protective equipment (and additional resources) before attempting patient assessment.

Detailed initial assessment information and interventions were presented in Chapter 2 and are not repeated here. Additional history, signs and symptoms, and interventions specific to each disorder are listed.

Additional History

The history provides critical information in the assessment of the patient with a suspected toxic exposure. In addition to the SAMPLE or CIAMPEDS history, consider the following questions when obtaining a focused history for a patient with a toxic exposure. This list will require modification on the basis of the patient's age and chief complaint.

Critical questions to ask in a toxic exposure situation include what, when, where, why, and how.

Knowing the time of ingestion is critical when considering gastric emptying and antidote administration.

- What is the poison?
  - Determine the exact name of the product, if possible (Figure 9-3).
  - Obtain histories from different family members to help confirm the type and dose of exposure.
  - Are there any pill bottles, commercial products, or plants to support the history?
- How was it taken (i.e., ingested, inhaled, absorbed, or injected)?
- When was it taken?

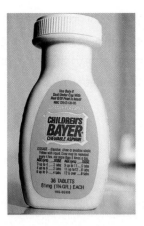

Figure 9-3   If the toxic exposure involves ingestion, obtain the bottle or container of the ingestant. If the specific substance is unknown or if there is any doubt as to the agent ingested, obtain all medicines from the home and transport them to the hospital with the child.

- Where was the child found? How long was the child alone? Any witnesses? Any other children around?
- How much was taken?
  - Number of pills, amount of liquid?
  - How many/amount available before ingestion?
  - How many/much now in the container?
- Where is the substance stored?
- What is the child's age? Weight?
- Has the child vomited? How many times?
- What home remedies have been attempted? (Ask specifically about herbal or folk remedies.)
- Has a PCC been contacted? If so, what instructions were received? What treatment has already been given?
- Has the child been depressed or experienced recent emotional stress?
  - Divorce, death in the family.
  - Possible suicide attempt in older school-age child or adolescent.

When performing a physical examination on a patient with a known or suspected toxic exposure, be vigilant in your search for information regarding the severity and cause of the exposure. Changes in the patient's mental status, vital signs, skin temperature and moisture, and pupil size may provide a constellation of physical findings that are typical of a specific toxin. Characteristic findings that are useful in recognizing a specific class of poisoning are called **toxidromes** (see Tables 9-1 and 9-2). Your physical examination findings may provide the only clues to the presence of a toxin if the patient is unresponsive. Familiarity with common toxidromes will enable you to recognize the diagnostic significance of your history and physical examination findings and implement an appropriate treatment plan.

Focused Physical Examination

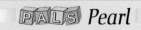
Pearl

It is important to note that a patient may not have all of the signs and symptoms associated with a single toxidrome and, when multiple substances are involved, it may be impossible to identify a specific toxidrome.

TABLE 9-1 *Clinical Presentations of Specific Toxidromes*

		Toxidrome
Anticholinergic	Signs/symptoms	Agitation or reduced responsiveness, tachypnea, tachycardia, slightly elevated temperature, blurred vision, dilated pupils, urinary retention, decreased bowel sounds; dry, flushed skin
	Typical agents	Atropine, diphenhydramine, scopolamine
	Primary antidote	Physostigmine
Cholinergic	Signs/symptoms	Altered mental status, tachypnea, bronchospasm, bradycardia or tachycardia, salivation, constricted pupils, polyuria, defecation, emesis, fever, lacrimation, seizures, diaphoresis
	Typical agents	Organophosphate insecticides (malathion), carbamate insecticides (carbaryl), some mushrooms, nerve agents
	Primary antidote	Atropine
Opioid	Signs/symptoms	Altered mental status, bradypnea or apnea, bradycardia, hypotension, pinpoint pupils, hypothermia
	Typical agents	Codeine, fentanyl, heroin, meperidine, methadone, oxycodone, dextromethorphan, propoxyphene
	Primary antidote	Naloxone
Sedative/hypnotic	Signs/symptoms	Slurred speech, confusion, hypotension, tachycardia, pupil dilation or constriction, dry mouth, respiratory depression, decreased temperature, delirium, hallucinations, coma, paresthesias, blurred vision, ataxia, nystagmus
	Typical agents	Ethanol, anticonvulsants, barbiturates, benzodiazepines
	Primary antidote	Benzodiazepines: flumazenil
Sympathomimetic	Signs/symptoms	Agitation, tachypnea, tachycardia, hypertension, excessive speech and motor activity, tremor, dilated pupils, disorientation, insomnia, psychosis, fever, seizures, diaphoresis
	Typical agents	Albuterol, amphetamines (e.g., "ecstasy"), caffeine, cocaine, epinephrine, ephedrine, methamphetamine, phencyclidine, pseudoephedrine
	Primary antidote	Benzodiazepines

TABLE 9-2 *Toxicology Memory Aids*

Anticholinergic syndrome (antihistamines, tricyclic antidepressants)	Mad as a hatter—confused delirium Red as a beet—flushed skin Dry as a bone—dry mouth Hot as Hades—hyperthermia Blind as a bat—dilated pupils
Cholinergic syndrome ("SLUDGE" or "DUMBELS")	**S**alivation, **L**acrimation, **U**rination, **D**efecation, **G**astrointestinal distress, **E**mesis **D**iarrhea, **U**rination, **M**iosis (pinpoint pupils), **B**ronchospasm/**B**ronchorrhea/**B**radycardia, **E**mesis, **L**acrimation, **S**alivation

Assessment of the patient with a possible toxic exposure includes the following objective measurements and clinical parameters:

Airway

- Look for signs of airway edema, burns, excessive crying, stridor, and drooling. If the child has any of these signs or refuses to eat or drink, suspect a significant airway injury.
- As you assess the patient's airway, note the presence of any odors that may help determine the cause of the patient's condition (Table 9–3).
- Use positioning or airway adjuncts as necessary to maintain patency and suction as needed.
- Perform tracheal intubation if the airway cannot be maintained by positioning or if prolonged assisted ventilation is anticipated. Consider the use of pharmacologic adjuncts to aid in intubation.
- Severe upper airway injury following a caustic ingestion may prevent routine tracheal intubation.
- The use of succinylcholine for rapid sequence intubation can result in prolonged paralysis in patients with organophosphate toxicity.

Breathing

- An increased ventilatory rate may result from theophylline or hydrocarbon ingestion or agents that cause metabolic acidosis such as

Because poisoned patients can deteriorate rapidly, frequent reassessment of the primary survey is necessary.

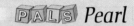 *Pearl*

The effects of toxins may result in altered mental status, emesis, or seizures, increasing the patient's risk of airway obstruction, aspiration, and lung damage. Be alert to potential airway problems and ensure suction is readily available.

TABLE 9-3 *Odors and Toxins*

Odor	Toxin
Acetone	Acetone, isopropyl alcohol, salicylates
Alcohol	Ethanol, isopropyl alcohol
Bitter almonds	Cyanide
Carrots	Water hemlock
Fishy	Zinc or aluminum phosphide
Fruity	Isopropyl alcohol, chlorinated hydrocarbons (e.g., chloroform)
Garlic	Arsenic, organophosphates, dimethyl sulfoxide, phosphorus, thallium
Glue	Toluene
Mothballs	Camphor
Pears	Chloral hydrate, paraldehyde
Rotten eggs	Sulfur dioxide, hydrogen sulfide
Shoe polish	Nitrobenzene
Vinyl	Ethchlorvynol
Wintergreen	Methyl salicylates

ethylene glycol, methanol, and salicylates (the increased ventilatory rate is a compensatory mechanism for acidosis).

- Noncardiogenic pulmonary edema is possible with any overdose that has led to apnea and has been associated with
  - Heroin, meperidine, methadone, barbiturates, cocaine, and salicylates.
  - After aspiration of chemicals such as kerosene and gasoline.
  - After exposure to toxic gases such as chlorine, phosgene, and carbon monoxide.
- Bradypnea may result from exposure to sedative/hypnotics, barbiturates, opioids, clonidine, alcohol, organophosphates, carbamates, strychnine, venom from the Mojave rattlesnake, and botulinum toxin.
- If ventilation is adequate, provide supplemental oxygen as necessary. Use a nonrebreather mask or blow-by as tolerated. If breathing is inadequate, assist ventilation using a bag-mask device with supplemental oxygen. If abdominal distention occurs, consider placing a nasogastric tube (if not contraindicated) to release air from stomach.

Circulation

- Place the child on a cardiac monitor.
- Sedative/hypnotics, opioids, β-blockers, calcium channel blockers, digoxin, clonidine, organophosphates, and carbamate insecticides, and some eye drops (e.g., Visine) cause bradycardia. Plants that contain cardiac glycosides such as lily of the valley, foxglove, and oleander also cause bradycardia.
- Examples of substances associated with an increased heart rate include amphetamines, caffeine, cocaine, ephedrine, phencyclidine, and theophylline.

Disability (Mental Status)

- Anticholinergic agents, cocaine, amphetamines, ethanol, sedative-hypnotic withdrawal, and hypoglycemic agents frequently cause central nervous system (CNS) stimulation, which is manifested as agitation and delirium.
- Benzodiazepines, sedative-hypnotics, barbiturates, and alcohols cause CNS depression. Agents such as ethanol and salicylates induce

Consider the possibility of a toxic exposure in an otherwise healthy patient with pulmonary edema.

Mental status is frequently affected by drugs and toxins.

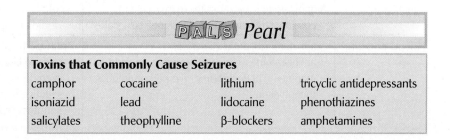

PALS Pearl

Toxins that Commonly Cause Seizures			
camphor	cocaine	lithium	tricyclic antidepressants
isoniazid	lead	lidocaine	phenothiazines
salicylates	theophylline	β-blockers	amphetamines

hypoglycemia, which may contribute to CNS depression. Some agents, such as tricyclic antidepressants, cause dose-related CNS excitation and depression.

Vital Signs

- Many toxins can produce changes in the patient's blood pressure, heart rate, ventilatory rate, and temperature (Table 9-4). The patient's mental status, skin temperature and moisture, and pupil size should also be assessed and documented. Frequent reassessment is important to note any trends or changes in the patient's condition.
- When assessing the patient's oxygen saturation, remember that:
  - Any condition that reduces the strength of the arterial pulse may interfere with the measurement of the SpO_2. This includes hypotension, hypothermia, vasoconstrictive drugs, or placement of the oximeter sensor distal to a blood pressure cuff.
  - Pulse oximeters may record falsely elevated amounts of oxyhemoglobin in patients with abnormal forms of hemoglobin, such as carboxyhemoglobin or methemoglobin.

Pupils

- Assessment of pupil size is important in the evaluation of a toxic patient.
- Agents such as opioids, clonidine, phencyclidine, and some sedative-hypnotics may cause constricted pupils (miosis).

TABLE 9-4 *Toxins and Vital Sign Changes*

Vital Sign	Increased	Decreased
Temperature	Amphetamines, anticholinergics, antihistamines, antipsychotic agents, cocaine, monoamine oxidase inhibitors, nicotine, phenothiazines, salicylates, sympathomimetics, theophylline, tricyclic antidepressants, serotonin reuptake inhibitors	Barbiturates, carbon monoxide, clonidine, ethanol, insulin, opiates, oral hypoglycemic agents, phenothiazines, sedative/hypnotics
Pulse	Amphetamines, anticholinergics, antihistamines, cocaine, phencyclidine, sympathomimetics, theophylline	Alcohol, β-blockers, calcium channel blockers, carbamates, clonidine, digoxin, opiates, organophosphates
Ventilations	Amphetamines, barbiturates (early), caffeine, cocaine, ethylene glycol, methanol, salicylates	Alcohols and ethanol, barbiturates (late), clonidine, opiates, sedative/hypnotics
Blood pressure	Amphetamines, anticholinergics, antihistamines, caffeine, clonidine, cocaine, marijuana, phencyclidine, sympathomimetics, theophylline	Antihypertensives, barbiturates, β-blockers, calcium channel blockers, clonidine, cyanide, opiates, phenothiazines, sedative/hypnotics, tricyclic antidepressants (late)

Pupil dilation is a less specific physical finding than pupil constriction.

- Meperidine (Demerol) is an opioid that may cause pupil *dilation*.
- Pupil dilation may result from sympathomimetics, anticholinergics, antihistamines, and hypoxia.
- Nystagmus (rapid, jerky eye movement) may be seen with exposure to anticonvulsants (especially carbamazepine and phenytoin), lithium, ethanol, barbiturates, sedative-hypnotics, monoamine oxidase inhibitors, isoniazid, and phencyclidine.

General Guidelines for Managing the Poisoned Patient

Most poisoned patients require only supportive therapy.

The poisoned patient can often be appropriately managed using the following general guidelines:

- Use personal protective equipment (PPE).
- Ensure adequate airway, ventilation, and circulation.
- If cervical spine trauma is suspected, manually stabilize the spine until the patient has been fully stabilized to a backboard or the cervical spine has been cleared.
- Obtain a thorough history and perform a focused physical examination.
- Consider hypoglycemia in an unresponsive or seizing patient. Check blood sugar.
- Initiate cardiac monitoring and obtain vascular access as indicated.
- Consult with a PCC as needed for specific treatment to prevent further absorption of the toxin (or antidotal therapy).
  - Decontamination procedures as indicated.
  - Opioid overdose: naloxone.
  - Organophosphates: high-dose atropine.
  - Tricyclic antidepressants: sodium bicarbonate.
  - β-Blockers: glucagon.
  - Dystonic reactions: diphenhydramine.
- Frequently monitor vital signs and electrocardiogram (ECG) findings.
- Safely obtain any substance or substance container of a suspected poison and transport it with the patient.

Decontamination methods used will depend on the toxin and type of exposure.

- Skin
  - If the toxic exposure involved absorption of the substance through the patient's skin, protect yourself by donning appropriate PPE. This may include specific clothing and respiratory gear designed to protect you while caring for the patient.
  - Remove the child's clothing and place it in plastic bags.
  - Flood exposed areas of the skin with water to remove residual material from the skin. Try to avoid contaminating uninvolved areas of skin on the patient.
  - Wash exposed areas with soap and water for 10 to 15 minutes with gentle sponging.
- Eyes
  - If the toxin has had direct contact with the eye, protect yourself by donning appropriate PPE.
  - Remove any contaminated clothing from the patient and place it in plastic bags.
  - Irrigate the exposed eye with saline or lukewarm water for at least 20 minutes, except in alkali exposures, which require 30 to 60 minutes of irrigation.
  - To minimize the risk of contaminating the unaffected eye, attach intravenous (IV) tubing to a bag of normal saline and use the end of the IV tubing to flush the eye. Make sure the eyes are open.
  - If a sink is used to decontaminate the eyes, do not use the full force of a faucet to irrigate the affected eye. Instead, use a pitcher or similar container to pour water into the eye.
- GI decontamination
  - The purpose of gastric decontamination is to prevent further absorption of the toxin by removing it from the GI tract or binding it to a nonabsorbable agent.
  - Activated charcoal
    - Treatment of choice for GI decontamination for substances that can adsorb onto charcoal (Figure 9–4).
    - Insertion of a tracheal tube is **essential** in a patient with a depressed gag reflex or altered mental status, especially in those undergoing gastric lavage.
    - Repeat dose charcoal is useful in the management of theophylline, phenobarbital, phenytoin, salicylates, and carbamazepine ingestions.
    - Cathartics are no longer recommended as a method of GI decontamination.

Decontamination

Gentle sponging should be used to avoid abrasions that would permit greater absorption of the toxin.

Airway protection is the primary concern during gastrointestinal (GI) decontamination procedures.

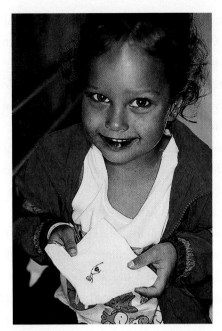

Figure 9-4   This young girl has brought a sample of the mushrooms she ate to the hospital to help identify them. She has been given activated charcoal.

- Gastric lavage
  - Indications
    - Orogastric lavage with a large-bore tube may be useful in patients who arrive within 1 hour after a life-threatening ingestion and/or those who are obtunded.
    - Decision to lavage should be made in consultation with a toxicologist or PCC.
  - Contraindications
    - Caustic or hydrocarbon ingestions.
    - Coingestion of sharp objects.
  - Insertion of a tracheal tube before gastric lavage should be performed in the patient with altered mental status or a depressed gag reflex to protect against aspiration of gastric contents.
  - Procedure
    - Position child on left side with the head slightly lower than the body.
    - Insert a large-bore orogastric tube (18 to 20 French).
    - Instill normal saline until gastric contents are clear.
    - Save initial return for toxicologic examination.

Watch the child closely for the development of gastric distention, which may interfere with ventilation.

- Complications may include aspiration, esophageal rupture, tracheal intubation, GI perforation, hypothermia, and electrolyte imbalances.
- Whole-bowel irrigation
  - Involves the administration, orally or via a gastric tube, of polyethylene glycol solution (Golytely, Colyte) in large volumes and at rapid rates to mechanically cleanse the GI tract.
    - Has been shown to be useful in certain ingestions when charcoal is not effective such as ingestion of toxic iron or lithium, or lead chips, or when there is ingestion of a large volume of toxic substance (cocaine swallowed in packages).
    - May also be useful in delayed therapy of enteric-coated or sustained-release preparations such as salicylates, calcium channel blockers, and β-blockers.
  - Contraindications: GI hemorrhage or obstruction, ileus, hemodynamically unstable patient, unresponsive patient, or patient with an altered mental status who is not intubated.

> At present, there is no conclusive evidence that whole-bowel irrigation improves the outcome of poisoned patients.

- pH alteration: urinary alkalinization.
  - Urinary alkalinization may be used to facilitate elimination of weak acids such as salicylates, barbiturates, and methotrexate from the body.
  - Sodium bicarbonate is given IV bolus and followed by a continuous infusion.
  - Goal is urinary pH of 7 to 8.
  - Monitor closely for electrolyte disturbances (e.g., hypocalcemia).
- Hemodialysis is useful for low-molecular-weight substances that have a low volume of distribution and low binding to plasma proteins, such as aspirin, theophylline, lithium, and alcohols.

Enhanced Elimination

Table 9-5 provides a list of commonly ingested substances, associated signs and symptoms, and possible interventions. Table 9-6 provides a list of substances that are particularly toxic, even in small doses.

TABLE 9-5 *Specific Drug Ingestions*

	Aspirin (Acetylsalicylic Acid)
Description	Common antipyretic, analgesic, antiinflammatory agent. More than 200 products contain aspirin. Metabolic acidosis common in children. Common products: Pepto-Bismol, Excedrin, Alka-Seltzer.
Signs/symptoms	Early signs and symptoms include tachypnea, diaphoresis, hyperpyrexia, vomiting, and tinnitus or deafness. Mild: nausea/vomiting. Moderate: tachypnea, tinnitus, dehydration, confusion, fever, metabolic acidosis, respiratory alkalosis. Severe: severe metabolic acidosis, coma, seizures, renal failure.
Interventions	ABCs, O$_2$ Activated charcoal appropriate for stable patients, but should not be given to moderately or severely ill patients; start IV for moderate to severe ingestion; fluid resuscitation if shock present. Alkalinization of urine with sodium bicarbonate; alkalinization is important in increasing the elimination of salicylate and decreasing the entry of salicylate into the CNS. Severe poisonings require hemodialysis.
	Acetaminophen
Description	Common analgesic with antipyretic properties. One of the five most common drugs ingested by children. Rapidly absorbed from GI tract and metabolized by liver. Common products: Nyquil, Percogesic, Comtrex.
Signs/symptoms	Initially, mild nausea or no symptoms. Does not usually present with altered mental status in the first 24 hours; mental status changes suggest polydrug overdose. Over several days, vomiting, abdominal pain, and jaundice occur caused by potentially fatal injury to the liver. Increased liver enzymes.
Interventions	ABCs, O$_2$, IV fluids, activated charcoal. Draw liver enzymes, acetaminophen/paracetamol level. Specific antidote is N-acetylcysteine (NAC or Mucomyst)—very effective; give within 8 hours of ingestion.
	Barbiturates
Description	Highly toxic agents that depress the CNS; anticonvulsant properties. High abuse potential; alcohol enhances toxicity. Common products: pentobarbital, phenobarbital, secobarbital, amobarbital.
Signs/symptoms	Dysrhythmias, hypotension, hypothermia; "Barb blisters"—hemorrhagic blisters over areas of pressure that develop about 4 hours after ingestion. Ataxia, slurred speech, flaccid muscle tone; respiratory depression and apnea may occur with severe overdoses. Infants born to addicted mothers will be physically dependent on the drug and will show signs of withdrawal within 72 hours of birth (e.g., high-pitched cry, tremors, vomiting, seizures).

Continued

TABLE 9-5, *cont'd*

	Barbiturates
Interventions	ABCs, O$_2$, IV, monitor. Activated charcoal; intubate if needed. Urine alkalinization with sodium bicarbonate can increase phenobarbital excretion; consider hemodialysis. Treat barb blisters as second-degree burns. Possible fluid challenges and vasopressors to maintain blood pressure.
	β-Blockers
Description	Small ingestions may cause serious toxicity in infant. Slow-release forms may lead to delayed and prolonged toxicity. Common products: propranolol, metoprolol, and atenolol.
Signs/symptoms	Bradycardia with variable degrees of AV block and hypotension. CNS depression, ranging from drowsiness to coma, is a relatively common effect of beta-blocker toxicity and generally reflects the severity of the poisoning.
Interventions	ABCs, O$_2$, IV, cardiac monitor. Glucagon is the treatment of choice for bradycardia and hypotension. Possible fluid challenges and vasopressors to maintain blood pressure.
	Calcium Channel Blockers
Description	Small ingestions may cause serious toxicity in infant. Slow-release forms may lead to delayed and prolonged toxicity. Common products: diltiazem (Cardizem), verapamil (Isoptin, Calan).
Signs/symptoms	Bradycardia with variable degrees of AV block and hypotension, prolongation of QT interval, widening of QRS complex, right bundle branch block. Altered mental status. Hyperglycemia (secondary to blockage of insulin release); seizures, coma.
Interventions	ABCs, O$_2$, IV, cardiac monitor. Treat bradycardia per resuscitation guidelines; have pacer at bedside. Possible calcium chloride. Possible fluid challenges and vasopressors to maintain blood pressure.
	Carbamate Insecticides
Description	Less toxic than organophosphates, although effects are similar. Toxicity is usually limited to muscarinic effects; nicotinic effects uncommon. Common products: flea and tick powders, ant killers.
Signs/symptoms	Muscarinic effects: vomiting, diarrhea, abdominal cramping, bradycardia, excessive salivation, and sweating.
Interventions	Protective equipment, remove contaminated clothing, ABCs, O$_2$, IV, cardiac monitor. Remove affected clothing. The benefits of gastrointestinal decontamination after ingestion are controversial because most patients have vomited before seeking medical assistance. Atropine is given until signs of muscarinic toxicity (e.g., symptomatic bradycardia, bronchorrhea, or wheezing) are reversed. Treat coma and seizures if they occur.

TABLE 9-5, *cont'd*

	Caustics (Acids, Alkalis)
Description	Alkaline agents cause liquefaction necrosis, a deep penetration injury that turns tissue, fats, and proteins to soap, damaging all tissue layers. Tissue destruction continues until the substance is significantly neutralized by tissue or the concentration is greatly reduced.
	Acids cause an immediate coagulation-type necrosis, which damages superficial layers of tissue and denatures protein, altering its structure in a process similar to cooking an egg white. This process creates an eschar, which tends to self-limit further damage. An acid injury may continue to evolve for up to 90 minutes after the ingestion.
	Common alkaline products: bleach, ammonia, dishwasher detergent, laundry detergent, drain and oven cleaners.
	Common acid products: sulfuric, hydrochloric, or hydrofluoric acid.
Signs/symptoms	Severe burns to the stomach or esophagus may be present with little external evidence of the severity of the injury.
	Upper airway obstruction with difficulty breathing, speaking, or swallowing.
	GI hemorrhage, esophageal or gastric perforation
	Vomiting, stridor, drooling—if two of these three symptoms are present, likelihood of GI burns is high. Of these signs, vomiting is the most powerful predictor of severe esophageal injury.
	Severity of injury due to caustics depends on nature, concentration, and volume of the caustic solution; duration of exposure, presence or absence of stomach contents, esophageal reflux after the ingestion, tone of pyloric sphincter.
Interventions	Protective equipment, ABCs, O_2, IV.
	Priority—airway management; flexible fiberoptic intubation over an endoscope is preferable to standard orotracheal intubation. Intubation may further traumatize damaged areas or perforate the pharynx; therefore, blind nasotracheal intubation is contraindicated. Emergent cricothyrotomy may be necessary.
	Do NOT induce vomiting—increased tissue damage as esophagus is reexposed to the substance. Activated charcoal is contraindicated because caustics are poorly adsorbed by charcoal; creates a problem with visualization during endoscopy.
	Controversy exists regarding whether attempts should be made to neutralize the caustic substance with water or milk.
	If a history of significant ingestion with oral lesions or if child is otherwise symptomatic, perform endoscopy to determine extent of injury.
	Clonidine
Description	Used for the treatment of hypertension and sometimes used to alleviate opioid and nicotine withdrawal symptoms.
	Available in pills and sustained-release transdermal patches.
	Several pediatric cases of clonidine toxicity have followed ingestion, mouthing, or inadvertent dermal application of clonidine transdermal patches; severe toxicity has been reported after ingestion of as little as 0.1 mg (one tablet) by a child.
Signs/symptoms	Altered mental status, pupil constriction, and respiratory depression. (Note: these symptoms can appear exactly like opiate toxicity making it difficult to distinguish clonidine ingestion from opiate overdose.)
	Hypotension, bradycardia, (may be initially hypertensive).
Interventions	ABCs, O_2, IV, cardiac monitor.
	Treat coma, hypotension, bradycardia, and hypothermia (usually resolve with supportive measures such as fluids, atropine, dopamine, and warming).
	Naloxone may be helpful in reversing effects (conflicting evidence).
	Gastric decontamination (lavage preferred).

Continued

TABLE 9-5, *cont'd*	
	Digoxin
Description	Used for treatment of congestive heart failure and supraventricular dysrhythmias.
	Several plants contain cardiac glycosides (digoxin-like substances) including foxglove, oleander, and lily of the valley.
Signs/symptoms	Altered mental status, nausea and vomiting, abdominal pain, headache.
	Almost any cardiac dysrhythmia may occur.
Interventions	ABCs, O$_2$, IV, cardiac monitor.
	Activated charcoal.
	Treat symptomatic or unstable dysrhythmias per resuscitation guidelines.
	Gastric aspiration or lavage may increase vagal tone and precipitate bradydysrhythmias.
	Administer antidote (digoxin immune Fab [Digibind]) for life-threatening dysrhythmias caused by digoxin overdose.
	Avoid calcium chloride and potassium when treating digoxin toxicity.
	Ethanol (Ethyl Alcohol, Alcohol)
Description	In young children, alcohol suppresses the liver's ability to manufacture glucose; alcohol intoxication increases susceptibility to hypoglycemia and altered mental status.
	As little as 30 to 60 mL of 40% ethanol can cause altered mental status and hypoglycemia in toddlers.
	Common products: Ethanol can be found in many household products including aftershave lotions, cold/allergy medications, cough preparations, glass cleaners, mouthwashes, and perfumes/colognes.
Signs/symptoms	Characteristic breath odor.
	Hypothermia, hypoglycemia in younger children.
	Respiratory depression, altered mental status, slurred speech, sedation.
	Gastric irritation, vomiting.
	Myocardial depression, hypotension due to vasodilation.
Interventions	ABCs, O$_2$.
	Treatment is primarily supportive.
	Administer glucose if hypoglycemia present.
	Ethylene Glycol (Antifreeze), Methanol (Methyl Alcohol, Wood Alcohol)
Description	Ethylene glycol is metabolized to oxalic and glycolic acids, leading to profound metabolic acidosis and coma; as little as 5 mL may be toxic to an infant.
	Methanol, found in window-washer fluid or gas-line antifreeze, is metabolized to formic acid, with the same effect as ethylene glycol; as little as 15 mL may be toxic to an infant.
Signs/symptoms	Altered mental status with appearance of inebriation or reduced responsiveness or coma.
	Tachypnea, tachycardia, nausea and emesis; abdominal pain, muscle incoordination, seizures; blurred vision possible with methanol.
Interventions	ABCs, O$_2$, IV.
	Administer glucose if hypoglycemia present.
	Fomepizole is an antidote for methanol and ethylene glycol poisoning. Iindications for use are levels 20 mg/dL or higher or high anion gap metabolic acidosis.
	Ethanol may be used when fomepizole is not available.
	Consider hemodialysis in severe cases (renal failure, blindness, and severe metabolic acidosis refractory to bicarbonate therapy).

TABLE 9-5, *cont'd*

	Heavy Metal Poisoning (Zinc, Lead, Mercury, Arsenic)
Description	Poisoning may affect every body system including CNS, heart, lungs, liver, and kidney. The metals deposit themselves in the body and are excreted slowly. 85% of arsenic exposures involve children younger than 6 years old.[4]
Signs/symptoms	Irritability, headaches, confusion, paresthesias around lips and mouth Nausea/vomiting, metallic taste, palpitations, ECG changes. Watery ricelike diarrhea with arsenic; garlic odor to breath or feces with arsenic. Burns, corneal changes with zinc. Metal fume fever—inhaling metal oxides causes fever, chills, vomiting. Lead poisoning—headaches, anorexia, abdominal pain, seizures.
Interventions	Protective equipment. ABCs, O$_2$, IV. Arsenic—chelation therapy; mercury—chelation therapy, treat seizures; zinc—chelation therapy, antipyretics, analgesics; lead—chelation therapy, treat seizures.
	Hydrocarbons (Petroleum Distillates)
Description	Toxic dose varies depending on agent involved and whether it was aspirated, ingested, or inhaled. Common products: lamp oil, gasoline, lighter fluid, kerosene, furniture polish, turpentine, pine oil, phenol.
Signs/symptoms	Coughing and choking on initial ingestion; gradual increase in work of breathing. Odor of hydrocarbon on breath. Dry, persistent cough; crackles, wheezes, diminished breath sounds, tachypnea. Nausea/vomiting. Dizziness, altered mental status. Dysrhythmias possible. May cause skin surface burns.
Interventions	Protective equipment, remove contaminated clothing, and wash skin with soap and water. ABCs, O$_2$, assist ventilations as necessary, anticipate need for intubation. Activated charcoal contraindicated; consult Poison Control.
	Iron
Description	In an infant, ingestion of 600 to 900 mg supplemental iron (generally two to three tablets) can cause severe toxicity. In survivors, severe scarring and obstruction of GI tract may develop. Common products: multivitamins, prenatal vitamins.
Signs/symptoms	Nausea (initial symptoms may appear flulike), emesis and diarrhea, possibly with blood; abdominal pain; severely poisoned child may present with lethargy or coma and signs of shock.
Interventions	ABCs, O$_2$, IV (aggressive IV fluids). NOT bound to activated charcoal. Antidote: deferoxamine (child's urine will turn pink, salmon, or rose in color). Obtain abdominal radiograph because most iron tablets are radiopaque (except chewable vitamins and children's liquid). Whole bowel irrigation if positive radiograph findings.

Continued

TABLE 9-5, *cont'd*

	Isoniazid
Description	Used in the treatment of tuberculosis; depletes vitamin B_6, which is required for synthesis of GABA, an inhibitory neurotransmitter. Reduced GABA concentration can lead to seizures. Initial signs of poisoning typically appear within 30 minutes to 2.5 hours of ingestion.
Signs/symptoms	Slurred speech, dizziness, ataxia, vomiting, and tachycardia may progress to seizures or coma; metabolic acidosis, altered mental status, tachypnea, hypotension.
Interventions	ABCs, O_2, IV. Activated charcoal. Treat coma, seizures, and metabolic acidosis if they occur. Pyridoxine (vitamin B_6) is specific antidote and usually terminates diazepam-resistant seizures.
	Isopropyl Alcohol (Rubbing Alcohol)
Description	Isopropyl alcohol is a potent CNS depressant (twice as potent as ethanol) and is metabolized to acetone, which may contribute to and prolong CNS depression. Adsorbs poorly to activated charcoal (approximately 1 g of charcoal will bind 1 mL of 70% alcohol). Widely used as a disinfectant and antiseptic.
Signs/symptoms	Altered mental status with the appearance of inebriation, slurred speech, reduced responsiveness, coma; tachycardia, hypotension, nausea and emesis, abdominal pain due to gastric irritation; hypoglycemia and hemorrhagic gastritis are possible. Distinct breath odor of acetone (because isopropyl alcohol is metabolized to acetone).
Interventions	ABCs, O_2, IV, monitor; monitor airway closely. Treatment is primarily supportive—observe for at least 6 to 12 hours. Administer glucose if hypoglycemia present. Do NOT induce vomiting (risk of rapidly developing coma). Large ingestion may require dialysis if coma or myocardial depression occurs.
	Opiates
Description	Common products: codeine, fentanyl, heroin, meperidine, methadone, oxycodone, dextromethorphan, and propoxyphene.
Signs/symptoms	Altered mental status, bradypnea or apnea, bradycardia, hypotension, pinpoint pupils, hypothermia. Suspect opioid toxicity when the clinical triad of CNS depression, respiratory depression, and miosis (pinpoint pupils) is present.
Interventions	ABCs, O_2, IV, cardiac monitor; cervical spine stabilization if trauma is suspected. Tracheal intubation is indicated in patients who cannot protect their airway. Obtain serum glucose level; give dextrose if indicated. Administer naloxone for significant CNS and/or respiratory depression. Assist breathing with a bag-mask device as necessary. If an IV cannot be established, administer naloxone IM. Larger than usual doses of naloxone may be required for diphenoxylate/atropine (Lomotil), methadone, propoxyphene, pentazocine, and the fentanyl derivatives.

TABLE 9-5, *cont'd*

	Organophosphates
Description	Widely used pesticides; signs and symptoms usually occur within 30 minutes to 2 hours of exposure but may be delayed up to several hours. In the acute phase, there is no test that can identify organophosphate toxicity; initial management based on clinical findings. Common products: No-Pest Strips, roach killers, diazinon, malathion, and parathion.
Signs/symptoms	Early signs are muscarinic: nausea, vomiting, abdominal cramps, urinary and fecal incontinence, increased bronchial secretions, cough, wheezing, dyspnea, sweating, salivation, miosis, blurred vision, and lacrimation. Nicotinic effects include twitching, fasciculations, weakness, hypertension, tachycardia, and in severe cases paralysis and respiratory failure; death is usually caused by respiratory muscle paralysis. There is frequently a solvent odor and some describe a garlic-like odor of the organophosphate. Pay careful attention to respiratory muscle weakness; sudden respiratory arrest may occur.
Interventions	Protective equipment, remove contaminated clothing, decontamination procedures; ABCs, O_2, IV, cardiac monitor. The benefits of gastrointestinal decontamination after ingestion are controversial because most patients have vomited before seeking medical assistance. Atropine is antidote for muscarinic effects; goal is drying of airway secretions to maintain oxygenation and ventilation—tachycardia is NOT a contraindication to its use; treatment must usually continue for at least 24 hours. Pralidoxime is antidote for nicotinic effects; treatment is generally necessary for at least 48 hours. If intubation is required, note potential interactions between neuromuscular blockers and organophosphates.
	Sedative/Hypnotics
Description	CNS depressants with primary effect of respiratory depression. Category includes barbiturates, benzodiazepines (e.g., alprazolam, clorazepate, chlordiazepoxide, clonazepam, diazepam, flurazepam, lorazepam, midazolam, oxazepam, temazepam, triazolam), and antihistamines.
Signs/symptoms	Slurred speech, confusion, hypotension, tachycardia, pupil dilation or constriction, decreased temperature. Overdose in children tends to cause excitation rather than CNS depression.
Interventions	ABCs, O_2. Activated charcoal. Benzodiazepine antidote (flumazenil) as directed; flumazenil should not be used routinely in setting of overdose—may be used as a diagnostic tool in pure benzodiazepine toxicity; contraindicated in patients with seizure disorders, chronic use of benzodiazepines, coingestion of substances that can cause seizures (includes tricyclic antidepressants, theophylline, chloral hydrate, isoniazid, and carbamazepine); may precipitate seizures that are difficult to control.

Continued

TABLE 9-5, *cont'd*

	Theophylline
Description	Widely used; narrow therapeutic index; many dosage forms.
	Many drug-drug, drug-disease, and drug-food interactions.
	Increased mortality associated with children younger than 2 years in acute overdoses.
Signs/symptoms	Agitation, tachycardia, nausea and emesis, depressed mental status.
	Hypotension possible, electrolyte disturbances common.
	Sinus tachycardia common, but SVT and other dysrhythmias possible.
	Seizures, status epilepticus.
Interventions	ABCs, O_2, IV, cardiac monitor.
	Well bound to activated charcoal; give if asymptomatic or minimally symptomatic.
	Dysrhythmias may respond to a short-acting β-blocker, such as esmolol.
	Seizures minimally responsive to conventional anticonvulsant agents.
	Serum theophylline level, electrolytes, glucose, ABG, 12-lead ECG.
	Tricyclic Antidepressants
Description	Toxicity causes direct effects on vascular tone (vasodilation), decreased cardiac contractility, intraventricular conduction delays, and serious dysrhythmias including VT (most common), torsades de pointes, and AV blocks (less common).
	Progression from early to late symptoms may be rapid.
	Common products: amitriptyline, desipramine, doxepin, trazodone, nortriptyline.
Signs/symptoms	Early signs: tachycardia, restlessness, anxiety, and increased temperature.
	Late signs (3 C's): Coma, Convulsions, Cardiac dysrhythmias (with widening of QRS complex, prolonged QT interval).
	Refractory hypotension, dilated pupils, slurred speech, dry mouth, urinary retention, seizures, altered mental status.
Interventions	ABCs, O_2, IV, cardiac monitor.
	Treat seizures, prevent injury.
	Continuous ECG monitoring, even in the patient who is asymptomatic at presentation.
	Treat symptomatic or unstable dysrhythmias per resuscitation guidelines; sodium bicarbonate is the primary treatment modality for severe intoxication.
	If hypotension present, IV fluid bolus of 10 mL/kg; monitor for pulmonary edema; vasopressors for persistent hypotension.
	Signs of significant toxicity (QRS prolongation, lethargy, or hypotension) mandate continuous monitoring until symptom free for 24 hours.

ABC, airway, breathing, circulation; ABGs, arterial blood gases; AV, atrioventricular; CBC, complete blood count; CNS, central nervous system; ECG, electrocardiogram; GABA, gamma-aminobutyric acid; GI, gastrointestinal; IM, intramuscular; IV, intravenous; O_2, oxygen; SVT, supraventricular tachycardia.

TABLE 9-6 *Toxicity in Small Doses*

	Benzocaine
Description	Found in many first aid ointments and infant teething formulas.
	Benzocaine is metabolized to aniline and nitrosobenzene, which can cause methemoglobinemia (especially in infants younger than 4 months). Methemoglobinemia has occurred in an infant after ingestion of 100 mg of benzocaine (amount in 1/4 teaspoon of Baby Orajel).
	Common products: Americaine Topical Anesthetic First Aid Ointment (20% benzocaine), Baby Orajel (7.5%), Baby Orajel Nighttime Formula (10%).
Signs/symptoms	Symptoms begin 30 minutes to 6 hours after ingestion.
	Tachycardia, tachypnea, and cyanosis that does not respond to oxygen.
	Agitation, hypoxia, metabolic acidosis, coma, seizures with more severe exposures.
Interventions	Gastric lavage if patient presents within 30 minutes of ingestion and has ingested less than 1/4 tsp of benzocaine-containing substance, followed by activated charcoal.
	Antidote is methylene blue. Indications for use are methemoglobin levels above 30% and symptoms of respiratory distress or altered mental status.
	Camphor
Description	Found in over-the-counter liniments and cold preparations.
	Rapid-acting neurotoxin that produces CNS excitation and depression
	Pediatric toxic dose: 1 g (equivalent to 10 mL of Campho-Phenique or 5 mL of camphorated oil).
	Rapid onset of symptoms 5 to 120 minutes after ingestion.
	Common products: Campho-Phenique (10.8% camphor), Vicks VapoRub (4.18%), camphorated oil (20% camphor), Mentholatum (9% camphor), Ben-Gay Children's Rub (5%).
Signs/symptoms	Initial feeling of generalized warmth that may be followed by altered mental status (confusion, delirium, restlessness, hallucinations).
	Muscle twitching and fasciculations may precede seizures, but seizures may occur without preceding symptoms.
Interventions	GI decontamination if it can be accomplished within 1 hour of ingestion followed by activated charcoal, seizures are managed with benzodiazepines, supportive care.
	Chloroquine
Description	Used for treatment and prophylaxis of malaria and specific connective tissue diseases.
	Powerful rapidly acting cardiotoxin capable of causing sudden cardiorespiratory collapse.
	One 300-mg tablet resulted in the death of a 3-year-old and 750 mg caused ventricular fibrillation in a 13-year-old.
Signs/symptoms	Bradycardia, ventricular tachycardia/fibrillation, torsades de pointes, profound hypotension, shock; drowsiness followed by excitability; dyspnea, sudden apnea; dysphagia, facial paresthesias, tremor, slurred speech, hyporeflexia, seizures, coma.
Interventions	Diazepam appears to have a cardioprotective effect in chloroquine poisoning.
	IV fluids and vasopressors as needed to manage hypotension, sodium bicarbonate for severe intoxication.
	Lomotil
Description	Antidiarrheal that is a combination opiate/anticholinergic preparation.
	Onset is biphasic—early anticholinergic toxicity, opiate toxicity delayed 8 to 30 hours.
	Respiratory depression can occur as late as 24 hours after ingestion and does not appear to be correlated with the dose ingested and severity of symptoms.

Continued

TABLE 9-6, *cont'd*	
Signs/symptoms	Signs and symptoms vary and depend on the time since the ingestion—manifestations may represent either anticholinergic or opioid intoxication; opioid effects often predominate. Opioid—constricted pupils, respiratory depression, and respiratory arrest. Anticholinergic—dilated pupils; warm, dry skin; tachycardia, flushed face.
Interventions	Naloxone—repeated doses may be necessary because duration of effect is much shorter than that of Lomotil; anticholinergic symptoms may appear when naloxone is given. Because of the risk of sudden respiratory arrest, admit and observe all children with Lomotil ingestion for at least 24 hours.
Description	**Methyl Salicylate** Mechanism: salicylate toxicity Oil of wintergreen contains 98% methyl salicylate; 1 tsp contains 7 g of salicylate (equivalent to 21 adult aspirin tablets). Amounts less than 1 tsp have resulted in a child's death. Common products: topical liniments (e.g., Ben Gay, Icy Hot Balm), oil of wintergreen food flavoring.
Signs/symptoms	Onset of symptoms typically within 2 hours of ingestion. Tachypnea, diaphoresis, hyperpyrexia, vomiting, tinnitus, hyperthermia, seizures, coma.
Interventions	Activated charcoal, urine alkalinization, hemodialysis, serum salicylate level (toxicity of salicylates correlates poorly with serum levels).
Description	**Tetrahydrozoline (Imidazolines)** Structurally similar to clonidine. Toxicity: 1-2 drops of 0.1% solution in infants. Onset of symptoms delayed 2 to 6 hours after ingestion. Common products: Visine (tetrahydrozoline), Afrin (oxymetolazine).
Signs/symptoms	Initial hypertension followed by hypotension, bradycardia, seizures, and coma.
Interventions	GI decontamination. If initial hypertension severe, consider titratable medication (e.g., esmolol, nitroprusside). Fluids, vasopressors may be necessary for treatment of hypotension.

CNS, central nervous system; GI, gastrointestinal; IV, intravenous.

Case Study Resolution

Quickly and carefully, assess the child to determine the patency of his airway. You find the child is acting normally for his age. Examination of the child's mouth reveals no signs of an exposure. His ventilatory rate is 26 breaths per minute, heart rate is 114 beats per minute, and the child has no signs of difficulty breathing, speaking, or swallowing. Wash off the bleach from the child's body. Contact poison control if additional advice is needed.

References

1. American Association of Poison Centers. http://www.1-800-222-1222.info/1800/home.asp (Accessed 9/16/2010).

2. Dart RC, Rumack BH. Poisoning. In: Hay Jr WW, Hayward AR, Levin MJ, et al., eds. *Current pediatric diagnosis and treatment*, 15th ed. 2000.

3. Watson WA, Litovitz TL, Rodgers Jr GC, et al. Annual report of the American Association of Poison Control Centers Toxic Exposure Surveillance System. *Am J Emerg Med* 2003;21:353–421.

4. Leikin JB. Arsenic. In Pediatric Emergency Medicine: A Comprehensive Study Guide, 2e. Strange GR, Ahrens WR, Lelyveld S, Schafermeyer RW (ed.), New York: McGraw-Hill, 2002, p 586-588.

Chapter Quiz

1. List five common toxidromes and provide an example of a typical agent in each category.

Toxidrome _____; example _____

Toxidrome _____; example _____

Toxidrome _____; example _____

Toxidrome _____; example _____

Toxidrome _____; example _____

Questions 2–8 refer to the following scenario.

A 3-year-old is found barely responsive by her babysitter. The babysitter was distracted "for just a minute" by a telephone call and lost track of the child. The child was located on the ground just outside the garage door. The patient's skin looks flushed and she is laboring to breathe. You note secretions are draining from the patient's mouth and she has been incontinent of urine. The child is unaware of your presence.

2. From the information provided, complete the following documentation regarding the Pediatric Assessment Triangle.
   Appearance:
   Breathing:
   Circulation:

3. Based on the information provided, your FIRST intervention should be to:
   A) Establish vascular access.
   B) Suction the airway.
   C) Perform a secondary (head-to-toe) survey.
   D) Perform tracheal intubation.

4. For each of the following, record the estimated values for a 3-year-old child.
   A) Weight:
   B) Ventilatory rate:
   C) Heart rate:
   D) Blood pressure:

5. Your assessment reveals the child will open her eyes and withdraw in response to a painful stimulus but makes incomprehensible sounds. Her Glasgow Coma Scale score is:
   A) 6
   B) 8
   C) 10
   D) 12

6. The child's ventilatory rate is 44/min, heart rate is 158/min, and blood pressure is 80/60. Her skin is warm and moist. Her pupils are equal and reactive at 2 mm. Auscultation of her lungs reveals bilateral diffuse wheezes. Excessive oral secretions are present. These findings are most consistent with the _____ toxidrome.

7. Further questioning of the babysitter reveals that the child may have been out of sight for 20 to 30 minutes before she was found. The babysitter recalls having seen an open bottle of white liquid on the floor of the garage. As you continue interviewing the babysitter, a coworker tells you that he smells garlic on the child's breath. This child was most likely exposed to:
   A) An organophosphate
   B) Camphor
   C) A narcotic
   D) A β-blocker

8. You are instructed to administer atropine to this patient. Which of the following statements is correct?
   A) Question the order. Atropine is indicated for symptomatic bradycardias. This patient is not bradycardic.
   B) Administer the atropine as instructed. Atropine is being ordered in this situation to increase the patient's blood pressure.
   C) Question the order. Although atropine may be used in situations such as this, the patient is tachycardic. Atropine is contraindicated if a tachycardia is present.
   D) Administer the atropine as instructed. In this situation, atropine is being given to dry the patient's airway of secretions.

Chapter Quiz Answers

1. Toxidromes are a group of signs and symptoms useful for recognizing a specific class of poisoning. Common toxidromes include anticholinergic, cholinergic, opiate, sedative/hypnotic, and sympathomimetic.
   Toxidrome *anticholinergic*; example *atropine, diphenhydramine, scopolamine*
   Toxidrome *cholinergic*; example *organophosphates, carbamate insecticides, some mushrooms, nerve agents*
   Toxidrome *opioid*; example *codeine, fentanyl, heroin, meperidine, methadone, oxycodone, dextromethorphan, propoxyphene*
   Toxidrome *sedative/hypnotic*; example *ethanol, anticonvulsants, barbiturates, benzodiazepines*
   Toxidrome *sympathomimetic*; example *albuterol, amphetamines, caffeine, cocaine, epinephrine, ephedrine, methamphetamine, phencyclidine, pseudoephedrine*

2. Pediatric Assessment Triangle (first impression) findings:
   Appearance: Barely responsive, incontinent of urine, unaware of your presence
   Breathing: Increased work of breathing evident
   Circulation: Skin is flushed; no evidence of bleeding

3.   B. The presence of secretions draining from the mouth of a child who is unaware of your presence requires **immediate** intervention. Clear the airway with suctioning.

4.   "Normal" values for a 3-year-old child:
   A) Weight: 14 kg (31 lb.)
   B) Ventilatory rate: 24 to 40
   C) Heart rate: 90 to 150
   D) Blood pressure: BP higher than 70 mm Hg
   Refer to the tables and formulas in Chapter 3 if you need to review this information.

5.   B. The patient's Glasgow Coma Scale score is 8.

Eyes:	To pain	2
Verbal:	Incomprehensible sounds	2
Motor:	Withdraws from pain	4

6.   This patient's physical findings are most consistent with the *cholinergic* toxidrome.

7.   A. The patient's physical findings and additional information regarding the events surrounding the exposure strongly suggest organophosphate exposure.

8.   D. Atropine is the antidote for the muscarinic effects of organophosphate exposure. The goal of atropine administration in this situation is drying of airway secretions to maintain oxygenation and ventilation. Tachycardia is NOT a contraindication to its use.

10 Death of an Infant or Child

Case Study

The mother of a 3-month-old infant has called you to her home. She says that she was laying her son down for a nap and noticed that his lips were blue and he was not breathing. She thinks the episode lasted about ten seconds. The infant has been sick with an upper respiratory infection and was seen by his pediatrician several days ago. The baby is acting normally now. The infant's father appears shortly after your arrival and says he will watch his son. He insists that his child not receive further care.

What would you do next?

Objectives

1. Define Sudden Infant Death Syndrome (SIDS).
2. Discuss the typical assessment findings associated with SIDS.
3. Define Apparent Life-Threatening Event (ALTE).
4. Identify common grief reactions demonstrated by parents immediately after the death of an infant or child.

Sudden Infant Death Syndrome

Description

SIDS is also called crib death or cot death.

Sudden infant death syndrome (SIDS) is the sudden and unexpected death of an infant that remains unexplained after a thorough case investigation, including performance of a complete autopsy, examination of the death scene, and review of the clinical history.[1]

Etiology

Significant controversy revolves around the cause(s) of SIDS. It has been suggested that that SIDS is the final common pathway of three coinciding factors: (1) an infant must first have an underlying vulnerability, (2) the infant is then stressed by an outside source (such as sleeping in a prone position), and (3) the stress must occur during a critical developmental period, as in the first year of life.[2]

Current SIDS research topics include defects in normal arousal mechanisms, gene mutations affecting autonomic nervous system development, prenatal and postnatal exposure to cigarette smoke and the effects of nicotine on the developing brain, and ion channel disorders, such as those that cause QT interval prolongation.

Epidemiology and Demographics

- SIDS is the third-leading cause of infant mortality in the United States and the most common cause of postneonatal infant mortality, accounting for 40% to 50% of all deaths between 1 month and 1 year of age).[3]
- The majority of SIDS deaths occur during the first 6 months of life, most between the ages of 2 and 4 months.
- SIDS occurs more often in infant boys than in girls.
- African-American and Native American infants are two to three times more likely to die from SIDS as other infants. A lower incidence is seen among Hispanic and Asian infants.
- The SIDS rate has declined by 42% since 1992, when the recommendation was issued to have infants sleep on their backs and sides rather than their stomachs.[4]

"Infants who have suffered such a near-miss death event (ALTE) show striking epidemiologic similarities to those who have died of SIDS. They are therefore widely regarded as a living model for SIDS and have hence been extensively studied. However, there are some problems with this approach.

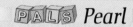 *Pearl*

SIDS and ALTE
The term near-SIDS or near-miss SIDS (now called an apparent life-threatening event or ALTE) has been applied to those infants who were about to die, but were found early enough for successful resuscitation.

TABLE 10-1 *Risk Factors for Sudden Infant Death Syndrome (SIDS)*

Maternal Risk Factors	Infant Risk Factors
• Smoking during pregnancy	• Male gender
• Drug use (cocaine, opiates)	• Prematurity
• Alcohol use	• Native American or African American ancestry
• Late or no prenatal care	• Low Apgar scores
• Low socioeconomic status	• Overheating
• Single parent status	• Prenatal and postnatal smoking exposure
• Nutritional deficiency	• Prone or side sleep position
• Young age (less than 20 y)	• Soft sleeping surface, soft bedding
• Shorter interpregnancy interval	• Recent febrile illness
	• Infant/caregiver bed sharing

- First, as is probably the case with SIDS, a large number of treatable disease entities can cause ALTE. These cannot always be identified from investigations performed after an event has occurred. A proportion of apparently idiopathic ALTE is caused by an identifiable mechanism (such as pneumonia or meningitis) that is temporary and, if identified, can be treated and therefore does not bear any relationship to SIDS itself.

- Second, it will always be impossible to say whether an infant who was resuscitated by his or her parents would indeed have died without this intervention.

- Third, certain "abnormalities" identified after ALTE (such as gastroesophageal reflux [GER]) may be coincidental and irrelevant to the ALTE themselves.

Therefore, there are some inherent ambiguities in the relationship between SIDS and ALTE, and this must be borne in mind if one draws conclusions from studies performed in infants with ALTE to the pathophysiology of SIDS."[5]

Autopsy Findings

Some SIDS victims will not have these findings.

- Multiple petechiae (most common finding) are typically present on the surfaces of the lungs, epicardium, and thymus.

- Lung congestion and vascular engorgement with or without pulmonary edema may be evident on microscopic examination

- Histologic evidence of a respiratory infection involving the larynx and trachea is present in some SIDS cases.

Apparent Life-Threatening Event

An apparent life-threatening event (ALTE) has been defined as "an episode that is frightening to the observer and that is characterized by some combination of apnea (central or occasionally obstructive), color change (usually cyanotic or pallid but occasionally erythematous or plethoric), marked change in muscle tone (usually marked limpness), choking, or gagging."[6] In clinical practice, the term ALTE has been restricted to events that fulfill the above criteria, but also involve vigorous stimulation or resuscitation.[5]

"Most idiopathic ALTEs appear to be caused by the progressive development of hypoxemia, which may progress until it becomes life-threatening or even fatal because of a failure of these infants to resuscitate themselves by arousal or gasping. This hypoxemia apparently does not, in most instances, result from a primary cessation of respiratory efforts, but is more likely to be caused by some form of upper or lower airway closure (such as obstructive apnea) and may also involve the sudden development of an intrapulmonary right-to-left shunt. The triggers eliciting these airway closures remain unknown."[5]

A wide spectrum of diseases and disorders has been found to precipitate an ALTE. The most frequent are digestive (about 50%), neurological (30%), respiratory (20%), cardiovascular (5%), metabolic and endocrine (under 5%), or diverse other problems, including abusive head injury. Fifty percent of ALTEs remain unexplained (Table 10-2).[7, 8]

Interventions for SIDS

- From a distance, use the Pediatric Assessment Triangle to form your general impression of the patient. Evaluate the child's appearance, work of breathing, and circulation to determine the severity of the child's illness or injury and assist you in determining the urgency for care.
- Perform a primary survey.
  - Assess the ABCs and determine the need for initiation/continuation of CPR.
  - Begin resuscitation using standard resuscitation guidelines if your assessment does not *clearly* indicate death, as in cases when the infant is still warm and flexible.
    - Rigor mortis is an obvious sign of death.
    - Dependent lividity is considered an obvious sign of death only when there are extensive areas of reddish-purple discoloration of the skin in dependent areas of an unresponsive, breathless, and pulseless patient.
    - In some areas, both lividity and rigor mortis must be present to be considered signs of obvious death.
  - If resuscitation is provided:
    - Calmly explain what you are doing. Explain the roles of each member of the resuscitation team. Keeping your explanations simple, provide frequent updates about what is happening and the infant's status, even if there is no change.
    - Permit the caregivers to remain within sight of the infant.
    - If possible, allow a caregiver to accompany the infant during transport to the emergency department.
    - If possible, allow caregivers to briefly touch the infant.

> If sufficient personnel are on the scene, assign one emergency medical services (EMS) professional to remain with the caregiver and provide comfort during the resuscitation effort.

- If the primary survey clearly indicates death or if the infant's response to resuscitation efforts was unsuccessful, follow local protocols regarding resuscitation and transport.
  - Some areas have an obvious death, field termination, death in the field, or similar protocol that is applicable to this type of situation.
  - In some areas, you may be required to leave the body at the scene pending the arrival of the medical examiner. In others, you may be asked to transport the body to a hospital or morgue.

> Do *not* express your own opinion about the cause of an infant's death in front of caregivers. Document your findings objectively.

TABLE 10-2 *Possible Underlying Diagnoses in Patients Presenting with ALTE*

Respiratory tract disorders	Gastrointestinal disorders
• Bronchiolitis • Pneumonia • Pertussis • Tracheoesophageal fistula • Aspiration • Laryngomalacia; tracheomalacia • Pierre Robin syndrome	• Gastroesophageal reflux • Toxic shock syndrome caused by gastroenteritis • Reye syndrome
Neurologic disorders	**Metabolic disorders**
• Meningitis • Epileptic seizures • Ondine's curse syndrome (central hypoventilation) • Spinal muscular atrophy (Werdnig Hoffmann) • Hyperexplexia (startle disease) • Joubert's syndrome • Arnold Chiari malformation • Myopathies	• Medium-chain acyl-coa deficiency • Biotinidase deficiency • Ornithine transcarbamylase deficiency • Glutaric aciduria type II • Systemic carnitine deficiency
Cardiovascular disorders	**Others**
• Long QT syndrome • Cardiac dysrhythmias • Aortic stenosis • Vascular ring	• Cyanotic breath-holding spells • Anemia • Intentional suffocation (smothering) • Munchausen syndrome by proxy

From Poets CF, Southhall DP. Sudden infant death syndrome and apparent life-threatening events. In: Taussig LM, Landau LI, eds. *Pediatric respiratory medicine.* St. Louis: Mosby, 1999:1079–1099.

- If the body must remain at the scene:
  ◦ Inform the caregivers in a sensitive manner and explain why.
  ◦ Explain that the infant is dead. Do not use euphemisms such as "expired" or "passed away."
  ◦ Initiate grief support for the family as soon as possible.
  ◦ Remain with the family until law enforcement personnel assume responsibility for the body and grief support personnel are on the scene to assist the family.
  ◦ While awaiting the arrival of grief support, law enforcement personnel, or the medical examiner, obtain the names of neighbors, relatives, or friends that you can contact to help care for other children in the home.

- If you are asked to transport the body to a hospital, encourage the caregivers to hold or touch the infant while you are on the scene.
  - Tell the caregivers the name and address of the hospital, and then write down the information for them. Do not assume they will remember.
  - If the caregivers cannot accompany you to the hospital, contact a family member or close friend who can arrive quickly and drive them.
  - En route to the hospital, allow the caregivers to touch and hold the infant.

Allowing the caregivers to hold the body enables them to focus on the reality of the death and provides an opportunity for them to say goodbye.

History and Documentation

A focused history must be obtained and the incident must be carefully documented, whether or not resuscitation efforts are initiated. Elicit the necessary information as tactfully as possible. Begin by asking the infant's name. After obtaining this information, use the baby's name when asking questions about the incident. Do not refer to the infant as "the baby," "it," or use other nonspecific words. The information in Table 10-3 should be obtained, if time permits.

SIDS Prevention

- Place an infant supine for sleep. The infant should sleep in the same room as his or her parents, but in his or her own crib or bassinette.
- The American Academy of Pediatrics recommends offering a pacifier at bedtime and naptime. The pacifier should be used when placing the infant down for sleep and not be reinserted once it falls out.[3] For breast-fed infants, delay introduction of the pacifier until breast-feeding is well established (i.e., after 1 month of age).
- Place an infant on a firm surface for sleep. Avoid placing the infant on soft or padded sleep surfaces (e.g., pillows, sheepskins, sofas, soft mattresses, waterbeds, beanbag cushions, quilts, comforters).
- Avoid the use of soft materials in the infant's sleep environment (over, under, or near the infant). This includes pillows, comforters, quilts, sheepskins, and stuffed toys. Blankets, if used, should be tucked in around the crib mattress.
- Do not overheat the infant (keep the room temperature comfortable, do not overdress the infant, use a light blanket).
- Avoid exposure to cigarette smoke.
- Do not sleep with a baby on a sofa or armchair.[9] Parents who smoke, are obese or especially tired, or have taken medicines, drugs, or alcohol that impairs their responsiveness should not share a bed with their infant.

TABLE 10-3 *SIDS History and Documentation*

Questions	Observations of the Scene
What is the baby's name?	Position and location of the infant on arrival
What happened?	General appearance of the home and other children, appearance of the room where the death occurred, condition and characteristics of the crib or sleep area
What is baby's* age?	
What does baby weigh?	
What time was baby put to bed?	Bedding (e.g., pillows, sheets, blankets, etc.), any objects in the crib (e.g., toys or bottles), or any unusual or dangerous items that could cause choking or suffocation
When did baby fall asleep?	
Who last saw baby alive?	
Who found baby? What did that person do?	
What position was baby in when he/she was found?	Medications
Was CPR attempted?	Electrical and mechanical devices in use in the room including vaporizers, space heaters, fans, and infant electronic monitors (e.g., apnea monitor or heart rate monitor)
Did baby share a bed with anyone else?	
What was the general health of baby?	
Had baby been ill recently?	
Was baby taking any medications?	Behavior of those present at the scene

*Substitute the infant's name for "baby."

Death of an Infant or Child

When communicating with the caregivers, be aware of your nonverbal communication.

Use the first name of the infant or child.

Be prepared for extremes in behavior ranging from screaming to no response.

Table 10-4 summarizes common caregiver reactions to the death of an infant or child.

- When communicating with caregivers about the death of a child, speak slowly in a quiet, calm voice. Pause every few seconds and ask the caregivers if they understand what is being said.

- Preface the bad news by saying, "This is hard to tell you, but..." Using simple terms (not medical jargon), explain that the infant or child is dead. Use the words "death," "dying," or "dead" instead of euphemisms such as "passed on," "no longer with us," or "has gone to a better place."

- Assume nothing as to how the news is going to be received. The caregiver's reaction to the disclosure of bad news may be anger, shock, withdrawal, disbelief, extreme agitation, guilt, or sorrow. In some cases, there may be no observable response, or the response may seem inappropriate.

TABLE 10-4 *Coping with the Death of an Infant or Child*

Caregiver Reaction	Intervention/Response
Shock, denial ("This can't be happening.") • Suddenness of the death left no time for preparation or goodbyes • Difficult to comprehend the death of an infant who did not appear to be sick • Inability or refusal to believe the reality of the event • Numbness, repression of emotional response	• Allow the caregivers to express their grief • Refer to the infant by name and encourage the caregivers to talk about the baby • Provide an opportunity for the caregivers to see and hold the infant's body • Do **not** say, "Time heals …"
Guilt ("If only I had …" "If only I had checked on the baby sooner." "If only I had taken the baby to the doctor with that slight cold.") • Caregiver often feels guilty about not being with the infant at the time of the incident occurred to prevent it from happening or that the infant's death was their fault	• Provide reassurance that the caregiver did not cause the infant's death • Encourage caregivers to ask questions • Keep answers to questions as brief as possible • Do **not** say, "This happened because …"
Anger ("Why my baby?") • Caregiver's anger is related to his or her inability to control or change the situation • Anger is displaced and projected to anything and everything	• Do not take anger or insults personally • Be tolerant and empathetic • Do not become defensive • Use good listening and communication skills • Do **not** say, "I know how you feel."
Helplessness, frustration ("What am I going to do?", "Why is this happening to me?") • Surfacing of painful feelings • Caregiver feels alone, disconnected, and alienated	• Ensure availability of a family friend, relative, or religious representative to provide further support • Encourage participation in local sudden infant death syndrome program support services • Do **not** say, "You can still have other children."

- Allow time for the shock to be absorbed and as much time as necessary for questions and discussion.
  - Questions frequently asked include, "Was I to blame?" "Did my baby suffer?" "Why did my baby die?" "What will happen next?" In the case of a SIDS death, common questions include, "What causes SIDS?" "What can I do to prevent another child from dying of SIDS?" "Are there symptoms I should have known about that could have prevented the death?"
  - It is important to provide adequate information to the caregivers. This may require repeating answers or explanations to make sure they are understood. Emphasize to the grieving caregivers that they were not responsible for the infant's death and that the death could not be prevented.
- An empathic response such as, "You have my (our) sincere sympathy" may be used to convey your feelings. However, there are times that silence is appropriate. Silence respects the family's feelings and allows them to regain composure at their own pace.

- Allow the family the opportunity to see and hold the infant or child. If equipment is still connected to the infant or child, prepare the family for what they will see. A child should be gowned and an infant should be gowned and diapered before the family views the body. Accompany them if necessary and assist them in relinquishing the infant's body when they are ready to do so. Some caregivers may prefer not to view the body. If this is their preference, do not attempt to force them to do so.
- Arrange for follow-up and continued support for the family during the grieving period.

Help for the Healthcare Professional

Although difficult for the family, the death of a child is also emotionally draining for healthcare professionals. Reactions suggesting a need for assistance include persistent feelings of anger, self-doubt, sadness, depression, or a desire to withdraw from others, identification with the infant's caregiver, avoidance of the caregiver, or feelings of blame toward the caregiver. It may be helpful for the healthcare team to meet with a qualified mental health professional and discuss the feelings that normally follow a pediatric death.

Case Study Resolution

This infant may have experienced an apparent life-threatening event. Attempt to convince the father that a medical evaluation is important and the baby should be transported for evaluation by a physician. If the father continues to refuse further treatment or transport for his son, seek the advice of medical direction. It may be helpful to have the physician speak directly with the baby's father by phone.

References

1. Willinger M, James LS, Catz C. Defining the sudden infant death syndrome (SIDS): deliberations of an expert panel convened by the National Institute of Health and Human Development. *Pediatr Pathol* 1991;11:677–684.

2. Filiano JJ, Kinney HC. A perspective on neuropathologic findings in victims of the sudden infant death syndrome: the triple-risk model. *Biol Neonate* 1994;65(3-4):194-197.

3. Hunt CE, Hauck FR. Sudden infant death syndrome. In: Kliegman RM, Behrman RE, Jenson HB, Stanton BF, eds. Nelson textbook of pediatrics, 18e. Philadelphia: WB Saunders, 2007.

4. Singh GK, Yu SM. Infant mortality in the United States: trends, differentials, and projections, 1950 through 2010. *Am J Public Health* 1995;85:957–964.

5. Poets CF, Southhall DP. Sudden infant death syndrome and apparent life-threatening events. In: Taussig LM, Landau LI, eds. *Pediatric respiratory medicine.* Philadelphia: Mosby, 1999:1079–1099.

6. National Institutes of Health consensus development conference on infantile apnea and home monitoring, Sept 29-Oct 1, 1986. *Pediatrics* 1987;79:292–299.

7. Kahn A. Recommended clinical evaluation of infants with apparent life-threatening event: consensus document of the European Society for the Study and Prevention of Infant Death, 2003. *Eur J Pediatr* 2004;163:108–115.

8. Altman RI, Brand DA, Forman S, et al. Abusive head injury as a cause of apparent life-threatening events in infancy. *Arch Pediatr Adolesc Med* 2003;157:1011–1015.

9. Fleming P, Blair PS. Sudden infant death syndrome. *Sleep Med Clin* 2007;2:463–476.

Chapter Quiz

You respond to a private residence for a 5-month-old male that is reportedly not breathing.

1. You are met by distraught parents who ask you to save their baby. You should first:
   A) Open the infant's airway.
   B) Perform a scene survey.
   C) Assess the infant's mental status.
   D) Ensure law enforcement personnel are en route to the scene.

2. Which of the following signs is consistent with sudden infant death syndrome (SIDS)?
   A) Bulging fontanelle
   B) Blood leaking from the ears
   C) Blood-tinged fluid in the mouth
   D) Multiple bruises on the chest and abdomen

3. Under which circumstances would you consider NOT beginning resuscitation efforts?
   A) The infant is cyanotic.
   B) Vomitus is present in the airway.
   C) The infant's torso is warm to the touch but his extremities are cool.
   D) The infant is cold to the touch and pooling of blood is evident where he was in contact with the bed.

4. SIDS is caused by:
   A) Malnutrition.
   B) Physical abuse.
   C) Airway obstruction.
   D) An unknown cause.

Chapter Quiz Answers

1. B. Rapidly survey the scene, examining the surroundings. Perform a primary survey. Begin the initial assessment by first assessing the child's mental status, then airway, breathing, circulation, and life-threatening conditions. A brief history will need to be obtained from the parents, but do not allow this to interfere with your efforts to save this patient.

2. C. A SIDS victim often has cold skin, frothy or blood-tinged fluid in the mouth and nose, lividity or dark, reddish-blue mottling on the dependent side of the body. Rigor mortis may be present. The child typically appears well nourished and healthy. Never discuss or imply child maltreatment as a possible cause of the infant's death.

3. D. Pooling in dependent areas of the body (also referred to as dependent lividity) is indicative of a "prolonged down time" (dead for a significant period). Follow local protocols regarding resuscitation and transport.

4. D. Although there are many theories about the possible causes of SIDS (second-hand smoke, sleeping position, mattress construction, etc.), the exact cause is yet unknown. SIDS is determined as the cause of death only after an autopsy is performed and all other possible causes are ruled out.

Children with Special Healthcare Needs

11

Case Study

An 18-month-old is exhibiting signs of respiratory distress. The child has a tracheostomy and has been ventilator dependent since birth. Your first impression reveals a pale, anxious child on a ventilator. You observe pale skin with cyanosis around the child's lips, nasal flaring, and minimal chest rise with ventilated breaths. You hear the sound of the high-pressure alarm on the ventilator.

What should you do next?

Objectives

1. Define children with special healthcare needs.
2. Define technology-assisted children.
3. Discuss specific assessment and management considerations for children with special healthcare needs.

Overview

- Children with special healthcare needs are those who have or who are at risk for chronic physical, developmental, behavioral, or emotional conditions that necessitate use of health and related services of a type and amount not usually required by typically developing children.[1,2]
- Technology-assisted children are a subgroup of children with special healthcare needs who depend on medical devices for their survival.
  - *Assistive technology* is a term used to describe devices used by children and adults with a disability to compensate for functional limitations and to enhance and increase learning, independence, mobility, communication, environmental control, and choice.
- The number of children with special healthcare needs is increasing. Children with gastrostomy tubes, indwelling central lines, tracheostomies, pacemakers, and home ventilators are frequently encountered by healthcare professionals.

- These children are particularly susceptible to medical problems involving the airway, breathing, and circulation.
- Vital signs may be controlled by the child's medical device.
  - Heart rate may be determined by a child's pacemaker.
  - Ventilator settings may determine the respiratory rate for a child on a home ventilator.
- Equipment failure may result in a medical emergency.
- Many children with special healthcare needs
  - Are small for age.
    - Weight or baseline vital signs may fall outside the typical range for the child's age.
    - May require equipment sizes that differ from those estimated by age.
  - Have sensory or motor deficits with or without normal cognitive function.
    - Physical and mental abilities may not be the same as those for other children of similar age.
  - Have a sensitivity or allergy to latex because of their repeated exposure to supplies and products made from latex.

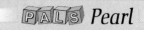

When communicating with a child in a wheelchair, keep in mind that the wheelchair is an extension of the child's personal space.

Treat each child with respect, compassion, and consideration when providing care.

Assessment and Management Considerations

- From a distance, use the Pediatric Assessment Triangle to form your general impression of the patient. Evaluate the child's appearance, work of breathing, and circulation to determine the severity of the child's illness or injury and assist you in determining the urgency for care.
  - The child's caregiver is often the best resource regarding the child's special healthcare needs. The caregiver can usually tell you what is "normal" for the child regarding his or her mental status, vital signs, normal assessment findings and level of activity, ongoing health problems, medications, and medical devices currently in use.
  - Look for a medical identification bracelet or necklace. A younger child may not have one because of the parent's fear that the child will pull it off, but an older child may wear one.
  - Ask the child's caregiver if an emergency information form (EIF) is available. The American Academy of Pediatrics (AAP) and the American College of Emergency Physicians (ACEP) advocate the use of this form for children with special healthcare needs. When completed, the form contains important information for use by healthcare personnel.

- If the child appears sick (unstable), proceed immediately with the primary survey and treat problems as you find them. If the child appears "not sick" (stable), complete the initial assessment.
- Perform a focused or detailed physical examination, based on the patient's presentation and chief complaint. Remember: your patient's condition can change at any time. A patient that initially appears "not sick" may rapidly deteriorate and appear "sick." Reassess frequently.

Airway and Breathing Considerations

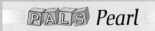 *Pearl*

A child with special healthcare needs who has any of the following conditions should be considered unstable or critical[3]:

- Partial or total airway obstruction in children with tracheostomies
- Respiratory difficulties in ventilator-dependent children
- Bradycardia, irregular pulses, or signs of compensated shock in children with pacemakers
- Fever, nausea, vomiting, headache, or a change in mental status in children with CSF shunts
- Signs of worsening illness despite appropriate home therapy in any child with a chronic health problem

Since ventilator-dependent children always require assisted ventilation, critical status applies only if one or more additional signs are present.

- Dyspnea is common in children with chronic illnesses because they have difficulty swallowing and handling their airway secretions. Excessive airway secretions and salivation may occur because of muscle weakness, brain stem injury, or other disease processes and increases the child's risk of aspiration.
- Children with tracheostomies or cerebrospinal fluid (CSF) shunts, children on home ventilators, and children with continuous positive airway pressure (CPAP) or bilevel positive airway pressure (BiPAP) devices are vulnerable to airway obstruction.
- Some congenital syndromes or diseases are associated with limited cervical motion, making intubation difficult.
  - An infant or child with Klippel-Feil syndrome has congenital fusion of the cervical vertebrae and severe shortness of the neck (Figure 11-1). Intubation can be difficult because of their inability to flex or extend their necks.
  - The child with Down syndrome is often difficult to intubate because neck rigidity and a large tongue obscure visualization of the glottis. Use of a curved blade may be more effective in displacing the large tongue to the left, permitting better visualization and easier intubation.
  - A child with juvenile-onset rheumatoid arthritis may have arthritis involving the temporomandibular joint, limiting mouth opening, and the cervical spine, limiting flexion and extension of the neck. It can be difficult or impossible to intubate these children because of their limited mouth opening and limited cervical flexion and extension.[4]
- The caregiver of an infant or child on a home apnea monitor may request evaluation of the patient after a monitor alarm. Evaluate each patient to determine life threats and the cause of the alarm.
  - When an apnea monitor is used, sensors are positioned on each side of the patient's chest. The monitor is intended to alarm primarily on the cessation of breathing timed from the last detected breath. Apnea monitors also use indirect methods to detect apnea, such as monitoring of heart rate. False alarms can occur because of a loose lead, low battery, or accidental shut off.

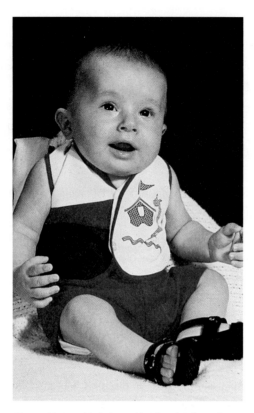

Figure 11-1   This infant with Klippel-Feil syndrome demonstrates a short neck because of fused cervical vertebrae.

- Because many apnea monitors contain a computer chip that can be downloaded to determine if the apnea or high/low heart rate alarms were accurate or caused by artifact, an apnea monitor should be transported with the patient.

Circulation Considerations

- Technology-assisted children may have a higher than normal resting heart rate, making assessment for signs of compensated shock difficult to detect.
- The infant or child with congenital heart disease (e.g., tetralogy of Fallot) may have chronic peripheral and/or central cyanosis. Consult the child's caregiver about the patient's baseline skin color.
- The infant or child with a vascular access device (VAD) (i.e., central venous catheter [CVC], implanted port, or peripherally inserted central catheter [PICC]) may require assistance because of a dislodged or damaged catheter, catheter obstruction or leakage from the catheter, or complications associated with these devices, such as a pneumothorax.

Disability (Mental Status)

Altered mental status and/or reduced responsiveness may be the normal baseline in a child with special healthcare needs. Compare your

AVPU and the pediatric Glasgow Coma Scale (GCS) may not be appropriate for these children.

assessment findings with the information provided by the patient's caregiver about the child's baseline mental status, behavior, and level of functioning.

Cerebrospinal Fluid Shunts

Purpose and Components

- CSF is produced in the choroid plexus located in the ventricles of the brain. CSF circulates through the ventricular system, around the spinal cord, and is then reabsorbed by vessels in the brain.
- Hydrocephalus ("water on the brain") develops when there is an interruption of this normal circulation due to an increase in CSF production, obstruction of CSF flow, or a decrease in CSF absorption (Figure 11-2).
  - Hydrocephalus often develops in infancy and coexists with many congenital and acquired brain disorders such as myelomeningocele, intraventricular hemorrhage, and CSF infection.
  - Signs and symptoms vary according to age. The young infant presents with a combination of irritability, lethargy, vomiting, a full fontanelle, and a head circumference that is larger than normal. After approximately 12 months of age, the head circumference changes more slowly, and the diagnosis becomes based on irritability, vomiting, lethargy, and ventriculomegaly detected by brain imaging. Older children usually complain of headache before other symptoms or signs of increased intracranial pressure.[5]

Shunts have a high complication rate.

- To drain excess CSF and reduce intracranial pressure, a shunting system is surgically implanted into the brain to drain (shunt) CSF from the ventricular system into another part of the body (Figure 11-3).

Complications

These are signs of increased ICP, as a result of fluid accumulation within the brain.

- The child with a malfunctioning shunt may present with irritability, headache, neck pain, vomiting, a bulging or full fontanelle in infants, new seizures or a change in the child's seizure pattern, behavioral

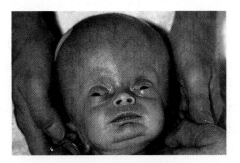

Figure 11-2   Hydrocephalus.

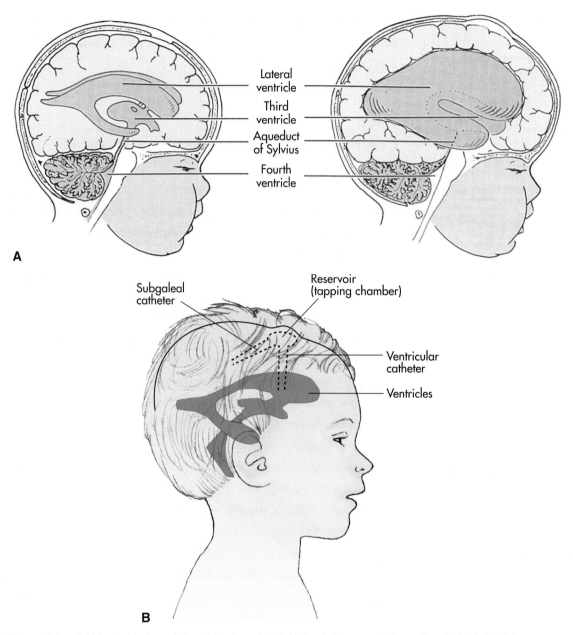

Figure 11-3   A, Untreated hydrocephalus. **B**, Cerebrospinal fluid shunt. The reservoir is usually palpable behind the ear.

changes, or "just not acting right." The child's caregiver is usually most familiar with the child's condition and can tell you if the shunt is the problem.

- In the first few months after surgery, misplacement, disconnection, or migration of the equipment can occur. These causes are identified in a "shunt series," which is a series of three radiographs including a skull film, chest film, and abdominal film.

- Infection usually occurs in the first few months after surgery and may be evidenced by obstruction, local wound problems, or unexplained fever.

Obstruction of the shunt system can occur at any time.

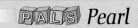 *Pearl*

Causes of Cerebrospinal Fluid Shunt Malfunction

D Displacement (catheter migration), disconnection of shunt components, drainage - overdrainage or inadequate drainage

O Obstructed or fractured catheter, kinking of distal catheter

P Perforated abdominal viscus, peritonitis, pseudocyst

E Erosion of the equipment through the skin

- Abdominal pain may be present because of infected CSF draining into the peritoneal cavity, causing peritoneal inflammation.
- If infection is present, redness, edema, or tenderness may be observed along the path of the shunt tubing. A child with a shunt infection is usually, but not always, febrile.
- Shunt failure that occurs after several years most often results from fractured tubing, overdrainage, or erosion of the equipment through the skin or into an abdominal viscus.
  - Overdrainage of the shunt can occur as the child spends more time in an upright position. A siphoning effect on the distal tubing can generate negative pressure across the valve, resulting in excessive drainage.
  - Perforation of the stomach or intestinal wall may result in peritonitis with signs and symptoms of shock. Surgical intervention is necessary.
- A pseudocyst may develop when bacteria and bacterial products enter the peritoneal cavity via the shunt catheter. This can cause an inflammatory response that involves a portion of the greater omentum, which wraps around the distal tip of the shunt catheter and seals off the catheter outlet. The resulting cyst fills with CSF, giving rise to abdominal pain and recurrence of the hydrocephalus.

Management

Maintenance of an adequate blood volume and blood pressure is critical for brain perfusion. If the blood pressure is reduced, so is cerebral perfusion pressure.

- A child with signs of increasing intracranial pressure may vomit, increasing his or her risk of aspiration.
  - Ensure suction equipment is readily available.
  - Administer supplemental oxygen, assist ventilation as necessary, and be prepared to intubate.
- If the child shows signs of shock or if hypotension is present, begin aggressive volume resuscitation using isotonic fluids. If necessary, administer a catecholamine via intravenous (IV) infusion to maintain blood pressure in the high-normal range.
- Check the child's blood sugar and administer IV dextrose if indicated.
- Treat seizures if indicated.
- Hospital management typically includes treatment of a CSF shunt infection with systemic antibiotics.
- Tapping the reservoir of the CSF shunt and aspirating fluid to temporarily lower intracranial pressure may be necessary and should be performed by a qualified and experienced healthcare professional.

Gastric Tubes and Gastrostomy Tubes

Gastric tubes and gastrostomy tube are used to provide nutrition to an infant or child who is unable to take food by mouth for an extended period. A gastric tube is a small tube passed through the nose (nasogastric) or mouth (orogastric) into the stomach. Although the diameter of the tube is small, it is uncomfortable for the patient and associated with irritation of the nasal and mucous membranes. Because of these limitations, a gastrostomy is performed when prolonged or permanent enteral nutrition is needed.

A gastrostomy feeding tube (G-tube) is either a tube or a button (skin-level device) that is surgically placed into the stomach through the abdominal wall (Figure 11-4). Initially, a full gastrostomy tube is placed (Figure 11-5), which is later replaced with a button (Figure 11-6). If the child has a gastrostomy button, ask the caregiver for the feeding tube adapter for it if the patient requires evaluation in the emergency department. A jejunostomy tube (J-tube) is another type of feeding tube that passes through the abdomen into the small intestine, bypassing the stomach.

All tubes have a balloon or mushroom-shaped tip on the inside of the stomach and a disk, clamp, or crossbar on the outside to keep them in place. If the balloon or mushroom sinks into the stomach or if the outside disk or clamp is too loose, stomach contents may leak out around the tube. After healing is complete (usually 2 to 3 weeks), a natural tract

Gastric Tubes

Many children with these tubes can eat, but they are unable to ingest sufficient calories so a G-tube is placed to supplement their feedings.

Gastrostomy Tubes

Feeding tube adapters are critical, expensive, and specific to the child's tube. Do not lose or throw away!

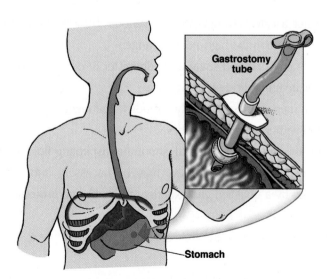

Figure 11-4 A gastrostomy tube is surgically placed into the stomach through the abdominal wall.

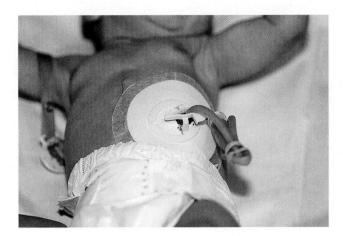

Figure 11-5   Gastrostomy tube.

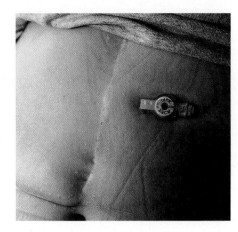

Figure 11-6   Gastrostomy button.

(fistula) is formed between the stomach and skin that helps hold the tube in place.

Complications

Common complications encountered with gastrostomy tubes include wound infection, obstruction of the tube, dislodgement of the tube, peritonitis, aspiration, leakage around the tube, bowel obstruction, electrolyte imbalance, dehydration, nausea, and diarrhea.

Management

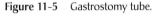

Gastric Tube

- If the child has an orogastric or nasogastric feeding tube in place and shows signs of possible aspiration (e.g., choking, coughing, and/or cyanosis), suction the airway and administer oxygen. Monitor the patient's oxygen saturation and cardiac rhythm and repeat the primary survey frequently.

- If the tube has become partially dislodged, it can be removed without harming the child. The tape should be removed from the child's face and the tube gently pulled out through the nose or mouth. When transferring care of the child, be certain to inform the receiving health–care provider of your actions so the tube can be replaced.

- If it is necessary to deliver positive-pressure ventilations to the child, the feeding tube can be used to decompress the stomach and relieve pressure on the diaphragm.

Gastrostomy Tube

- Look at the insertion site for signs of irritation, infection, or bleeding.
  - Skin irritation is not an emergent problem and can be evaluated by the child's physician.
  - If signs of infection are present, the child needs physician evaluation.
  - If bleeding is present, apply direct pressure with a sterile dressing.

- Inspect the insertion site to see if the tube has become dislodged.
  - If the tube is dislodged, you may observe a small amount of bleeding at the site and stomach contents may leak out of the hole. Cover the hole with a sterile dressing. Avoid using occlusive dressings because moisture accumulates under the dressing and can predispose the area to infection.
  - In the emergency department, assess the insertion site to determine if a temporary tube can be inserted.

Once the tube is out, the fistula will begin to close and may close completely within 4 to 6 hours.

Tracheostomy Tubes

A tracheostomy is a surgical opening into the trachea between the second through fourth tracheal rings (Figure 11-7). The opening (stoma) may be temporary or permanent.

Tracheostomy tubes have a neckplate (flange) that rests on the patient's neck over the stoma. Holes are present on each side of the neckplate through which soft tracheostomy tube ties are inserted and used to secure the tube in place.

Tracheostomy tubes range in size from 000 (for neonates) to 10 (for older adolescents). The size of the tube is marked on the sterile packaging and on the flange of the tube. A pediatric tracheostomy tube may be cuffed or uncuffed. If a cuff is present, it can be inflated with air or sterile water, depending on the brand of tube used (Figure 11-8).

Indications

Equipment

Some tracheostomy tubes are custom-made to accommodate unusual anatomy or pathology.

If it is necessary to replace a tracheostomy tube, try to use the same length and diameter tube as the one that is already in place.

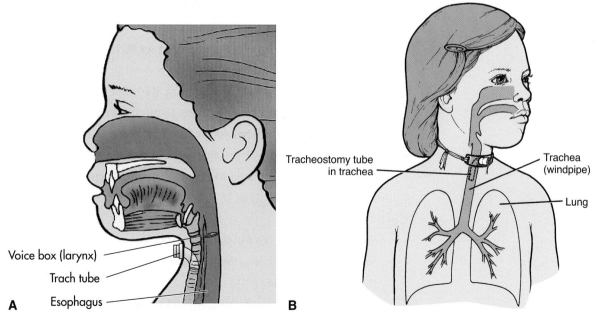

Voice box (larynx)
Trach tube
A   Esophagus

Tracheostomy tube in trachea — Trachea (windpipe)
Lung
B

Figure 11-7   A, Tracheostomy tube. **B,** Tracheostomy tube in position in the trachea and secured in place.

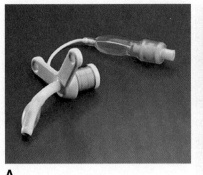 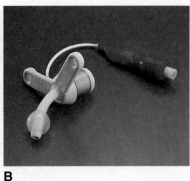 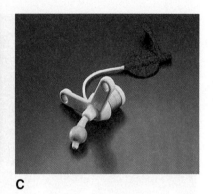

A   **B**   **C**

Figure 11-8   A, Cuffed TTS (tight to shaft) tracheostomy tube. When completely deflated, the cuff collapses tight to the shaft of the tube. **B,** Air-filled cuff. **C,** Foam cuff.

Types of Tracheostomy Tubes

All tracheostomy tubes have a standard-size opening or hub outside the patient's neck to enable attachment of a bag-mask device. Metal tracheostomy tubes require an adapter to make this connection.

- Single cannula
  - All neonatal tracheostomy tubes and most pediatric tubes are single-cannula tubes.
  - A single-cannula tracheostomy tube has one lumen that is used for airflow and suctioning of secretions (Figure 11-9). When it is necessary to change the tube, a new tube must be inserted quickly because there is nothing to keep the stoma open once the old tube is removed. When a new tube is inserted, an obturator is placed inside the tube to keep the flexible tube from kinking. After the new tube is in position, the obturator is quickly removed to permit ventilation.
- Double cannula
  - Consists of an outer cannula (main shaft), inner cannula, and an obturator (stylet) (Figure 11-10). The obturator is used only to guide the outer tube during insertion. When the outer cannula has been inserted, the obturator must be removed to permit ventilation.

When the inner tube is removed for cleaning, the outer tube keeps the child's airway open.

  - Once the outer tube is in place, the inner cannula is inserted and locked in place. The inner cannula may be disposable or reusable. A reusable inner cannula must be periodically removed for brief periods for cleaning.
- Fenestrated
  - A fenestrated tracheostomy tube helps the child learn to breathe through the upper airway and to expel secretions. It also allows the child to talk. A fenestrated tube has small holes (fenestrations) in the side of the tube (Figure 11-11). When a decannulation cap (plug) is attached to the tracheostomy tube, airflow through the stoma is blocked. Airflow is redirected through the holes in the tube, upward past the vocal cords, and out through the nose and mouth.
  - If the child cannot breathe through his or her nose or mouth, the decannulation cap **must** be removed to enable the child to breathe through the stoma.

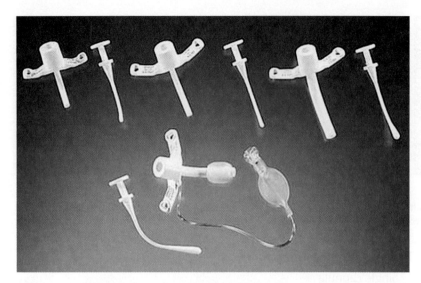

Figure 11-9 Neonatal and pediatric cuffed and uncuffed single-cannula tracheostomy tubes.

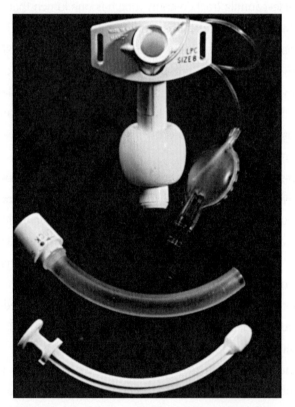

Figure 11-10 Double-cannula tracheostomy tube.
Tracheostomy tube (*top*) with inner cannula
(*middle*) and obturator (*bottom*).

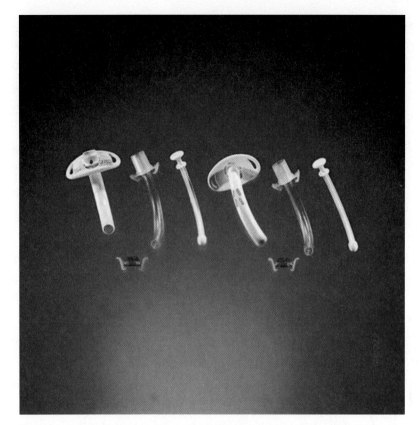

Figure 11-11 Disposable cannula cuffless fenestrated tracheostomy tubes with decannulation caps (shown in *red*).

PALS Pearl

Assume that any infant or child with a tracheostomy and signs of respiratory distress has an obstructed tube. Possible causes of the obstruction include increased secretions, a mucous plug, an obturator that was inadvertently left in the tracheostomy tube, or equipment failure, among other causes.

Complications

Although the child's caregiver is taught how to replace a tracheostomy tube at home, emergency care will be sought if the child is away from home or if the caregiver is unable to replace the tube.

Assessment and Management

An infant or child with a tracheostomy is often connected to an apnea monitor or pulse oximeter during periods when the caregiver is not present to provide direct supervision (e.g., bedtime).

The most common complications encountered with tracheostomies are dislodgement of the tube, obstruction of the tube, and infection. Incorrect reinsertion of a tracheostomy tube may result in bleeding, formation of a false tract, or perforation of the trachea or esophagus, with resulting inability to ventilate and development of subcutaneous emphysema, pneumothorax, and pneumomediastinum.[6]

Assess the child for signs of respiratory distress. If signs of respiratory distress are present, the child's history may help identify the cause of the problem.

- Consider a lower airway obstruction if the child has a history of fever and gradual worsening of his or her respiratory status.
- Consider a mucous plug, if the child's onset of symptoms was sudden and associated with a change in the consistency of his tracheostomy tube secretions.
- Consider a displaced or obstructed tracheostomy tube if the child has signs and symptoms consistent with a possible obstruction (see Box 11-4).
- In a ventilator-dependent child, a recent change in home ventilator settings or a ventilator malfunction may also cause worsening respiratory symptoms. Ask the child's caregiver about this possibility.

Clearing an Obstructed Tracheostomy Tube

- If a tracheostomy tube obstruction is suspected, attempt to ventilate through the tube with a bag-mask device with the mask removed to assess tube patency. If the child is on a home ventilator, disconnect the tracheostomy tube from the ventilator and attach the tube to the bag-mask device.

- If it is difficult to compress the bag, prepare to assess for tube obstruction.

  - Place the child in a supine position. Place a small towel roll beneath the shoulders to extend the neck and improve access to the tracheostomy tube.

  - Examine the tracheostomy tube. Ensure that the tube is properly positioned and the obturator has been removed. If the child has a fenestrated tube, make sure the decannulation cap has been removed from the tube.

  - If the child's condition has not improved, consider instilling 1 mL of normal saline into the tracheostomy tube.

- Select a suction catheter of appropriate size. The suction catheter should be no more than one half the internal diameter of the tube being suctioned. To determine the correct size suction catheter, use a length-based resuscitation tape or multiply the external diameter of the tracheostomy tube (in millimeters) by two. For example, if the tracheostomy tube is 4 mm in diameter, use an 8-French suction catheter.

- Set the suction pressure (portable or wall-mounted) to −100 mm Hg or less.

- If possible, preoxygenate the patient. Give blow-by oxygen by hold the oxygen tubing close to the opening of the tracheostomy tube. Set the oxygen flow rate to 10 to 15 L/min. If necessary, ventilate the child with a bag-mask device by attaching the bag to the tracheostomy tube.

- Gently insert the suction catheter into the tracheostomy tube (Figure 11-12).

  - The catheter should be inserted to 0.5 cm beyond or just to the end of the tracheostomy tube. Insertion of the suction catheter and suctioning should take no longer than 10 seconds per attempt. Insert the catheter without applying suction.

  - Once the catheter is in the tracheostomy tube, apply suction while slowly withdrawing the catheter, rolling it between your fingers to suction all sides of the tube.

- If suctioning equipment is not immediately available, attempt to clear the obstruction by quickly inserting and removing the obturator. This technique should *not* be used when suctioning equipment is available.

An infant or child with an obstructed tracheostomy tube will initially exhibit signs of respiratory distress that will progress to respiratory failure and arrest if the obstruction is not cleared.

In the field, ask the child's caregiver to provide you with suctioning equipment and supplies, because the items they use will be appropriate for the child's needs.

The upper airway filters and humidifies inspired air. Because a tracheostomy bypasses the upper airway, dried secretions can easily accumulate and occlude the tracheostomy, despite regular tracheostomy care.

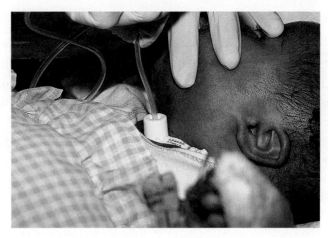

Figure 11-12 Suctioning a tracheostomy tube.

- Monitor the child's heart rate and color throughout the procedure. Stop suctioning immediately if the heart rate begins to slow or if the child becomes cyanotic.
- After suctioning, reassess the patient. Observe the child's rate and depth of breathing, skin color, heart rate, and mental status. Auscultate breath sounds and assess pulse oximetry, if available.
  - If breathing is adequate, administer oxygen.
  - If breathing is inadequate, suctioning must be repeated. Administer oxygen and allow the child to rest for 30 to 60 seconds (or provide assisted ventilation with oxygen) before beginning another attempt.
  - If there is no improvement, prepare to remove and replace the tracheostomy tube.

Removing and Replacing a Tracheostomy Tube

To remove a tracheostomy tube:

- Assemble and prepare the equipment.
  - Ensure oxygen, suction, and a bag-mask device are immediately available.
  - Ask the child's caregiver if a replacement tracheostomy tube is available. If the caregiver is not available, determine the size of the current tracheostomy tube by checking the wings (flanges) of the tube.
    - Attempt to locate the same size and model tracheostomy tube. If a similar tube is not available, use a tube of similar size. Select a tube with the same outer diameter as the child's tube or one half size smaller.
    - Inspect the new tube for cracks and tears. If the new tube has a cuff, inflate the cuff and check for leaks. Completely deflate the cuff. Avoid touching the portion of the tube that will be inserted into the trachea.

PALS Pearl

Signs of Possible Tracheostomy Tube Obstruction

- Altered mental status with restlessness, agitation
- Increased work of breathing
- Raspy noises from tracheostomy tube during breathing
- Change in sounds during breathing
- Diminished breath sounds
- Nasal flaring, retractions
- Difficulty eating or sucking
- Decreased oxygen saturation

- Marked use of accessory muscles
- Poor peripheral perfusion; mottling
- Tachycardia (bradycardia is a late sign)
- Inadequate chest rise during spontaneous or assisted ventilation
- High peak pressure alarm on ventilator
- Difficulty ventilating when providing assisted ventilation
- Cyanosis, bradycardia, and unresponsiveness (late findings)

PALS Pearl

Because the mouth and pharynx normally harbor more bacteria than the trachea does, suction the trachea (i.e., the lower airway) before suctioning the mouth or nose; however, if excessive oral secretions are present, clear the mouth with suctioning first.

- ○ Insert the obturator into the new tube and ensure that it slides in and out easily. The obturator serves as a stylet to guide the tube during insertion. Its blunt tip helps to protect the stoma from trauma during insertion.
- ○ Moisten the new tracheostomy tube with normal saline or a small amount water-soluble lubricant to ease insertion.
- ○ If time permits, cut tracheostomy ties to the appropriate length and thread the tracheostomy tie through the flange on one side of the new tube.
  - Some patients may use a tracheostomy tube holder that uses Velcro or nylon hooks to secure the tube in place instead of ties.
- ○ If a tracheostomy tube is unavailable, an endotracheal tube with an *outer* diameter equivalent to the child's tracheostomy tube can be inserted though the stoma in an emergency.
  - An endotracheal tube and tracheostomy tube that are designated as the same size may not actually be equivalent.
- Using age-appropriate language, explain the procedure to the child.
- Suction the tracheostomy tube to minimize secretions.
- If the existing tube has a deflatable cuff, deflate the cuff by connecting a 5- to 10-mL syringe to the valve on the pilot balloon. With the syringe, aspirate air or water until the pilot balloon collapses.
- While holding onto the tracheostomy tube with one hand, cut or untie the cloth ties that hold the tube in place with the other.
- Removing the tube:
  - If the child has a single-cannula tracheostomy tube, slowly withdraw the tube (Figure 11-13).

Indications for Tracheostomy Tube Suctioning

- Indication by the patient that suctioning is necessary
- Suspected aspiration of gastric or upper airway secretions
- Visible secretions in the airway; secretions bubbling in the tracheostomy tube
- Wheezes, crackles, or gurgling on inspiration or expiration audible to the patient and/or caregiver with or without auscultation
- More frequent or congested-sounding cough
- Patient unable to clear secretions by coughing
- Altered mental status, restlessness or irritability
- Unexplained increase in work of breathing, ventilatory rate, or heart rate
- Decrease in vital capacity and/or oxygen saturation
- Unilateral or bilateral absent or diminished breath sounds
- Cyanosis

Cutting the pilot balloon will not reliably deflate the cuff.

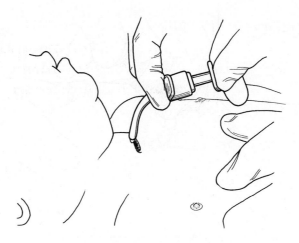

Figure 11-13 Slowly withdraw the tracheostomy tube.

Because a cough can dislodge the tracheostomy tube, be sure to hold on to the tube when the ties are not secure.

The inner cannula of a reusable tube is cleaned with hydrogen peroxide and rinsed with normal saline.

In most patients with a tracheostomy, the upper airway connected to their trachea is patent, enabling bag-mask ventilation and standard orotracheal intubation if necessary. If oxygen is administered through the mouth and nose, cover the stoma with sterile gauze.

- If the child has a double-cannula tracheostomy tube, remove the inner cannula. If the inner cannula is reusable, clean it and reinsert it. If the inner cannula is disposable, remove and discard it, and insert a new inner cannula.
- If replacing the inner cannula fails to clear the airway, remove the outer cannula as well, administer oxygen, and replace both tubes at the same time.
- Administer oxygen until the new tracheostomy tube is inserted.
  - Oxygen can be administered directly through the stoma.
  - If airflow can be heard and felt through the upper airway, oxygen can be administered by mask.
  - If there is a significant delay in replacing the tracheostomy tube, the child may require positive-pressure ventilation. If the upper airway is obstructed, deliver positive-pressure ventilation by ventilating the stoma with a bag-mask device using a neonatal mask.
- With the obturator in place inside the new tube, gently insert the tube into the stoma using a downward and forward motion that follows the curve of the trachea (Figure 11-14). If necessary, place gentle traction on the skin above or below the stoma to ease insertion. If the tracheostomy tube cannot be inserted easily, withdraw the tube, administer oxygen, and begin again. If the second attempt is unsuccessful, try a smaller tube. **Never force the tube**. Forcing the tube can create a false tract.
- After insertion, remove the obturator from the tracheostomy tube.
- Connect a bag-mask device with the mask removed to the tracheostomy tube and ventilate the child. *Do not let go of the tracheostomy tube* until it has been secured with tracheostomy ties or a tracheostomy tube holder.
- Check for proper placement of the tracheostomy tube.

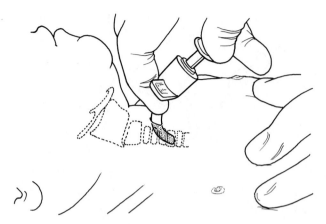

Figure 11-14 With the obturator in place inside the new tracheostomy tube, gently insert the tube into the stoma using a downward motion, following the curve of the trachea.

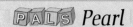 *Pearl*

A suction catheter or feeding tube may be used as a guide to facilitate insertion of a new tracheostomy tube. Insert the suction catheter through the new tracheostomy tube, and then insert the suction catheter into the stoma without applying suction. Slide the tracheostomy tube along the suction catheter and into the stoma, until it is in the proper position. *Do not let go of the suction catheter at any time before removing it from the tracheostomy tube.* Withdraw the suction catheter from the tracheostomy tube. Assess the patient.

- Signs of proper placement include equal bilateral chest rise, equal breath sounds (either spontaneous or with assisted ventilation), and improvement in mental status, heart rate, and decreased work of breathing.

- Signs of improper placement include resistance during insertion of the tube, bleeding from the stoma, lack of chest rise or poor compliance during assisted ventilation, or development of subcutaneous air in the tissues surrounding the stoma.

- After confirming proper placement of the tracheostomy tube, secure the tube using tracheostomy ties or a tracheostomy tube holder. The ties or holder should be snug enough that you can place only one finger between the fastening device and the patient's skin.

Placing a Tracheal Tube in a Tracheostomy

- If a new tracheostomy tube is not available or if replacement attempts are unsuccessful, try to insert a tracheal tube. Insertion of a tracheal tube is a temporizing measure until a tracheostomy tube of the proper size can be replaced.

- To place a tracheal tube through the stoma:

  - Select a tracheal tube that is the same or slightly smaller size than the child's tracheostomy tube. If the tracheal tube has a cuff, inflate the cuff and check for leaks. Completely deflate the cuff. Avoid touching the portion of the tube that will be inserted into the trachea. Moisten the distal end of the tracheal tube with a saline or a small amount of water-soluble lubricant.

  - Place the child in a supine position. Place a small towel roll beneath the shoulders to extend the neck.

  - Oxygenate the patient if possible just before inserting the tracheal tube.

A child with a tracheostomy may have some airway narrowing, requiring a smaller tracheal tube than usual for his or her age and size.

Note the length of the original tracheostomy tube and use it as a guide for depth of insertion of the tracheal tube.

- - Gently slide the tracheal tube through the stoma and into the airway, directing the tip downward after passing it through the stoma.
  - The insertion depth of the tracheal tube should equal the distance between the flange and the distal tip of the tracheostomy tube.
- If the tracheal tube is cuffed, inflate the cuff to stabilize the tube and minimize air leakage. Secure the tube in place.
- Tracheal intubation
  - If a tracheostomy tube or tracheal tube cannot be inserted through the stoma, orotracheal intubation can be performed unless an upper airway obstruction in present.
  - If the patient's condition does not improve or if a tracheal tube cannot be inserted, attempt assisted ventilation through the stoma.
    - For best results, attach a neonatal mask to the bag-mask device and place the mask over the stoma.
    - Alternatively, deliver positive-pressure ventilation with a mask placed over the patient's mouth and nose while covering the stoma with a gloved hand to prevent the escape of air.

Home Ventilators

A child may require long-term mechanical ventilation for many reasons including the following:
- Inadequate respiratory drive secondary to a congenital brain abnormality or brainstem damage.
- Weak respiratory muscles due to neuromuscular disease.
- Cervical spinal cord injury or other conditions that impair the conduction of nerve impulses to respiratory muscles.
- Severe chronic pulmonary disease, such as bronchopulmonary dysplasia or cystic fibrosis.

Some children require continuous mechanical ventilation; others require intermittent ventilatory support (e.g., during sleep).

Ventilator Emergencies

If signs of respiratory distress are present in a child on a ventilator, identification and treatment of possible causes are important. The DOPE mnemonic can be used to recall possible reversible causes of acute deterioration in an intubated child.
- **D**isplaced tube (e.g., right mainstem or esophageal intubation) or **D**isconnection of the tube or ventilator circuit–Reassess tube position, ventilator connections.
- **O**bstructed tube (e.g., blood or secretions are obstructing air flow)–Suction.
- **P**neumothorax (tension)–Needle thoracostomy.

- *E*quipment problem/failure (e.g., empty oxygen source, inadvertent change in ventilator settings, low battery)—Check equipment and oxygen source.

If you suspect ventilator malfunction and you cannot quickly find and correct the problem, proceed with the following:

- Disconnect the ventilator tubing from the tracheostomy tube.
- Attach a bag-valve device to the tracheostomy tube and provide manual ventilation with supplemental oxygen.
- Watch for equal chest rise and listen for equal breath sounds.
- If the patient's chest rise is shallow, ensure that the bag-valve device is securely connected to the tracheostomy tube. If chest rise does not improve, assess the tracheostomy tube for obstruction as previously described.

Continuous Positive Airway Pressure

CPAP is the delivery of slight positive pressure (like blowing through a straw) to prevent airway collapse and improve oxygenation and ventilation in spontaneously breathing patients. When using CPAP, the child wears a mask that covers the mouth and nose, providing continuous increased airway pressure throughout the ventilatory cycle as the child breathes. CPAP may be used to assist ventilation in children with neuromuscular weakness, chronic pulmonary edema, tracheomalacia, or obstructive sleep apnea. Some children use the device continuously, whereas others require it only at night when airway obstruction is most likely.

Bilevel Positive Airway Pressure

Like CPAP, BiPAP is delivered through a tight-fitting mask that fits over either the patient's nose or the mouth and nose. In BiPAP therapy, two (bi) levels of positive pressure are delivered; one during inspiration (to keep the airway open as the patient inhales) and the other (lower) pressure during expiration to reduce the work of exhalation. The BiPap device can be set to deliver pressure at a set rate or to sense when an inspiratory effort is being made by the patient and deliver a higher pressure during inspiration. BiPAP is used in the treatment of patients with chronic respiratory failure and may be helpful in the transition from invasive to noninvasive respiratory support.

Assessment and Management

A child who requires noninvasive mechanical ventilation has a higher-than-average risk for partial or total airway obstruction. The patient may be removed from a CPAP or BiPAP device if it interferes significantly with assessment and interventions. The child will be still able to breathe but may tire easily. If the patient exhibits signs of respiratory distress, administer supplemental oxygen or provide assisted ventilation as necessary.

Noninvasive Mechanical Ventilation

CPAP and BiPAP are noninvasive methods of ventilatory assistance used in spontaneously breathing patients. They do not require a tracheal tube or tracheostomy.

Vascular Access Devices

VADs are catheters placed in children who require frequent blood withdrawal, prolonged or frequent IV fluid or drug administration, and/or nutritional support. The catheters are inserted into the central circulation for long-term use, usually for weeks or months. VADs have allowed many patients to be treated as outpatients rather than have prolonged hospital stays.

Although several types of VADs are available, they can be classified into three general categories:

- Central venous catheters (CVCs)
- Implanted ports
- PICCs

Central Venous Catheters

These catheters are also referred to as "tunneled catheters."

- CVCs implanted for long-term use are typically referred to by the individual that created them (e.g., Broviac, Hickman).
- The catheter is surgically inserted into the external jugular, subclavian, or cephalic veins, with the catheter tip in the superior vena cava, just above the right atrium. The other end of the catheter is tunneled subcutaneously and exits the skin on the anterior chest wall.
- A small cuff is located around the catheter about 1 inch inside the point where the catheter enters the patient's skin. Fibrous tissue grows around the cuff, anchoring the catheter in place and creating a barrier against infection (Figure 11-15A).
- The external portion of a tunneled catheter may have a single, double, or triple lumen, depending on the patient's treatment needs. A small cap covers each lumen and is filled with heparin or saline solution to keep blood clots from occluding the catheter (Figure 11-15B).

Implanted Ports

Implanted ports are known by their brand names (e.g., Portacath, Mediport, or Infusaport).

- An implanted (or subcutaneous) port is surgically placed completely below the skin, with no parts external to the skin. Like the tunneled catheters, a silastic catheter is inserted into a central vein and advanced so that the tip lies at the junction of the superior vena cava and the right atrium. However the other end is tunneled subcutaneously and is attached to a port (reservoir).
- The port can be palpated as a raised disk under the skin. To administer medications or draw blood, a needle is inserted through the skin overlying the port. The port has titanium or plastic housing and a hard silicone septum that is self-sealing. To extend the life of the septum, a special "Huber" needle is used to access it (Figure 11-16).

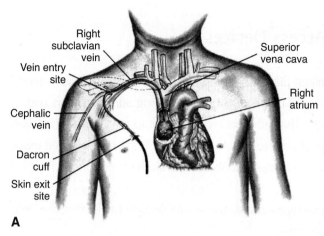

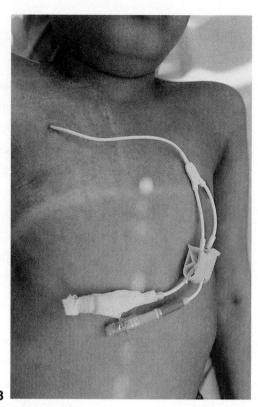

Figure 11-15 A, Central venous catheter insertion and exit site. **B,** External venous catheter (note the redness from the dressing site).

- PICCs are not inserted directly into a central vein. Instead, a PICC line is inserted into an antecubital vein and then advanced into the subclavian vein so that the tip lies in the superior vena cava or right atrium.
- PICC lines are small (23 to 16 gauge) single-lumen or double-lumen catheters. Their small size is advantageous for use in infants and small children (Figure 11-17).
- A PICC line does not require surgical placement; it can be inserted at the bedside, usually by a specially trained nurse.
- PICC lines are less expensive and are associated with fewer complications than CVCs.

Peripherally Inserted Central Catheters

PICC lines are also called nontunneled catheters because they enter the skin near the point at which they enter the vein.

Emergencies from CVCs may result from local or systemic complications associated with their use:

- Infection or allergic reaction
- Breakage and leakage
- Air embolism
- Infusion errors
- Catheter migration
- Catheter obstruction

If a CVC is dislodged or damaged, apply direct pressure as needed to control hemorrhage. Clamp the exposed catheter to prevent further blood loss and treat for shock, if indicated.

Vascular Access Device Emergencies

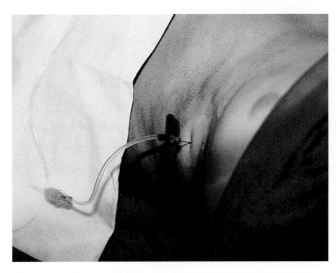

Figure 11-16 To administer medications or draw blood through an implanted port, a special Huber needle is used to access the septum of the device.

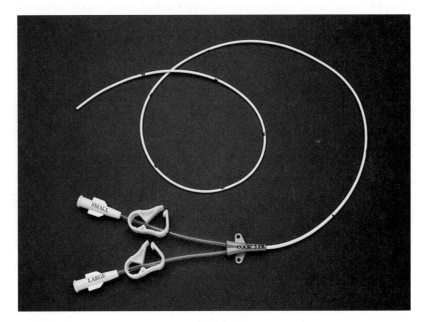

Figure 11-17 A peripherally inserted central catheter (PICC).

Emergent Use of Vascular Access Devices

Do not administer medications or fluids through a CVC unless other methods of vascular access cannot be obtained (e.g., peripheral or central line access), you have received special training to access central catheters, and an emergent condition exists.

Case Study Resolution

This child is exhibiting clear signs of respiratory distress while on a ventilator. Use the DOPE mnemonic to recall the possible reversible causes of acute deterioration in an intubated child.

- **D**isplaced tube (e.g., right mainstem or esophageal intubation) or **D**isconnection of the tube or ventilator circuit—Reassess tube position, ventilator connections.
- **O**bstructed tube (e.g., blood or secretions are obstructing air flow)—Suction.
- **P**neumothorax (tension)—Needle thoracostomy.
- **E**quipment problem/failure (e.g., empty oxygen source, inadvertent change in ventilator settings, low battery)—Check equipment and oxygen source.

A high-pressure ventilator alarm often indicates a mechanical or medical problem that has increased airflow resistance, such as an obstructed tracheostomy tube or worsening pulmonary disease. If you suspect ventilator malfunction and cannot quickly find and correct the problem, disconnect the ventilator tubing from the tracheostomy tube. Attach a bag-valve device to the tracheostomy tube and provide manual ventilation with supplemental oxygen. Watch for equal chest rise and listen for equal breath sounds. If the patient's chest rise is shallow, ensure that the bag-valve device is securely connected to the tracheostomy tube. If chest rise does not improve, assess the tracheostomy tube for obstruction. Provide additional interventions as necessary.

References

1. McPherson M, Arango P, Fox H, et al. A new definition of children with special health care needs. *Pediatrics* 1998:102(Pt 1):137–140.

2. Newacheck PW, Strickland B, Shonkoff JP, et al. An epidemiologic profile of children with special health care needs. *Pediatrics* 1998;102(Pt 1):117–123.

3. Foltin GL, Tunik MG, Cooper A, et al. *Teaching resource for instructors in prehospital pediatrics for paramedics.* New York: Center for Pediatric Emergency Medicine, 2002.

4. Infosino A. Pediatric upper airway and congenital anomalies. *Anesthesiol Clin North America* 2002;20:747–766.

5. Kestle JRW. Pediatric hydrocephalus: current management. *Neurol Clin* 2003;21:883–895.

6. Bower CM. The surgical airway. In: Dieckmann RA, Fiser DH, Selbst SM, eds. *Illustrated textbook of pediatric emergency & critical care procedures.* St. Louis: Mosby, 1997:116–122.

Chapter Quiz

1. List three categories of vascular access devices.

    1.

    2.

    3.

2. Suctioning should be performed for no longer than _____ seconds per attempt.
    A) 5
    B) 10
    C) 15
    D) 20

3. Which of the following tubes or catheters do not require surgical insertion?
    A) Gastric feeding tube, peripherally inserted central catheter
    B) Gastrostomy tube, tracheostomy tube
    C) Tunneled central venous catheter, implanted port
    D) Peripherally inserted central catheter, tunneled central venous catheter

4. Select the **incorrect** statement regarding CPAP and BiPap.
    A) CPAP and BiPAP may be used in spontaneously breathing patients.
    B) Use of CPAP or BiPAP does not require a tracheal tube or tracheostomy.
    C) CPAP provides two levels of positive pressure are delivered; one level of positive pressure during inspiration and a lower pressure during expiration
    D) BiPAP is used in the treatment of patients with chronic respiratory failure.

Chapter Quiz Answers

1. Although many types of vascular access devices exist, they can be classified into one of these three general categories:
    A) Central venous catheters (CVC)
    B) Implanted ports
    C) Peripherally inserted central catheters (PICC)

2. B. Insertion of the suction catheter and suctioning should take no longer than 10 seconds per attempt.

3. A. A gastric feeding tube and peripherally inserted central catheter (PICC) do not require surgical insertion. A gastrostomy tube, tracheostomy tube, tunneled central venous catheter, and implanted port require surgical placement.

4. C. CPAP and BiPAP may be used in spontaneously breathing patients. Use of CPAP or BiPAP does not require a tracheal tube or tracheostomy. BiPap (not CPAP) provides two levels of positive pressure are delivered; one level of positive pressure during inspiration and a lower pressure during expiration. BiPAP is used in the treatment of patients with chronic respiratory failure and may be helpful in the transition from invasive to noninvasive respiratory support.

Resuscitation of the Newly Born Outside the Delivery Room

12

Case Study

A 19-year-old-woman has just given birth. Your patient is the term infant.

During your visual assessment of the newborn, what questions should you ask yourself to determine if routine care is appropriate or if resuscitation must be initiated?

Objectives

1. Discuss the physiologic changes that occur in the transition from intrauterine life to extrauterine life.
2. Discuss antepartum and intrapartum factors associated with an increased risk for neonatal resuscitation.
3. Discuss the assessment findings associated with primary and secondary apnea in the neonate.
4. Discuss the treatment plan for apnea in the neonate.
5. Differentiate when a woman in labor should be transported and when to prepare for delivery in the field.
6. Describe the steps for performing a vaginal delivery and the steps performed immediately after delivery for every newborn.
7. Identify equipment that should be readily available for resuscitation of the newly born.
8. Identify the primary signs used for evaluating a newborn during resuscitation.
9. Formulate an appropriate treatment plan for providing initial care to a newborn.
10. Determine when the following interventions are appropriate for a newborn:
    a. Blow-by oxygen delivery
    b. Ventilatory assistance
    c. Chest compressions
    d. Tracheal intubation
    e. Vascular access
11. Discuss the routes of medication administration for a newborn.

Principles of Resuscitation of the Newly Born

Successful resuscitation of the newly born presents a challenge that requires the following:

- An understanding of the newborn transitional physiology.
- The ability to anticipate high-risk situations in which the newborn may require resuscitation.
- Adequate preparation with appropriate equipment and medications for newborn resuscitation.
- The ability to initiate resuscitative efforts in a timely and effective manner.

The term *newly born* refers to the infant in the first minutes to hours after birth. *Neonate* and *newborn* are terms that apply to any infant during the initial hospitalization.

Newborn Transitional Physiology (Adjustments to Extrauterine Life)

In utero, all of the oxygen used by the fetus diffuses across the placenta from the mother's blood to the baby's blood. The alveoli of the fetus are open and filled with fetal lung liquid instead of air and the pulmonary blood vessels are constricted. Before labor, the production of fetal lung fluid decreases dramatically, decreasing the volume by about one third. During vaginal delivery, the baby's thorax is squeezed, further reducing the volume of fetal lung fluid by approximately one third.

With the first breath, the newborn must pull air into his or her fluid-filled airways and alveoli. When the alveoli begin to fill with air for the first time, surfactant helps them remain partially open and keeps the walls of the alveoli from sticking together when the newborn exhales. As air enters the lungs, pressure drives the remaining fetal lung fluid into the interstitium, where one half is absorbed by pulmonary lymphatics and the other half is absorbed by the interstitium and then carried away by the pulmonary vasculature. Breathing becomes easier and easier as the air sacs fill even more and then remain full of air.

Unless the lungs are immature, absorption of fetal lung liquid is usually complete within 24 hours of birth.

As the lungs fill with air, the pulmonary blood vessels relax, significantly increasing blood flow to the lungs. At about the same time, the umbilical arteries and vein constrict, increasing systemic blood pressure. Blood flow through the ductus arteriosus decreases and the newborn's skin turns from gray-blue to pink as oxygen-enriched blood enters the newborn's systemic circulation. Possible problems that may disrupt the newborn's transition to extrauterine life are shown in Table 12-1.

The newborn's initial cries and deep breaths help move the fetal lung fluid out of his or her airways.

During the birth process, a newborn may experience some asphyxia. A variety of circumstances can exaggerate the degree of asphyxia, resulting in a depressed newborn and the need for neonatal resuscitation (Table 12-2). Identifying patients who may require intervention at birth based on the antepartum or intrapartum history is important and facilitates having the appropriate equipment and trained personnel available at the time of

Factors Associated with Increased Risk for Neonatal Resuscitation

TABLE 12-1 *Problems that may Disrupt the Normal Transition to Extrauterine Life*

Problem	Possible Result
Newborn does not breathe sufficiently to force fluid from alveoli	Lungs do not fill with air; oxygen is not available to blood circulating through the lungs → hypoxia, cyanosis
Meconium blocks air from entering alveoli	
Insufficient blood return from placenta before or during birth	Systemic hypotension
Poor cardiac contractility	
Bradycardia due to insufficient delivery of oxygen to heart or brainstem	
Lack of oxygen or failure to distend lungs with air may result in sustained constriction of pulmonary arterioles	Persistent pulmonary hypertension
Insufficient oxygen delivery to brain	Depressed respiratory drive
Insufficient oxygen delivery to brain and muscles	Poor muscle tone

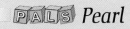 *Pearl*

It is estimated that about 5% to 10% of newborns require some form of active resuscitation at birth.[1]

Ventilations are the first vital sign to cease when a newborn is deprived of oxygen.

In animal studies, this initial period of apnea typically lasts about 30 to 60 seconds.

delivery. However a detailed maternal history is impractical when delivery is imminent in the field or emergency department. Answers to the questions in Table 12-3 may be helpful in preparing for the birth.

Depending on gestational age, a premature baby may not have sufficient lung development for survival. Premature babies are at higher risk of needing resuscitative efforts because:

- The lungs may lack sufficient surfactant and be more difficult to ventilate.
- The brain substance is soft, gelatinous, easily torn and has fragile capillaries that may bleed during stress.
- They are more likely to be born with an infection.
- They are predisposed to problems with temperature regulation due to their thin skin, large surface area to body mass ratio, and lack of subcutaneous fat.

When deprived of oxygen, a newborn's response follows a predictable pattern.

- Primary apnea
  - The newly born will initially respond to asphyxia by breathing faster in an attempt to maintain perfusion and oxygen delivery to vital organs.
  - The heart rate drops abruptly and skin color typically becomes progressively cyanotic and then blotchy because of vasoconstriction in an effort to maintain systemic blood pressure (blood pressure increases slightly).
  - If oxygen levels do not improve, ventilatory efforts slow and eventually cease. This is called **primary apnea**.

TABLE 12-2 *Factors Associated with Increased Risk for Neonatal Resuscitation*

Antepartum Risk Factors	Intrapartum Risk Factors
• Maternal age above 35 y or less than 16 y • Maternal diabetes • Maternal bleeding in second or third trimester • Maternal drug therapy (e.g., magnesium, adrenergic-blocking drugs, lithium carbonate) • Maternal substance abuse (e.g., heroin, methadone) • Chronic or pregnancy-induced hypertension • Chronic maternal illness (e.g., cardiovascular, thyroid, neurologic, pulmonary, renal) • Maternal anemia or isoimmunization • Maternal infection • Polyhydramnios • Oligohydramnios • Premature rupture of membranes • Previous fetal or neonatal death • Postterm gestation • Multiple gestation • Size-dates discrepancy • No prenatal care • Diminished fetal activity • Fetal malformation	• Abruptio placentae • Placenta previa • Premature labor • Precipitous labor • Chorioamnionitis • Prolonged rupture of membranes (more than 18 h before delivery) • Prolonged labor (more than 24 h) • Prolonged second stage of labor (more than 2 h) • Use of general anesthesia • Emergency cesarean delivery • Forceps or vacuum-assisted delivery • Uterine tetany • Narcotics administered to mother within 4 h of delivery • Breech or other abnormal presentation • Fetal bradycardia • Nonreassuring fetal heart rate patterns • Prolapsed cord • Meconium-stained amniotic fluid

- If gently stimulated (e.g., drying, gently rubbing the back) during this period, the newborn will respond by resuming spontaneous breathing.
- Secondary apnea
  - Oxygen deprivation continues.
  - The newborn takes several gasping ventilations.
  - The skin is cyanotic, bradycardia ensues, and blood pressure falls.
  - Gasping ventilations become weaker and slower and then stop (**secondary apnea**).
    - During secondary apnea, the newborn will not respond to stimulation.
    - More vigorous and prolonged resuscitation is needed to reverse the process and restore adequate ventilation and circulation. Death will ensue unless resuscitation begins immediately.
    - Intervention requires bag-mask ventilation with supplemental oxygen.
  - "If gasping has already ceased, the first sign of recovery with initiation of positive-pressure ventilation is an increase in heart rate. The blood pressure then rises, rapidly if the last gasp has only just passed, but more slowly if the duration of asphyxia has been longer.

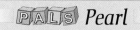 *Pearl*

Because there is no definitive way to differentiate primary apnea from secondary apnea in the field or clinical setting, assume that any newborn who does not respond immediately to gentle stimulation and blow-by oxygen is experiencing secondary apnea. Provide positive-pressure ventilation with a bag-mask and supplemental oxygen immediately.

Unlike adults, who develop tachycardia in response to hypoxia, the newly born responds initially with a reflex bradycardia.

TABLE 12-3 *Focused Maternal History*

Risk Factor	Question	Possible Risk	Preparation/Action
Estimate gestational age	When is your baby due?	Prematurity	Assisted ventilation Ensure availability of size-appropriate equipment
Multiple gestation	How many babies are there?	If more than one, newborns at greater risk for prematurity	Additional personnel and equipment needed
Meconium in amniotic fluid	Did your bag of waters rupture? What was the color of the water?	Respiratory distress Hypoxemia Aspiration pneumonia	Immediate suction Possible tracheal intubation
Maternal medications	Have you taken any medications or drugs?	Narcotic use within 4 h of delivery may result in neonatal respiratory depression	Assisted ventilation
Maternal diabetes	Do you have high blood sugar or diabetes?	Neonatal hypoglycemia Congenital anomalies Large for gestational age	Assisted ventilation Vascular access
Breech position	Has your doctor told you if the baby is coming head first or feet first?	Birth trauma Prematurity Umbilical cord prolapse	Assisted ventilation Additional personnel and equipment needed
Vaginal bleeding	Have you experienced any vaginal bleeding? How long ago? Did you have any pain with the bleeding?	Maternal/placental hemorrhage: increased likelihood of hypovolemic shock and respiratory distress in neonate	Vascular access Fluid/blood administration
Fetal movement	When was the last time you felt the baby move?	Fetal distress	Assisted ventilation

The skin then becomes pink, and gasping ensues. Rhythmic spontaneous respiratory efforts become established after a further interval. For each 1 minute past the last gasp, 2 minutes of positive-pressure breathing is required before gasping begins and 4 minutes to reach rhythmic breathing. Not until some time later do the spinal and corneal reflexes return. Muscle tone gradually improves over the course of several hours."[2]

Preparation for Delivery

Equipment

Table 12-4 presents a list of suggested supplies, medications, and equipment that should be readily available during delivery of a newborn. The availability of properly sized equipment is essential, particularly equipment used for airway management and ventilation, because it is most likely to be used.

TABLE 12-4 *Prehospital and Emergency Department Equipment List for Newborn Delivery*

Obstetrics Kit

- Sterile gloves
- Scalpel or surgical scissors
- Two hemostats or cord clamps
- Bulb syringe
- Four or more clean, dry towels
- Gauze sponges
- Two or more baby blankets
- Sanitary napkins
- Identification bands for mother and neonate (hospital)
- Footprint kit (optional—hospital)

Suction Equipment

- Bulb syringe
- Suction source and tubing
- 8-French feeding tube and 20-mL syringe
- Suction catheters in sizes 5 or 6 French, 8 French, and 10 or 12 French
- Meconium aspirator

Bag-Mask Equipment

- Oxygen source and tubing
- Bag-mask (200 to 750 mL) with pressure-release valve; must have oxygen reservoir
- Anesthesia bag (hospital)
- Transparent face mask with soft inflatable rim (sizes for preterm and term babies)

Tracheal Intubation Equipment

- Pediatric laryngoscope handle with extra batteries
- Straight laryngoscope blades in sizes 0 (preterm) and 1 (term) with extra bulbs
- Tracheal tubes in sizes 2.5, 3, 3.5, and 4 mm
- Tracheal tube stylets (small)
- Tape or securing device for tracheal tube
- End-tidal carbon dioxide detector (optional)
- Laryngeal mask airway (optional)
- Stethoscope
- 5-French feeding tube (optional: for tracheal medications)

Intraosseous Equipment

- 18-gauge intraosseous needle and syringe
- Normal saline

Umbilical Vessel Catheterization Equipment

- Povidone-iodine solution
- Scalpel with blade
- Sterile gauze sponges, 5 cm or 10 cm square
- 3.5-French and 5-French umbilical catheters
- Three-way stopcock
- Mosquito clamp
- Fine forceps without teeth
- Umbilical tape

Medications

- Epinephrine 1:10,000
- Sodium bicarbonate 4.2%
- Naloxone 0.4 mg/mL
- Dextrose 10%, 250 mL
- Normal saline for flushes and sterile water if dilution of bicarbonate or hypertonic glucose solutions is necessary
- Normal saline for volume expansion

Gastric Decompression Equipment

- 8-French gastric or feeding catheter
- 20-mL syringe

Additional Supplies

- Personal protective equipment
- Oral airways (0, 00, and 000 sizes)
- Cardiac monitor + electrodes (optional)
- Clock
- 18-, 21-, and 25-gauge needles or puncture device for needleless systems
- Tape (1/2 or 3/4 inch)
- 1-, 3-, 5-, 10-, 20-, and 50-mL syringes
- Pulse oximeter and probe (optional)

Prehospital Predelivery Considerations

- Generally, transporting a woman in labor to the hospital is best unless delivery is expected within a few minutes.
- Signs of imminent delivery.
  - Consider delivering at the scene when:
    ○ Delivery can be expected in a few minutes.
    ○ The patient feels the urge to push, bear down, or have a bowel movement.

- ◦ Crowning is present.
- ◦ Contractions are regular, lasting 45 to 60 seconds, and are 1 to 2 minutes apart.
    - Intervals are measured from the beginning of one contraction to the beginning of the next.
    - If contractions are more than 5 minutes apart, there is generally time to transport the mother to an appropriate receiving facility.
- ◦ No suitable transportation is available.
- ◦ The hospital cannot be reached (e.g., heavy traffic, bad weather, natural disaster).
- • If there is time to transport the patient to the hospital:
    - ◦ Place the patient on her left side.
    - ◦ Remove any undergarments that might obstruct delivery.
    - ◦ Transport promptly.
- • If the decision is made to deliver on the scene:
    - • Consider the need for additional personnel and equipment (e.g., multiple birth).
    - • Use personal protective equipment, including gloves, mask, eye protection, and a gown. Blood and amniotic fluid are expected and may splash.
    - • Contact medical direction:
        - ◦ If complications are anticipated. Medical direction may recommend expedited transport of the patient to an appropriate receiving facility.
        - ◦ If delivery does not occur within 10 minutes.
    - • Do not let the mother go to the bathroom. The mother will feel as if she needs to move her bowels. This sensation is caused by the head of the fetus in the vagina pressing against the walls of the patient's rectum.
    - • Do not hold the mother's legs together or attempt to delay or restrain delivery.

Delivery Procedure

- • Use appropriate personal protective equipment (e.g., gloves, mask, gown, eye protection).
- • Position the patient.
    - • Remove the patient's undergarments.
    - • The mother may be positioned in one of three ways for delivery:
        - ◦ Supine with good support for her head and a firm, stable surface under her lower body (e.g., bed) (Figure 12-1). Position the mother with her knees drawn up and spread apart. Elevate the patient's

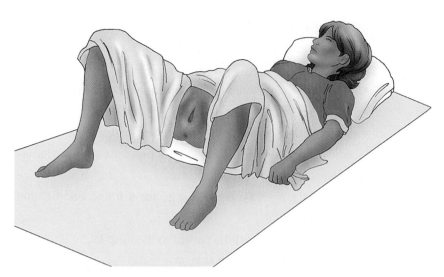

Figure 12-1   Position the mother with her knees drawn up and spread apart. Elevate the patient's buttocks with a towel or blanket. Make sure sufficient space exists in front of the mother, at the end of the stretcher or bed, to accommodate the newborn after delivery.

    buttocks with a towel or blanket. Make sure sufficient space exists in front of the mother, at the end of the stretcher or bed, to accommodate the newborn after delivery. This position provides easy access to the infant's mouth and nares for suctioning.

- ◦ Recumbent on her left side with her back toward you and her knees drawn up to her chest (Sims position). This position also provides easy access to the infant's mouth and nares for suctioning.

- ◦ Supine with her buttocks at the edge of the bed or stretcher, legs apart, and her feet supported on chairs positioned at either side of her body. This position provides less support for the mother, lacks a stable surface under the perineum for the newborn, and increases the risk of dropping the infant as delivery progresses.

- Organize the obstetric (OB) kit and create a sterile field around the vaginal opening using sterile towels or sterile packaged paper drapes. Prepare oxygen and blankets for the newborn.

- Controlling the head:
  - When the infant's head appears:
    - ◦ Place your gloved fingers on the bony part of the infant's skull and apply very gentle palm pressure to prevent an explosive delivery (Figure 12-2). Do not apply pressure to the infant's face or fontanelles.
    - ◦ If the amniotic sac does not break or has not broken, use a clamp or your gloved fingers to puncture the sac and push it away from the infant's head and mouth as they appear.
  - As the infant's head appears, determine if the umbilical cord is around the infant's neck ("nuchal cord") (Figure 12-3).

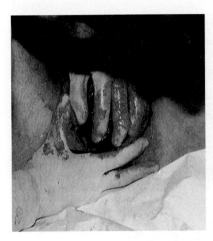

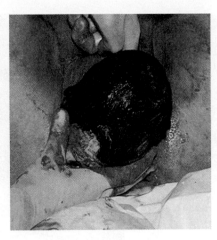

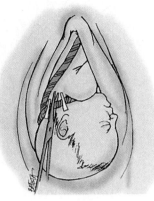

Figure 12-2   When the infant's head appears during crowning, place your gloved fingers on the bony part of the infant's skull and apply very gentle palm pressure to prevent an explosive delivery.

Figure 12-3   As the infant's head appears, determine if the umbilical cord is around the infant's neck.

Figure 12-4   If the umbilical cord is around the baby's neck and cannot be removed, clamp the cord in two places, and carefully cut the cord between the two clamps. Remove the cord from the infant's neck.

The primary purpose of suctioning the airway is to remove secretions and reduce the risk of airway obstruction, enabling effective oxygenation and ventilation.

- ○ If the cord is around the neck, try to free it by gently pushing it over the newborn's head. If the cord cannot be removed, place two umbilical clamps on the cord, carefully cut the cord between the two clamps with sterile scissors, and remove the cord from the infant's neck (Figure 12-4).
- ○ If the cord is *not* wrapped around the infant's neck, or if it can be freed easily, do not cut it until the infant is fully delivered.
- When the infant's head is delivered, support the head with one hand and suction the mouth and then the nose with a bulb syringe (Figure 12-5).
- After the head is delivered:
  - Support the baby's head as it rotates to line up with the shoulders (Figure 12-6). Guide the head downward to deliver the anterior (top) shoulder (Figure 12-7). Guide the head upward to deliver the posterior (bottom) shoulder (Figure 12-8). Tell the mother not to push during this time.
  - As the torso and full body are born, support the newborn with both hands. As the feet are born, grasp the feet.
  - Wipe blood and mucus from the newborn's mouth and nose with sterile gauze. Suction the mouth and nose again with a bulb syringe as necessary.
- Dry, warm, and position the newborn (see Initial Steps of Resuscitation of the Newly Born).

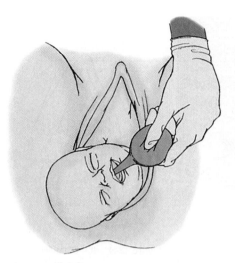

Figure 12-5 After the head is delivered, support the head and suction the baby's mouth, and then the nose, with a bulb syringe.

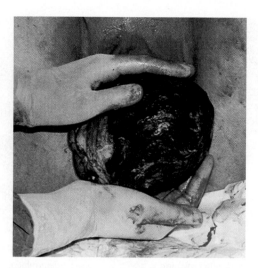

Figure 12-6 Support the baby's head as it rotates to line up with the shoulders.

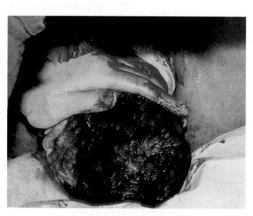

Figure 12-7 Guide the infant's head downward to deliver the anterior (top) shoulder.

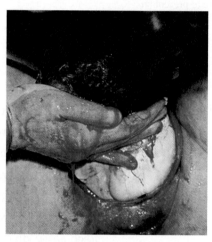

Figure 12-8 Guide the infant's head upward to deliver the posterior (bottom) shoulder.

- It is important to position the newborn at the same level as the mother's vaginal opening until the cord has been clamped because blood can continue to flow between the newborn and the placenta.
- If the infant is positioned above the level of the mother's vaginal opening (as when the baby is placed on the mother's abdomen or chest), blood may drain from the newborn's circulation into the placenta, decreasing the newborn's blood volume.
- Clamp and cut the umbilical cord after the cord stops pulsating.
  - Place the first clamp approximately 4 inches from the newborn's belly. Place the second clamp approximately 2 inches distally from the first. If the clamps are firmly in place, cut the cord between the two clamps with sterile scissors (Figure 12-9).
  - Periodically check the cut ends of the cord for bleeding. If the cut end of the cord attached to the newborn is bleeding, clamp the cord

The umbilical cord usually stops pulsating 3 to 5 minutes after delivery of the newborn.

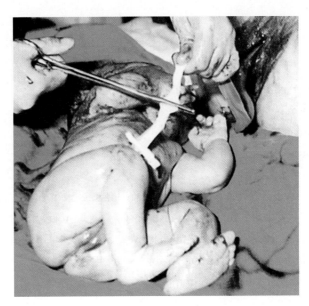

Figure 12-9   Clamp and cut the umbilical cord after the cord stops pulsating. Place the first clamp approximately 4 inches from the newborn's belly. Place the second clamp approximately 2 inches distally from the first. If the clamps are firmly in place, cut the cord between the two clamps with sterile scissors.

proximal to the existing clamps. Do not remove the first clamp.

The placenta is usually delivered within 20 minutes of the newborn.

- Observe for delivery of the placenta.
  - While preparing mother and newborn for transport, continue to warm and assess the newborn and watch for delivery of the placenta. (It is not necessary to wait for the placenta to deliver before transporting the mother and newborn.)
  - Signs of placental separation include a gush of blood, lengthening of the umbilical cord, contraction of the uterus, and an urge to push.
  - Encourage the mother to push to help deliver the placenta. Do **not** pull on the umbilical cord to deliver the placenta. Pulling can cause the uterus to invert.

Retained pieces of placenta in the uterus will cause persistent bleeding.

- After delivery of the placenta
  - Put the newborn to the mother's breast to nurse. This stimulates the uterus to contract, thus constricting blood vessels within its walls and decreasing bleeding.
  - Wrap the placenta in a towel and put in a plastic bag or in an appropriate container with a lid. Transport the placenta to the hospital with the mother. Hospital personnel will examine the placenta for completeness.
- Examine the skin between the anus and the vagina (the perineum) for tears. Apply pressure to any bleeding tears with a sanitary napkin.
- Record the time of delivery and transport the mother, newborn, and placenta to the hospital.

Initial Steps of Resuscitation of the Newly Born

Ask yourself three questions at the time of birth:

1. Term gestation?
2. Breathing or crying?
3. Good muscle tone?

These questions can be answered by visual assessment of the newborn. If the answer to *all* of these questions is "Yes," proceed with routine newborn care (i.e., provide warmth, clear the airway, dry). If the answer to *any* question is "No," continue to the initial steps of resuscitation (see Newborn Resuscitation Algorithm).

- Whenever possible, deliver the newborn in a warm, draft-free area.
- Methods to minimize heat loss:
  - Placing the newborn under a radiant warmer (ideal).
  - Rapidly drying the skin.
  - Removing wet linens immediately from the newborn.
  - Wrapping the newborn in prewarmed blankets or towels insulating film blankets or using an infant chemical warming mattress.
  - Covering the newborn's body and top of the head.
  - Placing the dried newborn against the mother's chest (skin-to-skin contact).
  - Increasing room temperature.

- Positioning
  - Dry the newborn quickly and place supine with the head in a "sniffing" position.
    - The newborn has a relatively large occiput and anterior airway. Hyperextension or flexion of the neck may produce airway obstruction.
    - Proper positioning may be facilitated by placing a rolled washcloth, blanket, or towel under the newborn's shoulders.
  - If copious secretions are present, place the newborn on his/her side.
- Suctioning
  - If the amniotic fluid is clear of meconium and signs of infection, suctioning should be reserved for babies who have obvious obstruction to spontaneous breathing or who require positive pressure ventilation.[3]

General Impression

Provide Warmth

Care must be taken to maintain the newborn's body temperature.

Position and Suction

Mouth before nose—M comes before N in the alphabet. Suctioning of the mouth and nose is associated with risks such as bradycardia, apnea, and delays in normal oxygenation.

NEWBORN RESUSCITATION ALGORITHM

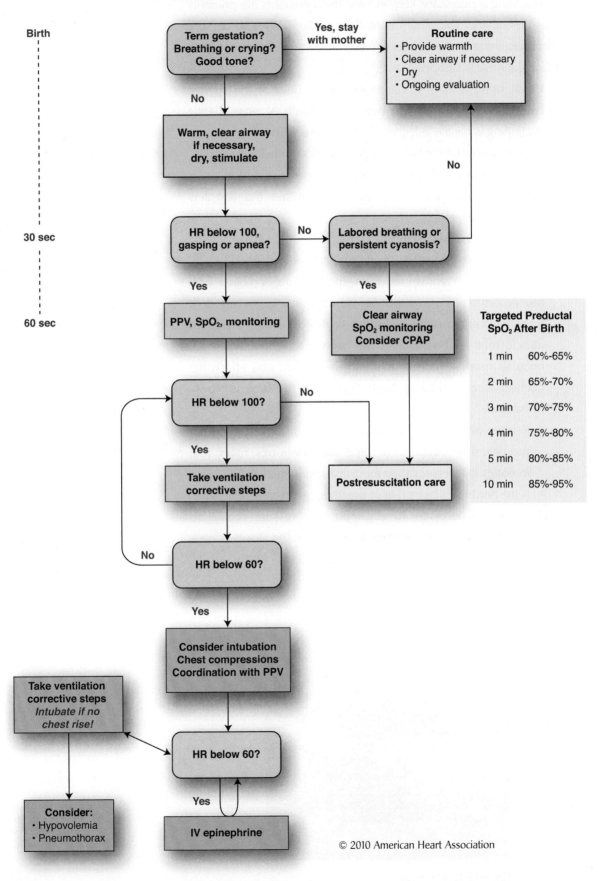

© 2010 American Heart Association

- If suctioning is necessary, keep in mind that newborns are primarily "nose breathers." The mouth should be suctioned first to be sure there is nothing for the newborn to aspirate if he or she should gasp when the nose is suctioned.
  - When using a bulb syringe, squeeze the bulb of the syringe before inserting it into the newborn's mouth or nose. Gentle suctioning is usually adequate to remove secretions.
  - Be careful how far the bulb syringe or suction catheter is inserted. Stimulation of the back of the throat can cause severe reflex bradycardia or apnea when performed within the first few minutes of delivery.
- Meconium stained fluid (Figure 12-11)
  - If the newborn is vigorous (strong ventilatory effort, good muscle tone, heart rate above 100 beats per minute), proceed with routine newborn care (i.e, provide warmth, clear the airway, dry).
  - If the newborn is depressed (poor ventilatory effort, decreased muscle tone, and/or a heart rate slower than 100 beats per minute), insert a tracheal tube into the trachea and attach the tracheal tube to suction. Apply suction as the tube is slowly withdrawn.
    - Repeat intubation and suctioning until little additional meconium is obtained or until the newborn's heart rate indicates that resuscitation must proceed immediately.
    - If the newborn's heart rate or breathing is severely depressed, it may be necessary to begin positive-pressure ventilation despite the presence of some meconium in the airway.

Meconium staining of the amniotic fluid occurs in 7% to 22% of live births.[4-7] Meconium is found below the vocal cords in 10% to 40% of infants born through meconium-stained amniotic fluid.[4, 5, 8] Meconium aspiration can occur in utero or immediately after delivery when the infant takes his or her first breaths.

Do not suction for more than 3 to 5 seconds per attempt. Administer blow-by oxygen throughout the suctioning procedure.

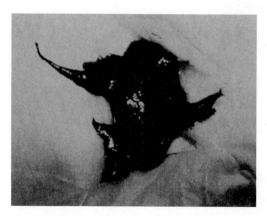

Figure 12-11 Meconium.

PALS *Pearl*

The newly born infant is at risk for heat loss because of its relatively large surface-to-volume area, wet amniotic fluid covering, and exposure to a relatively cool environment, especially in contrast to intrauterine temperature. Further, the newly born cannot generate heat by shivering and cannot retain heat because of low fat stores. Preventing heat loss in the newly born is important because cold stress can lead to increased oxygen consumption, metabolic acidosis, hypoglycemia, and apnea. Increased oxygen consumption in a poorly oxygenated newborn can precipitate a change from aerobic to anaerobic metabolism. This change may lead to tissue hypoxia and acidosis because of the buildup of metabolic byproducts, such as lactate.

Hypoglycemia may develop in response to cold stress because the infant uses up glucose and glycogen reserves rapidly during anaerobic metabolism. Signs and symptoms of hypoglycemia include apnea, color changes, respiratory distress, lethargy, jitteriness, and seizures.

Stimulate

- In most cases, the stimulation received during drying, warming, and suctioning is sufficient to cause the newborn to breathe effectively and may be the only resuscitative measures needed. However, if adequate ventilations are not present, provide additional stimulation by rubbing the newborn's back, trunk, or extremities or tapping or flicking the soles of the feet. These methods may be tried for 5 to 10 seconds to stimulate breathing.

- If a brief period of tactile stimulation is not effective in initiating ventilations, the newborn is in secondary apnea and positive-pressure ventilation with a bag–mask device is required.

Oxygen Administration

Studies have revealed conflicting evidence regarding the use of room air versus supplemental oxygen during resuscitation. Tissue damage may occur because of oxygen deprivation during and after asphyxia. Conversely, cell and tissue injury may increase if hypoxic tissue is exposed to high concentrations of oxygen. Supplemental oxygen should be available for use if resuscitation is begun with room air and there is no appreciable improvement within 90 seconds after birth. If the infant's heart rate is slower than 60 beats per minute after 90 seconds of resuscitation with a lower concentration of oxygen, increase the oxygen concentration to 100% until recovery of a normal heart rate.[3]

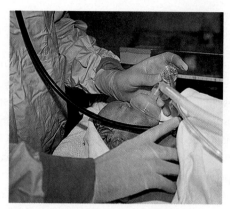

Figure 12-12 Blow-by oxygen can be delivered by means of a face mask and flow-inflating (anesthesia) bag (as shown here), simple face mask held firmly to the newborn's face, or by means of a hand cupped around oxygen tubing. The oxygen source should be set to deliver at least 5 L per minute and held close to the face to maximize oxygen flow to the newborn's nose and mouth.

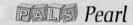

PALS Pearl

When stimulating a newborn, avoid methods that are too vigorous because they will not help initiate ventilations and may harm the newborn. Examples of methods that should **not** be used include the following:

- Slapping the back
- Forcing the thighs onto the abdomen
- Using hot or cold compresses
- Blowing cold oxygen onto the face or body
- Squeezing the rib cage
- Dilating the anal sphincter
- Shaking
- Putting the newborn into a hot or cold bath

Blow-by oxygen can be delivered by means of a face mask and flow-inflating (anesthesia) bag (Figure 12-12), simple face mask held firmly (but not too tightly) to the newborn's face, or by means of a hand cupped around oxygen tubing. The oxygen source should be set to deliver at least 5 L per minute and held close to the face to maximize oxygen flow to the newborn's nose and mouth. Avoid administering unheated and un-humidified oxygen to a newborn at high flow rates (i.e., more than 10 L per minute) because convective heat loss can become a problem.

Blow-by oxygen refers to the administration of oxygen over the newborn's nose to enhance breathing of oxygen-enriched air.

Assessment of the newborn begins immediately after birth (Figure 12-13). Further resuscitative efforts are required if the newborn's ventilatory effort is inadequate, or the heart rate is less than 100 beats/minute.

- Ventilatory rate and effort (e.g., crying, adequate, gasping, apneic).
  - The term newborn's ventilatory rate is normally between 30 and 60 breaths per minute in the first 12 hours of life.
  - The presence of gasping breathing or apnea requires intervention with positive-pressure ventilation.
- Heart rate
  - The term newborn's heart rate is normally 100 to 180 beats per minute in the first 12 hours of life.

Evaluate Ventilations and Heart Rate

In an uncompromised newborn, the heart rate should be consistently above 100 beats per minute. An increase or decrease in heart rate can provide evidence of improvement or deterioration in the newborn's condition.

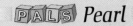

Many bag-mask devices will not passively deliver sufficient oxygen flow (i.e., when not being squeezed) for effective use in blow-by oxygen administration.

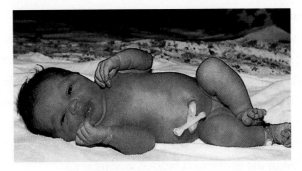

Figure 12-13 Assessment of the newborn begins immediately after birth.

Pulse oximetry can be used to measure heart rate and provide a continuous heart rate reading. Until the pulse oximeter provides stable readings, clinical assessment of heart rate is required.

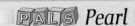

Count the heart rate for 6 seconds and multiply by 10 to estimate the beats per minute. Because the rate is rapid, it may be helpful to tap out the newborn's heart rate as you count it. This technique also enables an assistant to help listen for changes in the rate.

- Heart rate may be evaluated by:
  - Listening to the apical beat with a stethoscope.
  - Feeling the pulse by lightly grasping the base of the umbilical cord.
    - Palpation of the umbilical pulse allows assessment of heart rate without interruption of ventilation for auscultation.
    - If pulsations cannot be felt at the base of the cord, auscultate the apical pulse.
- In general, a spontaneously breathing newborn with effective ventilations, pink color, and a heart rate over 100 beats per minute will require no further intervention.
- If the heart rate is less than 100 beats per minute, begin positive-pressure ventilation. A heart rate below 60 beats per minute indicates that additional resuscitative measures are needed.
- Color
  - Acrocyanosis (cyanosis of the extremities) is a common finding immediately after delivery and is not a reliable indicator of hypoxemia. Acrocyanosis may be an indicator of cold stress.
  - Pallor may indicate decreased cardiac output, severe anemia, hypothermia, acidosis, or hypovolemia.
  - Studies have shown that clinical assessment of skin color is a very poor indicator of oxyhemoglobin saturation during the immediate neonatal period and that lack of cyanosis appears to be a very poor indicator of the state of oxygenation of an uncompromised newborn following birth. It is normal for the oxygen saturation level to remain in the 70% to 80% range for several minutes following birth with the appearance of cyanosis during this period.[3]

Apgar Scoring System

An Apgar scoring system is a numerical method of rating five specific signs pertaining to the newborn's condition after birth. Each sign is assigned a value of 0, 1, or 2 and added for a total Apgar score (Table 12-5). In general, the higher the score, the better the condition of the newborn.

Although the Apgar score is an important tool used in the assessment of a newborn, it is not recorded until 1 and 5 minutes after birth. If resuscitation of the newborn is needed, waiting until the first Apgar score (which reflects the need for immediate resuscitation) is obtained could be disastrous. The decision to begin resuscitative efforts and the newborn's response to resuscitation can be more accurately determined by evaluating the newborn's ventilatory effort and heart rate.

Do not delay resuscitative efforts to obtain an Apgar score.

- Components of the Apgar scoring system.
  - **A**ppearance (color).
  - **P**ulse (heart rate).
  - **G**rimace (irritability).
  - **A**ctivity (muscle tone).
  - **R**espirations.

- Indications for positive-pressure ventilation.
  - Apnea or gasping ventilations.
  - Heart rate less than 100 beats per minute despite initial steps of resuscitation.
- Face mask and resuscitation bag size.
  - Select a properly sized face mask.
    - Face masks are available in a variety of sizes and shapes. The preferred mask is equipped with a cushioned rim and is anatomically shaped. This type of mask offers several advantages.
      - Low dead space (less than 5 mL).

Ventilation

TABLE 12-5 *The Apgar Scoring System*

	0	1	2
Appearance	Blue, pale	Body pink Extremities blue	Completely pink
Pulse	Absent	Less than 100	100 or more
Grimace/reflex irritability	No response	Grimaces, cries	Cough, sneeze, vigorous cry
Activity/muscle tone	Limp, flaccid	Some flexion of extremities	Active motion
Respiratory effort	Absent	Slow, irregular	Good, crying

- Less pressure required to maintain a tight seal than with a round or noncushioned mask.
- Less chance of injury to the newborn's eyes if the mask is improperly positioned.
  - A properly sized mask avoids the eyes, and covers the nose, mouth, and tip of the chin. Masks fitting preterm, term, and large newborns should be available. A mask that is too large will not seal well and may damage the newborn's eyes. A mask that is too small will not cover the mouth and nose (and may occlude the nose).
- For a term newborn, select a resuscitation bag with a minimum volume of 450 to 500 mL and a maximum volume of 750 mL.
  - A term newborn requires approximately 15 to 25 mL with each ventilation (5 to 8 mL/kg). A preterm baby requires even less volume—some require as little as 5 to 10 mL per ventilation. Using a 750 mL volume (or larger) bag makes it difficult to provide such small tidal volumes and increases the risk of complications (e.g., hyperinflation).
  - If the bag-mask has a pop-off valve, it should release at approximately 30 to 35 cm H_2O pressure and should have an override feature to permit delivery of higher pressures if necessary to achieve good chest expansion.
  - To open the alveoli in the newly born, pressures of 30 to 40 cm H_2O may be needed during the first few ventilations. This may necessitate temporary disabling of the pop-off valve. After the first few breaths, pressure requirements typically drop to 20 to 30 cm H_2O.

Breathe, two, three = Squeeze, release, release.

- Assisting ventilation.
  - Ventilate the newborn at a rate of 40 to 60 breaths per minute (i.e., slightly less than 1 breath per second) to achieve or maintain a heart rate above 100 beats per minute. (The rate is 30 breaths per minute when chest compressions are also being delivered).

A rapid improvement in heart rate is considered the primary measure of adequate initial ventilation. Reassess movement of the chest wall if the heart rate does not improve.

- Signs of adequate ventilation.
  - Gentle chest rise.
  - Presence of bilateral breath sounds.
  - Improvement in color and heart rate.
- A poor response to ventilation efforts may be the result of
  - A poor seal between the newborn's face and the mask. Corrective action: Reapply the mask to the face. Check the seal when you reapply the mask, particularly between the cheek and the bridge of the nose.
  - Poor alignment of the head and neck. Corrective action: Reposition the head.

- Insufficient ventilation pressure. Corrective action: Increased inflation pressure may be required. If adequate chest rise is still not achieved, tracheal intubation may be required.
- Improper tracheal tube position (if intubated). Corrective action: Reassess tube placement; remove if the tube is improperly positioned or position is uncertain.
- Blocked airway. Corrective action: Reposition the head, suction as needed, ventilate with the mouth slightly open.
- Gastric distention. Corrective action: Insert an 8-French or 10-French orogastric tube and leave the end open to air. Periodically aspirate the tube with a syringe.

- Once adequate ventilation has been established for 30 seconds, reassess the newborn's heart rate and ventilatory effort.
  - If the newborn is spontaneously breathing and the heart rate is greater than 100 beats per minute, positive-pressure ventilation may be gradually discontinued.
    - Observe the newborn for signs of adequate spontaneous breathing before ceasing ventilation.
    - Gentle tactile stimulation may help maintain spontaneous breathing.
  - If spontaneous breathing is inadequate, continue assisted ventilation.
  - If the newborn is unresponsive to positive-pressure ventilation and the heart rate is less than 60 beats per minute, continue positive-pressure ventilation and begin chest compressions. Consider tracheal intubation.

Chest Compressions

- Indications
  - Chest compressions are indicated if the newborn's heart rate is less than 60 beats per minute despite adequate ventilation with supplemental oxygen for 30 seconds.[3]
  - Because chest compressions may diminish the effectiveness of ventilation, they should not be initiated until ventilation has been established.
- Compression technique
  - Two compression techniques can be used, both of which should be delivered on the lower third of the sternum.
  - Thumb technique (preferred)
    - The thumbs are placed on the sternum side by side just below the nipple line unless the infant is small (or the rescuer's hands are extremely large), in which case the thumbs may be placed one

Inadequate lung inflation or severe hypoxemia are the most common causes of bradycardia in a newborn, which can corrected by ensuring adequate ventilation.

Allow the newborn's chest to fully recoil during relaxation while keeping your fingers or thumbs (depending on the technique used) in contact with the chest.

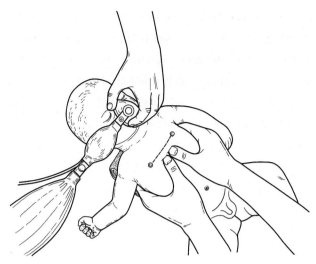

Figure 12-14 Newborn cardiopulmonary resuscitation using the thumb technique. The thumbs are placed on the sternum side by side just below the nipple line unless the infant is small (or the rescuer's hands are extremely large), in which case the thumbs may be placed one over the other. The fingers encircle the chest and support the back .

over the other (Figure 12-14). The fingers encircle the chest and support the back.

- This technique may be used in newly born infants and older infants whose size permits its use.
- Studies suggest that this technique may offer some advantages in generating peak systolic and coronary perfusion pressure.
- Two-finger method
  - The ring and middle fingers of one hand are placed on the sternum just below the nipple line (Figure 12-15). The other hand should support the infant's back.

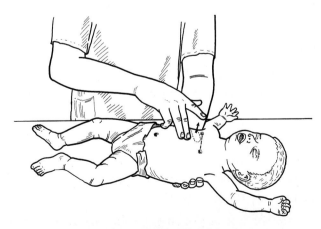

Figure 12-15 Two-finger method of cardiopulmonary resuscitation. The ring and middle fingers of one hand are placed on the sternum just below the nipple line. The other hand should support the baby's back.

- Compression-ventilation ratio
  - Compressions and ventilations must be coordinated to avoid simultaneous delivery. Deliver compressions smoothly, compressing approximately one third the depth of the chest.
  - The compression to ventilation ratio is 3:1. Three chest compressions should be followed by a brief pause to deliver one ventilation.
  - Provide one complete cycle (three compressions and one ventilation) every 2 seconds. This results in 90 compressions and 30 breaths (approximately 120 events) per minute.
- Periodically reassess oxygenation, ventilation, and heart rate.
  - Myocardial blood flow is dependent on coronary perfusion pressure, which is generated when performing external chest compressions. Because it takes time to build up cerebral and coronary perfusion pressures, interrupting chest compressions causes cerebral and coronary perfusion pressures to fall quickly and dramatically, reducing flow to the brain and heart. Even after compressions are resumed, several chest compressions are needed to restore coronary perfusion pressure. Therefore, it is important to minimize interruptions in chest compressions during resuscitation.
- Discontinue chest compressions when the heart rate reaches 60 beats per minute or more.
- If the heart rate remains slower than 60 beats per minute, continue compressions.

- Tracheal intubation may be indicated at several points during neonatal resuscitation:[3]
  - When tracheal suctioning for meconium is required.
  - If bag-mask ventilation is ineffective (i.e., inadequate chest expansion, persistent low heart rate) or prolonged.
  - When chest compressions are performed.
  - Special resuscitation circumstances (e.g., congenital diaphragmatic hernia or extremely low birth weight).
- Blade size
  - A straight blade should be used for tracheal intubation of the newborn.
  - Use size 0 for a preterm infant and size 1 for a term newborn.
- Tracheal tube size (Table 12-6).
- Vocal cord guide.
  - Most tracheal tubes intended for newborn use have a vocal cord line (a black line) near the distal tip of the tracheal tube. The tip of the tracheal tube should be inserted until the vocal cord guide is at

Compression to ventilation ratio is 3:1. Unlike adults, newborns have no or minimally established functional residual capacity. Resuscitation efforts attempt to replenish oxygen with effective ventilation and deliver proportionally more ventilations over a specific period in relation to chest compressions. The 3:1 ratio is a consensus opinion of experts that is based on the likelihood that newborns who require cardiac compressions are asphyxiated and that newborns have higher ventilatory rates adults and older children even when not asphyxiated. Consider using a compression to ventilation ratio of 15:2 if the arrest is believed to be of cardiac origin.

Tracheal Intubation

Intubation attempts should be limited to 20 seconds to minimize the risk of hypoxia.

Changes in the newborn's head position will alter the depth of insertion and may predispose to unintentional extubation or right primary bronchus intubation.

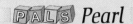 *Pearl*

Possible causes for a newborn's failure to respond to intubation and ventilation include mechanical difficulties, profound asphyxia with myocardial depression, or an inadequate circulating blood volume. If the patient acutely deteriorates after intubation, quickly check the equipment. If no explanation is obvious, remove the tracheal tube and ventilate the patient with a bag-mask.

the level of the cords. In this position, the tip of the tube should be between the vocal cords and carina.

- After placement of the tube, note the centimeter marking on the tube at the newborn's upper lip. The tube should be located 7 cm at the lip for a 1000-g infant, 8 cm for a 2000-g infant, and 9 cm for a 3000-g infant. After proper tube position is confirmed, document and maintain this depth of insertion.
- Confirm the position of the tube.
  - Watch for symmetric rise and fall of the chest.
  - Listen high in the axillae for equal breath sounds and for an absence of sounds over the stomach.
  - Confirm absence of gastric distention with ventilation.
  - Note improvement in color, heart rate, and activity of the newborn.
  - Detection of exhaled carbon dioxide.
    - In all resuscitation settings (prehospital, emergency departments, intensive care units, operating rooms), confirmation of tracheal tube placement should be achieved using detection of exhaled CO_2 in intubated infants and children with a perfusing cardiac rhythm. A colorimetric detector or capnometry should be used for this purpose.
    - If exhaled CO_2 is not detected during cardiac arrest, confirm tube position using direct laryngoscopy.
    - An esophageal detector device may be considered for confirmation of tracheal tube placement in children weighing more than 20 kg.
- Chest radiograph.

TABLE 12-6 *Estimation of Laryngoscope Blade and Tracheal Tube Size Based on Infant Gestational Age and Weight*

Weight (g)	Gestational Age (wk)	Laryngoscope Blade Size	Laryngoscope Blade Type	Tracheal Tube Size (mm)	Depth of Tracheal Tube Insertion from Upper Lip (cm)
Less than 1000	Less than 28	0	Straight	2.5	6.5 to 7.0
1000 to 2000	28 to 34	0	Straight	2.5 to 3.0	7.0 to 8.0
2000 to 3000	34 to 38	0 to 1	Straight	3.0 to 3.5	8.0 to 9.0
More than 3000	More than 38	1	Straight	3.5 to 4.0	More than 9.0

- Acute deterioration (bradycardia, decreased oxygen saturation) after intubation suggests one of the following problems (DOPE):
  - *D*islodgement: The tube is no longer in the trachea (right primary bronchus or esophagus).
  - *O*bstruction: Secretions are obstructing airflow through the tube. Suspect obstruction of the tube when there is resistance to bagging and no chest wall movement.
  - *P*neumothorax.
  - *E*quipment: Oxygen is not being delivered to the patient (check equipment).

PALS Pearl

The laryngeal mask airway (LMA) has been shown to be effective for ventilating infants weighing more than 2000 g or delivered 34 weeks or longer gestation. When used by appropriately trained professionals, use of an LMA should be considered during resuscitation of a newly born infant, especially in the case of unsuccessful bag-mask ventilation or failed tracheal intubation".[3]

Routes of Medication Administration

If timely assessment and rapid response to a newborn with cardiopulmonary compromise are initiated, medications are rarely indicated for resuscitation. Bradycardia in the newborn is usually secondary to inadequate lung inflation and hypoxia, so ensuring adequate ventilation is an essential step in correcting a low heart rate. However, epinephrine administration or volume expansion, or both, may be necessary if the heart rate remains slower than 60 beats per minute despite adequate ventilation with 100% oxygen and chest compressions.

- Tracheal
  - In the past, it was recommended that the tracheal route be used for epinephrine administration because this route was often the most rapidly accessible route for newborn resuscitation. Studies have shown that epinephrine has no effect when administered tracheally using the currently recommended intravenous (IV) dose (0.01 to 0.03 mg/kg of 1:10,000 solution).[3]
  - Current resuscitation guidelines recommend that epinephrine be administered IV as soon as venous access is available. Administration of tracheal epinephrine (0.05 to 0.1 mg/kg of 1/10,000 solution) can be considered while attempting to obtain venous access, but the safety and efficacy of this practice have not been evaluated.[3]

Medications and Fluids

The Broselow tape has a section for newborns that can be used to determine equipment size and medication dosages for newborn resuscitation.

- Umbilical vein
    - Rarely used as a means of vascular access outside the delivery room.
    - Should only be attempted by those specially trained in this technique.
    - Anatomy
        ◦ Two arteries and one vein readily identified in the umbilical cord stump.
        ◦ The vein is a thin-walled vessel. The arteries are thicker-walled, paired, and often constricted.
    - Cannulation
        ◦ A 3.5-French or 5-French umbilical catheter is attached to a 3-way stopcock flushed with heparinized saline.
        ◦ The catheter is inserted into the umbilical vein until the tip of the catheter is just below the skin and there is a good blood return (Figure 12-16).
    - Complications
        ◦ Infection.
        ◦ A fatal air embolus can result if air enters the umbilical venous catheter.
        ◦ Advancing the catheter too far into the umbilical vein may cause infusion of medications directly into the liver with the potential for hepatic damage.
- Peripheral vascular access
    - Veins of the scalp and extremities are acceptable routes for administration of fluids and medications but are difficult to access during resuscitation.

Volume Expanders

Suspect hypovolemia in any infant who fails to respond to resuscitation.

- Indications
    - Volume expanders should be considered when acute blood loss is known or suspected with signs of hypovolemia:
        ◦ Pallor that persists despite oxygenation.
        ◦ Poor perfusion.
        ◦ Weak pulses with a heart rate faster than 100 beats per minute.
        ◦ Poor response to resuscitative efforts, including effective ventilation.
- Fluid choice
    - Fluid of choice for volume expansion is an isotonic crystalloid solution (e.g., normal saline or Ringer lactate).
- Dosage
    - Initial volume expander dosage is 10 mL/kg given slow IV push over 5 to 10 minutes.
    - Boluses may be repeated several times, guided by patient assessment.

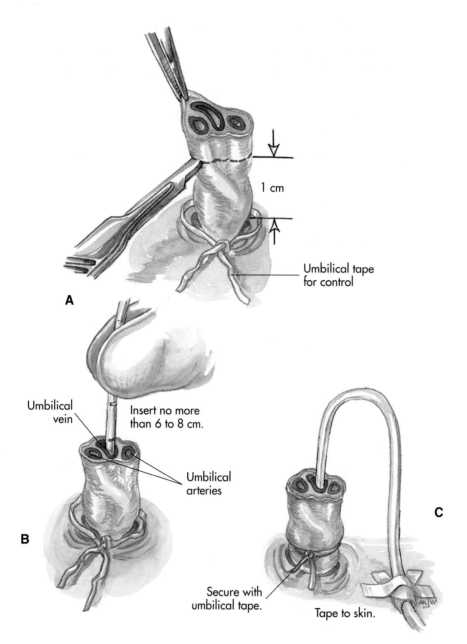

1 cm

Umbilical tape
for control

A

Umbilical
vein

Insert no more
than 6 to 8 cm.

Umbilical
arteries

B

C

Secure with
umbilical tape.

Tape to skin.

Figure 12-16 **Cannulation of the umbilical vein. A,** Identify the umbilical vein after trimming the cord. **B,** Insert the umbilical catheter into the vein. **C,** Secure the base of the cord to hold the catheter in place and stabilize the catheter with tape.

- Care must be taken to minimize the use of rapid boluses of volume expanders or hyperosmolar solutions (e.g., sodium bicarbonate), when administering medications to a preterm newborn because portions of the brain are particularly vulnerable to bleeding when subjected to rapid changes in vascular pressure and osmolarity.

Medications

Table 12-7 lists medications that may be used during newborn resuscitation. Table 12-8 lists other medications that may be administered to newborns.

TABLE 12-7 *Medications Used in Neonatal Resuscitation*

Epinephrine

- **Indications**: Asystole or when the heart rate remains less than 60 beats per minute despite adequate ventilation with 100% oxygen and chest compressions
- **Mechanism of Action**: Has both α-adrenergic and β-adrenergic stimulating properties. In cardiac arrest, α-adrenergic–mediated vasoconstriction may be the more important action. Vasoconstriction elevates the perfusion pressure during chest compressions, enhancing delivery of oxygen to the heart and brain. Epinephrine also enhances myocardial contractility, stimulates spontaneous contractions, and increases heart rate.
- **Dosage**: IV 0.01 to 0.03 mg/kg of 1:10,000 solution: tracheal dose 0.05 to 0.1 mg/kg of 1:10,000 solution.[3]

IV, intravenous.

TABLE 12-8 *Other Medications*

Glucose

- **Notes**: There are currently no neonatal studies that have addressed whether early supplemental glucose during and/or following delivery room resuscitation can or will improve outcome.

Naloxone

- **Notes**: Current resuscitation guidelines do not recommend administration of naloxone as part of the initial resuscitative efforts in the delivery room for newborns with respiratory depression. Support of ventilation should be the primary means used to restore oxygenation and heart rate.

Postresuscitation Care

Continued monitoring, supportive care, and appropriate diagnostic evaluation are indicated in any newly born infant requiring stabilization and resuscitation. Postresuscitation monitoring should include the following:

- Monitoring of heart rate, ventilatory rate, blood pressure, temperature, and oxygen saturation.
- Determination of blood sugar and treatment of hypoglycemia
- Consider induced therapeutic hypothermia for infants born at 36 weeks gestation or longer with evolving moderate to severe hypoxic-ischemic encephalopathy.[3]
- Obtaining a chest radiograph to evaluate lung expansion, placement of tubes and catheters, identify possible underlying causes of the arrest, or detect complications, such as pneumothorax.
- Treatment of hypotension with volume expanders, vasopressors, or both.
- Treatment of possible infection or seizures.
- Initiation of vascular access and appropriate fluid therapy.
- Documentation of observations and actions.
- Transport of the infant to the most appropriate unit (newborn nursery, level II nursery, or neonatal intensive care unit) for further care. A transport team with personnel skilled in neonatal resuscitation should be used.

Case Study Resolution

Ask yourself three questions at the time of birth:
1. Term gestation?
2. Breathing or crying?
3. Good muscle tone?

These questions can be answered by visual assessment of the newborn. If the answer to *all* of these questions is "Yes," proceed with routine newborn care (i.e., provide warmth, clear the airway, dry). If the answer to *any* question is "No," begin the initial steps of resuscitation.

References

1. Zideman DA, Hazinski MF. Background and epidemiology of pediatric cardiac arrest. *Pediatr Clin North Am* 2008;Aug;55(4):847–59, ix. Review.

2. Rosenberg AA. Abnormalities of the cardiopulmonary transition. In: Gabbe SG, Niebyl JR, Simpson JR, eds. *Obstetrics–Normal and Problem Pregnancies*, 4th ed. New York: Churchill Livingstone, 2002;661–662.

3. Kattwinkel J, Perlman JM, Aziz K, et al. Part 15: Neonatal resuscitation: 2010 American Heart Association Guidelines for Cardiopulmonary Resuscitation and Emergency Cardiovascular Care. *Circulation* 2010;122(suppl 3):S909–S919.

4. Davis RO, Harris BA Jr, Wilson ER, Huddleston JF. Fatal meconium aspiration syndrome occurring despite airway management considered appropriate. *Am J Obstet Gynecol* 1985;Mar 15;151(6):731–736.

5. Dooley SL, Pesavento DJ, Depp R, et al. Meconium below the vocal cords at delivery: correlation with intrapartum events. *Am J Obstet Gynecol* 1985;Dec 1;153(7):767–770.

6. Falciglia HS. Failure to prevent meconium aspiration syndrome. *Obstet Gynecol* 1988;71:349–353.

7. Wiswell TE, Henley MA. Intratracheal suctioning, systemic infection, and the meconium aspiration syndrome. *Pediatrics* 1992; 89:203–206.

8. Peng TC, Gutcher GR, Van Dorsten JP. A selective aggressive approach to the neonate exposed to meconium-stained fluid. *Am J Obstet Gynecol* 1996;175:296–301.

Chapter Quiz

1. Which of the following signs are associated with secondary apnea?
   A) Pink skin, increasing heart rate, normal blood pressure
   B) Cyanotic skin, falling heart rate, falling blood pressure
   C) Pink skin, falling heart rate, falling blood pressure
   D) Cyanotic skin, increasing heart rate, normal blood pressure

2. The heart rate of the newly born should be assessed by:
   A) Palpating the umbilical or carotid pulse.
   B) Ausculating the apical pulse or palpating the femoral pulse.
   C) Ausculating the apical pulse or palpating the umbilical pulse.
   D) Palpating the femoral or brachial pulse.

3. When delivering positive-pressure ventilations with a bag-mask device to a newborn, the assisted ventilation rate should be _____ breaths/minute and _____ breaths/minute when chest compressions are also being delivered.
   A) 10 to 20; 30
   B) 20 to 40; 20
   C) 30 to 40; 40
   D) 40 to 60; 30

4. Assessment of a newly born infant one minute after delivery reveals the infant is crying vigorously on light tapping of the foot. Her heart rate is 130 beats/minute and some flexion of the extremities is noted. Ventilations are regular at approximately 40 breaths/minute. The body is pink and the extremities are blue. You would assign an Apgar score of:
   A) 7
   B) 8
   C) 9
   D) 10

5. Volume expansion with normal saline or lactated Ringer's solution should begin with an initial bolus of _____ in a newborn and _____ in an infant or child.
   A) 10 mL/kg; 20 mL/kg
   B) 20 mL/kg; 30 mL/kg
   C) 10 mL/kg; 10 mL/kg
   D) 20 mL/kg; 40 mL/kg

6. When delivering blow-by oxygen during resuscitation of the newly born, the oxygen flow rate should be at least _____ L/min.
   A) 3
   B) 5
   C) 10
   D) 15

7. True or False: Neonates often demonstrate tachycardia in response to hypoxemia; older children will initially demonstrate bradycardia.

8. Acceptable methods of stimulating the newly born include:
   A) Squeezing the rib cage
   B) Dilating the anal sphincter
   C) Rubbing the back
   D) Shaking the infant

Chapter Quiz Answers

1. B. In secondary apnea, oxygen deprivation persists. The newborn takes several gasping ventilations. The skin is cyanotic, bradycardia ensues, and blood pressure falls. Gasping ventilations become weaker and then stop (secondary apnea).

2. C. Because central and peripheral pulses in the neck and extremities are often difficult to feel in newborns, heart rate should be assessed either by auscultating the apical pulse with a stethoscope or by palpating the base of the umbilical cord. The umbilical pulse is readily accessible in the newly born and permits assessment of heart rate without interruption of ventilation for auscultation.

3. D. The assisted ventilation rate should be 40 to 60 breaths per minute and 30 breaths per minute when chest compressions are also being delivered.

4. B. An Apgar score of 8 is assigned based on the following: Some flexion of the extremities (1 point), regular ventilations (2 points), blue extremities/pink body (1 point), heart rate faster than 100 (2 points), and vigorous crying on stimulation (2 points).

5. A. Volume expansion with normal saline or lactated Ringer's solution should begin with an initial bolus of **10 mL/kg** in a newborn and **20 mL/kg** in an infant or child.

6. B. When delivering blow-by oxygen during resuscitation of the newly born, the oxygen flow rate should be at least 5 L/min.

7. False. Neonates often demonstrate **bradycardia** in response to hypoxemia; older children may initially demonstrate **tachycardia**.

8. C. If adequate ventilations are not present, stimulate the newly born infant by rubbing the infant's back, trunk, or extremities or tapping the soles of the feet. These methods may be tried for 5 to 10 seconds to stimulate breathing. Avoid methods that are too vigorous because they will not help initiate ventilations and may harm the newborn. Examples of methods that should **not** be used include slapping the back, squeezing the rib cage, forcing the thighs onto the abdomen, dilating the anal sphincter, using hot or cold compresses, shaking, blowing cold oxygen onto the newborn's face or body, and putting the newborn into a hot or cold bath.

Posttest

1. Which of the following correctly reflects the sequence of steps in the pediatric Chain of Survival?
   A) Early CPR, prevention of illness or injury, early advanced life support (ALS), early EMS activation, and integration of post-cardiac arrest care.
   B) Early ALS, early EMS activation, early CPR, integration of post-cardiac arrest care, and prevention of illness or injury.
   C) Prevention, early CPR, early EMS activation, rapid ALS, and integration of post-cardiac arrest care.
   D) Early EMS activation, early ALS, integration of post-cardiac arrest care, prevention, and early CPR.

2. Which of the following is the most useful for removing thick secretions and particulate matter from the pharynx?
   A) Oropharyngeal airway.
   B) Rigid plastic suction catheter.
   C) Flexible plastic suction catheter.
   D) Nonrebreather mask.

3. Under optimum conditions, blow-by oxygen administered by means of a facemask can deliver an oxygen concentration of _____ at a flow rate of 10 L/min.
   A) 25% to 45%
   B) 30% to 40%
   C) 50% to 60%
   D) 60% to 95%

4. The initial energy dose for synchronized cardioversion for an infant or child is:
   A) 0.2 to 0.4 J/kg
   B) 0.5 to 1 J/kg
   C) 2 to 4 J/kg
   D) 5 to 10 J/kg

5. In which of the following situations would chest compressions be indicated?
   A) A 3-year-old with a pulse rate of 100.
   B) An apneic18-month-old with a pulse rate of 50.
   C) An apneic 4-year-old with a pulse rate of 84.
   D) An 11-year-old with a pulse rate of 78.

6. When performing chest compressions on an infant, compress the chest approximately _____ at a rate of _____ times per minute.
   A) $1/2$ to 1 inch, at least 100
   B) $1 1/2$ inches, at least 100
   C) 2 inches, at least 120
   D) $2 1/2$ inches, at least 120

7. What is the formula used to estimate cuffed tracheal tube size?
   A) 3.5 + (age in years/4)
   B) 4 + (age in years/4)
   C) (12 + age in years) ÷ 2
   D) Age in years x 2.2

8. Bradycardia that causes severe cardiopulmonary compromise in an infant or child is initially treated with:
   A) Effective oxygenation and ventilation.
   B) Transcutaneous pacing.
   C) Synchronized cardioversion.
   D) Administration of atropine.

9. Synchronized cardioversion:
   A) Is used in the treatment of pulseless ventricular tachycardia.
   B) Delivers a shock between the peak and end of the T wave.
   C) Is timed to avoid the vulnerable period of the cardiac cycle.
   D) Is used only for rhythms with a ventricular response of less than 100 beats/min.

10. Which of the following signs are the MOST important when determining if additional resuscitative efforts are needed in the newly born?
    A) Color and muscle tone
    B) Ventilations and heart rate
    C) Reflexes and ventilations
    D) Capillary refill and muscle tone

11. A patient with a malfunctioning VP shunt may present with irritability, headache, neck pain, vomiting, a bulging or full fontanelle in infants, new seizures or a change in the child's seizure pattern, behavioral changes, or "just not acting right." These signs are most suggestive of:
    A) Congenital heart disease.
    B) Chronic pulmonary disease.
    C) Increased intracranial pressure.
    D) Congenital neuromuscular disease.

12. The patient who has ingested a toxic dose of a tricyclic antidepressant should receive:
    A) Sodium bicarbonate
    B) Amiodarone
    C) Procainamide
    D) Glucagon

13. A 7-year-old is experiencing anaphylaxis after a bee sting. In this situation, epinephrine should be administered by which of the following routes?
    A) Tracheal
    B) Intravenous
    C) Subcutaneous
    D) Intramuscular

14. Which of the following are the most common causes of shock in the pediatric patient?
    A) Hypovolemia and sepsis
    B) Anaphylaxis and tension pneumothorax
    C) Spinal cord injury and cardiac tamponade
    D) Impaired cardiac muscle function and sepsis

15. What is meant by the term *pulseless electrical activity* (PEA)?
    A) PEA refers to a flat line on the cardiac monitor.
    B) PEA refers to a chaotic dysrhythmia that is likely to degenerate into cardiac arrest.
    C) PEA refers to an organized rhythm on the cardiac monitor, though a pulse is not present.
    D) PEA refers to a slow, wide-QRS ventricular rhythm.

16. Volume expansion with normal saline or lactated Ringer's solution should begin with an initial bolus of _____ in a newborn and _____ in an infant or child.
    A) 10 mL/kg; 20 mL/kg
    B) 20 mL/kg; 30 mL/kg
    C) 10 mL/kg; 10 mL/kg
    D) 20 mL/kg; 40 mL/kg

17. Assessment of a term newly born infant reveals a heart rate of 80 beats/min and shallow, spontaneous ventilations at a rate of 40/min. Your best course of action will be to:
    A) Perform immediate tracheal intubation and administer epinephrine
    B) Observe and reassess in 5 minutes
    C) Clear the airway and begin chest compressions
    D) Assess oxygen saturation and begin positive-pressure ventilation

18. The lower limit of a normal systolic blood pressure for a 5-year-old should be:
    A) 80 mm Hg
    B) 90 mm Hg
    C) 100 mm Hg
    D) 120 mm Hg

Questions 19-24 pertain to the following scenario:

A 9-month-old infant has a history of poor feeding. You note that the infant appears pale and limp in her mother's arms. Intercostal retractions are present. She does not respond when her mother speaks her name.

19. From the information provided, complete the following documentation regarding the Pediatric Assessment Triangle.
    Appearance:
    Breathing:
    Circulation:

20. The normal ventilatory rate range for an infant at rest is:
    A) 15 to 30 breaths/min.
    B) 20 to 40 breaths/min.
    C) 30 to 60 breaths/min.
    D) 40 to 70 breaths/min.

21. The normal heart rate range for an infant at rest is:
    A) 80 to 140 beats/min.
    B) 100 to 160 beats/min.
    C) 120 to 220 beats/min.
    D) 150 to 250 beats/min.

22. Your initial assessment reveals clear lung sounds and a ventilatory rate of 40/min. Peripheral pulses are difficult to palpate. Capillary refill is longer than 5 seconds. The infant's heart rate is 250 beats/min. Oxygen saturation on room air is 88%. Based on this information, your **first** action should be to:

    A) Begin chest compressions.

    B) Establish vascular access.

    C) Administer supplemental oxygen.

    D) Place the infant in a position of comfort.

23. The infant responds only to painful stimulation, and has no history of fever, vomiting, or diarrhea. The cardiac monitor displays the following rhythm.

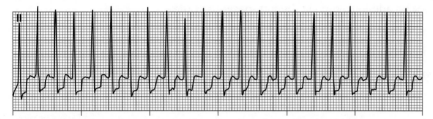

    This rhythm is:

    A) Sinus tachycardia.

    B) Supraventricular tachycardia.

    C) Ventricular tachycardia.

    D) Ventricular fibrillation.

24. Vascular access has not been established. Your best course of action will be to:

    A) Defibrillate immediately with 0.5 J/kg.

    B) Insert an IV and administer atropine.

    C) Insert an IV and administer adenosine.

    D) Perform synchronized cardioversion with 0.5 to 1 J/kg.

25. Select the **incorrect** statement regarding defibrillation and synchronized cardioversion.

    A) Before delivering a shock, ensure that everyone is clear of the patient, bed, and any equipment connected to the patient.

    B) Defibrillation is indicated for pulseless ventricular tachycardia, ventricular fibrillation, and supraventricular tachycardia.

    C) If VF occurs during the course of synchronization, check the patient's pulse and rhythm, turn off the sync control, and defibrillate.

    D) Before delivering a shock, ensure that oxygen is not flowing over the patient's torso.

26. Select the **incorrect** statement regarding vagal maneuvers and the pediatric patient.
    A) Application of external ocular pressure is the preferred vagal maneuver for terminating dysrhythmias in the pediatric patient.
    B) If the child is able to follow instructions, ask the child to blow through a straw or take a deep breath and bear down as if having a bowel movement.
    C) Ensure that oxygen, suction, a defibrillator, and emergency medications are available before attempting the procedure.
    D) In general, a vagal maneuver should not be continued for more than 10 seconds.

27. Which of the following is true regarding intraosseous access?
    a. Viscous drugs cannot be administered via the intraosseous route.
    b. The intraosseous route may be used in infants but not in children.
    c. The intraosseous route may be used as the initial method of vascular access in cardiac arrest.
    d. Although blood products can be administered intravenously, they cannot be administered intraosseously.

28. True or False: To insert an oropharyngeal airway in a child properly, insert the airway upside down until it reaches the back of the throat. Then rotate the device 180° until the flange rests on the patient's lips or teeth.

29. A 6-year-old suffered burns to his anterior chest, abdomen, and the anterior portion of both legs. What percentage of body surface area was burned?
    A) 18%
    B) 27%
    C) 32%
    D) 36%

30. Which of the following findings would **NOT** be expected in the early (hyperdynamic) phase of septic shock?
    A) Bounding peripheral pulses.
    B) Mottled, cool extremities.
    C) Brisk capillary refill.
    D) Tachycardia.

31. Select the **incorrect** statement regarding pain management and the pediatric patient.
    A) In general, healthcare professionals adequately treat pain in the pediatric patient.
    B) Some healthcare professionals do not view pain relief as important or do not want to "waste time" assessing pain.
    C) The *patient*, not the healthcare professional, is the authority regarding his or her pain.
    D) Methods for assessing pain in the pediatric patient will vary according to the age of the child.

32. The preferred intramuscular injection site in infants and children under 3 years of age is the:
    A) Vastus lateralis.
    B) Ventrogluteal.
    C) Dorsogluteal.
    D) Deltoid.

33. True or False: When you suspect cervical spine injury, traction should be applied to the neck while waiting to immobilize the child to a spine board.

34. Select the **incorrect** statement regarding bag-mask ventilation.
    A) The bag-mask device is most effectively applied by a single, experienced rescuer.
    B) Ventilate the patient at an age-appropriate rate and with just enough volume to see the patient's chest rise gently.
    C) In cardiac arrest, ventilate the intubated infant or child at a rate of about 1 breath 8 to 10 times per minute.
    D) Ventilate the infant or child with a perfusing rhythm but absent or inadequate ventilatory effort at a rate of 12 to 20 breaths per minute.

35. True or False: There is no evidence that cricoid pressure prevents aspiration during rapid sequence or emergency tracheal intubation in infants or children.

36. Shockable cardiac arrest rhythms include:
    A) Asystole and pulseless electrical activity.
    B) Pulseless ventricular tachycardia and asystole.
    C) Pulseless electrical activity and ventricular fibrillation.
    D) Ventricular fibrillation and pulseless ventricular tachycardia.

37. Which of the following statements is **incorrect** when assessing the abdomen of a pediatric patient?
    A) The abdomen of a young child is naturally protuberant and may appear somewhat distended.
    B) A toddler may scream throughout the examination.
    C) It is abnormal for an infant to tense his or her abdominal muscles when palpated.
    D) It may be necessary to evaluate the abdomen more than once for a more accurate assessment.

38. A 10-year-old is unresponsive with spontaneous ventilations at a rate of 4/min. Chest movement is barely visible with each breath. A pulse is present and the patient's heart rate is 90 beats/min. Which of the following oxygen delivery devices would be most appropriate to use in this situation?
    A) A nasal cannula at 4 L/min.
    B) A simple face mask at 4 L/min.
    C) A nonrebreather mask at 15 L/min.
    D) A bag-mask device with a reservoir at 15 L/min.

39. True or False: Spontaneous emesis in the first 30 to 60 minutes after head injury is common in children.

40. Which of the following may result from a sudden impact to the anterior chest wall and cause cessation of normal cardiac function?
    A) Pericardial tamponade.
    B) Traumatic asphyxia.
    C) Beck's triad.
    D) Commotio cordis.

41. If a properly fitting rigid cervical collar is not available, which of the following items should NOT be used when one is stabilizing the head and neck of a pediatric patient?
    A) Towels
    B) Blanket rolls
    C) Wash cloths
    D) Sandbags

42. True or False. Neurogenic shock is characterized by a decreased blood pressure (BP) and normal or decreased heart rate. Hypovolemic shock is characterized by a decreased BP and increased heart rate.

43. True or False. Analgesics used to manage severe pain usually cause sedation, but most sedatives do not provide analgesia.

44. True or False. If you observe a change in mental status in a febrile child (inconsolable, unable to recognize parents, unarousable), *immediately* consider the possibility of septic shock.

45. True or False. Medications administered via a peripheral vein during CPR should be followed with a saline flush of 15 to 20 ml to facilitate delivery of the medication to the central circulation.

46. True or False. In the pediatric patient, a QRS complex is considered wide if it exceeds 0.06 second.

47. A 5-year-old has been intubated. You note that there is an absence of chest wall movement when ventilating with a bag-valve device. You are unable to auscultate breath sounds on either side of the chest. What is the most likely cause of this situation?
    A) A mucus plug in the tracheal tube.
    B) Esophageal intubation.
    C) Right primary bronchus intubation.
    D) Left primary bronchus intubation.

48. Which of the following statements is true regarding hypovolemic shock?
    A) Initial management of hypovolemic shock includes aggressive administration of vasopressors.
    B) Signs of shock should be treated with a bolus of 20 mL/kg of isotonic crystalloid even if blood pressure is normal.
    C) Albumin, a colloid, is the preferred solution for volume expansion during the early phase of resuscitation.
    D) Administration of normal saline is preferred over Ringer's lactate solution during the early phase of resuscitation.

49. Which of the following statements is **incorrect** regarding PICC lines?
    A) A PICC line is inserted directly into a central vein.
    B) PICC lines are small single or double lumen catheters.
    C) A PICC line does not require surgical placement; it can be inserted at the bedside.
    D) PICC lines are less expensive and are associated with fewer complications than central venous catheters.

50. Which of the following statements is **incorrect** regarding cerebrospinal fluid shunts?
    A) The proximal catheter is usually inserted into one of the ventricles of the brain.
    B) The distal catheter is tunneled under the skin and is most often placed in the peritoneal cavity (ventriculoperitoneal [VP] shunt).
    C) Shunts are named for the position of their proximal and distal catheters.
    D) A child with a malfunctioning shunt will always present with a fever.

Posttest Answers

1. C. The pediatric Chain of Survival represents a sequential series of events to assess, support, or restore effective ventilation and circulation to the infant or child experiencing a respiratory or cardiorespiratory arrest. The sequence consists of five important steps: 1) Prevention of illness or injury, 2) Early CPR, 3) Early EMS activation, 4) Rapid advanced life support (ALS), and 5) Integration of post-cardiac arrest care.

2. B. A rigid (also called a "hard," "tonsil tip," or "Yankauer") suction catheter is made of hard plastic and is angled to aid in the removal of thick secretions and particulate matter from the mouth and oropharynx.

3. B. Under optimum conditions, blow-by oxygen administered by means of a face mask can deliver an oxygen concentration of 30 to 40% at a flow rate of 10 L/min.

4. B. The initial energy dose for synchronized cardioversion for an infant and child is 0.5 to 1 J/kg.

5. B. Begin chest compressions if there is no pulse (or you are unsure if there is a pulse) or a pulse is present but the rate is slower than 60 beats per minute with signs of poor perfusion (e.g., pallor, mottling, cyanosis).

6. B. When performing chest compressions on an infant, deliver compressions at a rate of at least 100 per minute. Apply firm pressure, depressing the sternum at least 1/3 the depth of the chest (about 1.5 inches or 4 cm).

7. A. If a cuffed tracheal tube is used for intubation of an infant, use of a 3-mm ID tube is considered reasonable. Use of a 3.5-mm ID tube for children between 1 and 2 years of age is considered reasonable. After age 2, the following formula can be used to estimate cuffed tracheal tube size: Cuffed tracheal tube ID (mm) = 3.5 + (age in years/4).

8. A. A bradycardia that causes severe cardiopulmonary compromise in an infant or child is initially treated with effective oxygenation and ventilation. If the heart rate is slower than 60/min and poor systemic perfusion persists despite oxygenation and ventilation, establish vascular access, identify and treat possible causes, and give epinephrine. Synchronized cardioversion is not indicated in the treatment of a bradycardia. Give atropine before epinephrine if the bradycardia is due to suspected increased vagal tone or any type of AV block. If no response, consider pacing.

9. C. Synchronized cardioversion is the delivery of a shock to the heart to terminate a rapid dysrhythmia that is timed to avoid the vulnerable period during the cardiac cycle. On the ECG, this period occurs during the peak of the T wave to approximately the end of the T wave. Synchronized cardioversion may be used to treat the "sick" (unstable) patient in supraventricular tachycardia due to reentry, atrial fibrillation, atrial flutter, atrial tachycardia, or monomorphic ventricular tachycardia with a pulse. Signs of hemodynamic compromise include poor perfusion, hypotension, or heart failure. This procedure

may also be performed electively in a child with stable SVT or VT at the direction of a pediatric cardiologist.

10. B. Assessment of the newborn begins immediately after birth and focuses on ventilations and heart rate. Further resuscitative efforts are required if the newborn's ventilatory effort is inadequate (apnea, gasping, or labored breathing), or the heart rate is less than 100 beats/minute.

11. C. Irritability, headache, neck pain, vomiting, a bulging or full fontanelle in infants, new seizures or a change in the child's seizure pattern, behavioral changes, or "just not acting right" are signs suggestive of increased intracranial pressure.

12. A. Tricyclic antidepressant toxicity causes direct effects on vascular tone (vasodilation), decreased cardiac contractility, intraventricular conduction delays, and serious dysrhythmias including VT (most common), torsades de pointes, and AV blocks (less common). Sodium bicarbonate is the primary treatment modality for severe intoxication. Medications such as amiodarone and procainamide may worsen cardiac toxicity and should be avoided. Glucagon administration is not indicated.

13. D. Give epinephrine via intramuscular injection (site of choice is the lateral aspect of the thigh).

14. A. Hypovolemia and sepsis are the most common causes of shock in the pediatric patient.

15. C. In pulseless electrical activity (PEA), organized electrical activity is visible on the ECG, but central pulses are absent. PEA has a poor prognosis unless the underlying cause can be rapidly identified and appropriately managed.

16. A. Volume expansion with normal saline or lactated Ringer's solution should begin with an initial bolus of *10 mL/kg* in a newborn and *20 mL/kg* in an infant or child.

17. D. In this situation, you should assist ventilation using positive-pressure at a rate of 40 to 60 breaths per minute to achieve or maintain a heart rate 100 per minute.

18. A. Using the formula 70 + (2 x age in years), the lower limit of a normal systolic blood pressure for a 5-year-old should be 80 mm Hg.

19. Appearance: Unresponsive to verbal stimuli, limp.
    Breathing: Increased work of breathing evident.
    Circulation: Pale.

20. C. The normal ventilatory rate range for an infant at rest is 30 to 60 breaths/minute.

21. B. The normal heart rate range for an infant at rest is 100 to 160 beats/minute.

22. C. Your first action must be to ensure effective oxygenation and ventilation. Administer supplemental oxygen.

23. B. The rhythm displayed is supraventricular tachycardia.

24. D. Because vascular access has not been established, perform synchronized cardioversion beginning with 0.5 to 1 J/kg. If cardioversion does not terminate the dysrhythmia, increase the energy level to 2 J/kg.

25. B. Before delivering a shock, ensure everyone is clear of the patient, bed, and any equipment connected to the patient. Ensure oxygen is not flowing over the patient's torso (oxygen flow over the patient's torso during electrical therapy increases the risk of spark/fire). Defibrillation is indicated for pulseless ventricular tachycardia and ventricular fibrillation. Synchronized cardioversion may be used to treat the unstable patient in supraventricular tachycardia due to reentry, atrial fibrillation, atrial flutter, atrial tachycardia, or monomorphic ventricular tachycardia with a pulse. If VF occurs during the course of synchronization, check the patient's pulse and rhythm (verify all electrodes and cable connections are secure), turn off the sync control, and defibrillate.

26. A. Application of external ocular pressure may be dangerous and should not be used because of the risk of retinal detachment. Ensure oxygen, suction, a defibrillator, and crash cart are available before attempting the procedure. Obtain a 12-lead ECG before and after the vagal maneuver. Continuous monitoring of the patient's ECG essential. Note the onset and end of the vagal maneuver on the ECG rhythm strip. In general, a vagal maneuver should not be continued for more than 10 seconds. Application of a cold stimulus to the face (e.g., a washcloth soaked in iced water, cold pack, or crushed ice mixed with water in a plastic bag or glove) is often effective in infants and young children. When using this method, do not obstruct the patient's mouth or nose or apply pressure to the eyes. Valsalva's maneuver is also an effective vagal maneuver. Instruct the child to blow through a straw or take a deep breath and bear down as if having a bowel movement for 10 seconds. This strains the abdominal muscles and increases intrathoracic pressure.

27. C. The intraosseous route is an acceptable means of vascular access in infants and children and may be used as the initial method of vascular access in cardiac arrest. Any medication, fluid, or blood product that can be administered intravenously can be administered intraosseously. Administration of viscous drugs or rapid fluid boluses often requires the use of manual pressure or an infusion pump.

28. False. The preferred technique for oropharyngeal airway insertion in an infant or child requires the use of a tongue blade. Depress the tongue with a tongue blade and gently insert the oropharyngeal airway with the curve downward. Place the airway over the tongue down into the mouth until the flange of the airway rests against the patient's teeth or lips.

29. C. Using the rule of nines, the child's anterior chest is 9%, abdomen 9%, and the anterior portion of each leg is approximately 7% (14% for the anterior portion of both legs).

30. B. Septic shock occurs in two clinical stages. The early (hyperdynamic) phase is characterized by peripheral vasodilation (warm shock) due to endotoxins that prevent catecholamine-induced vaso-constriction. The late (hypodynamic or decompensated) phase is characterized by cool extremities (cold shock) and resembles hypovolemic shock.

31. A. Pain is a subjective experience that is underestimated and inadequately treated by many healthcare professionals despite the availability of effective medications and other therapies. Many factors contribute to the inadequate treatment of pain including the attitudes, beliefs, and behaviors of healthcare professionals. Some do not view pain relief as important or do not want to "waste time" assessing pain. The safe and effective relief of pain should be a priority in the management of a patient of *any* age.

32. A. The vastus lateralis is the preferred intramuscular injection site for infants and children younger than 3 years, but may be used in all ages.

33. False. Do NOT apply traction to the neck. In a child with possible cervical spine trauma, the application of traction can exacerbate an existing injury or convert a stable cervical fracture to an unstable fracture.

34. A. Two-person bag-mask ventilation may be more effective than ventilation with a single rescuer. Ventilate a patient in cardiac arrest at an age-appropriate rate and with just enough volume to see the patient's chest rise gently. Ventilating a cardiac arrest patient too fast or with too much volume results in excessive intrathoracic pressure, which results in decreased venous return into the chest, decreased coronary and cerebral perfusion pressures, diminished cardiac output, and decreased rates of survival. It also increases the risk of stomach inflation, regurgitation, and aspiration. Ventilate the infant or child with a perfusing rhythm but absent or inadequate ventilatory effort at a rate of 1 breath every 3 to 5 seconds (12 to 20 breaths per minute), using the higher rate for the younger child. In cardiac arrest, ventilate the intubated infant or child at a rate of about 1 breath every 6 to 8 seconds (8 to 10 times per minute) without interrupting chest compressions.

35. True. There is no evidence that cricoid pressure prevents aspiration during rapid sequence or emergency tracheal intubation in infants or children.

36. D. There are four cardiac arrest rhythms: 1) Ventricular fibrillation, 2) ventricular tachycardia, 3) asystole, and 4) pulseless electrical activity. Shockable cardiac arrest rhythms include ventricular fibrillation and ventricular tachycardia. Defibrillation is not indicated for asystole or pulseless electrical activity.

37. C. Assessment of an infant or young child's abdomen can be difficult. The abdomen of a young child is naturally protuberant and may appear somewhat distended. An infant will naturally tense his or her abdominal muscles when palpated, simulating guarding. A toddler may scream throughout the examination. It may be necessary to evaluate the abdomen more than once for a more accurate assessment.

38. D. Remember that an open airway does not ensure adequate ventilation. This patient's breathing is inadequate as evidenced by his rate and depth of ventilations. The patient with inadequate breathing requires positive-pressure ventilation with supplemental oxygen. Of the choices listed, the only device that can provide positive-pressure ventilation is the bag–mask. If readily available, an oral airway should be inserted before beginning bag–mask ventilation (if the patient does not have a gag or cough reflex).

39. True. Spontaneous emesis in the first 30 to 60 minutes following head injury is common in children.

40. D. Commotio cordis is a disorder described in the pediatric population that results from sudden impact to the anterior chest wall (e.g., baseball injury) that causes cessation of normal cardiac function. The patient may have an immediate dysrhythmia or ventricular fibrillation that is refractory to resuscitation efforts.

41. D. If a properly fitting device is not available, use towels, washcloths, or blanket rolls (depending on the child's size) and adhesive tape across the forehead to stabilize the head as best as possible. Avoid the use of IV bags or sand bags; their weight may push the cervical spine out of alignment.

42. True. Neurogenic shock is characterized by a decreased BP and normal or decreased heart rate. Hypovolemic shock is characterized by a decreased BP and increased heart rate.

43. True. Analgesics used to manage severe pain usually cause sedation, but most sedatives do not provide analgesia.

44. True. If you observe a change in mental status in a febrile child (inconsolable, inability to recognize parents, unarousable), *immediately* consider the possibility of septic shock.

45. False. Medications administered via a peripheral vein during CPR should be followed with a saline flush of 5 to 10 mL to facilitate delivery of the medication to the central circulation.

46. False. In the pediatric patient, a QRS complex is considered wide if it exceeds 0.09 second.

47. B. If breath sounds are absent on both sides of the chest after placing a tracheal tube, assume esophageal intubation. Deflate the tracheal tube cuff and remove the tube. If breath sounds are diminished on the left after intubation but present on the right, assume right primary bronchus intubation. Deflate the tracheal tube cuff, pull back the tube slightly, reinflate the cuff, and reevaluate breath sounds. Once placement is confirmed, note and record the depth (centimeter marking) of the tube at the patient's teeth and secure the tube in place.

48. B. Signs of shock should be treated with a bolus of 20 mL/kg of isotonic crystalloid even if blood pressure is normal. Consider the use of vasopressors if poor perfusion persists despite adequate oxygenation, ventilation, and volume expansion. Studies have shown no added benefit in using colloid solutions, such as albumin, for volume expansion during the early phase of resuscitation. There is no evidence to support the use of a specific isotonic crystalloid.

49. A. Peripherally inserted central catheters (PICC) are not inserted directly into a central vein. Instead, a PICC line is inserted into an antecubital vein and then advanced into the subclavian vein so that the tip lies in the superior vena cava or right atrium.

50. D. The child with a malfunctioning shunt may present with irritability, headache, neck pain, vomiting, a bulging or full fontanelle in infants, new seizures or a change in the child's seizure pattern, behavioral changes, or "just not acting right." These are signs of increased intracranial pressure, due to fluid accumulation within the brain. Abdominal pain may be present because of infected CSF draining into the peritoneal cavity, causing peritoneal inflammation. If infection is present, redness, edema, or tenderness may be observed along the path of the shunt tubing. A child with a shunt infection is usually, but not always, febrile.

Illustration Credits

Chapter One

Fig 1-1. EMSC Slide Set (CD-ROM). 1996. Courtesy of the Emergency Medical Services for Children Program, administered by the U.S. Department of Health and Human Service's Health Resources and Services Administration, Maternal and Child Health Bureau.

Chapter Two

Figs. 2-2, 2-4. Zitelli B, Davis H: *Atlas of pediatric physical diagnosis,* 5e, St. Louis, 2007, Mosby.

Figs. 2-3, 2-5, 2-11. Hockenberry M, Wilson D, Winkelstein M, Kline N: *Wong's nursing care of infants and children,* 7e, St. Louis, 2002, Mosby.

Figs. 2-6, 2-8, 2-15, 2-16. Seidel H, Ball J, Dains J, Benedict GW: *Mosby's guide to physical examination,* 5e, St. Louis, 2003, Mosby.

Fig. 2-7. Courtesy Mead Johnson & Co., Evansville, Indiana.

Fig. 2-9. From Beattie T: *Pediatric emergencies,* London, 1997, Mosby-Wolfe.

Figs. 2-12, 2-14. EMSC Slide Set (CD-ROM). 1996. Courtesy of the Emergency Medical Services for Children Program, administered by the U.S. Department of Health and Human Service's Health Resources and Services Administration, Maternal and Child Health Bureau.

Fig. 2-13. Courtesy Gary Quick, MD.

Chapter Three

Figs. 3-1, 3-2, 3-3, 3-11. EMSC Slide Set (CD-ROM). 1996. Courtesy of the Emergency Medical Services for Children Program, administered by the U.S. Department of Health and Human Service's Health Resources and Services Administration, Maternal and Child Health Bureau.

Figs. 3-4, 3-6, 3-9. Zitelli B, Davis H: *Atlas of pediatric physical diagnosis,* 5e, St. Louis, 2007, Mosby.

Fig. 3-5. Hockenberry M, Wilson D, Winkelstein M, Kline N: *Wong's nursing care of infants and children,* 7e, St. Louis, 2002, Mosby.

Figs. 3-7, 3-10. Behrman R, Kliegman R, Jenson H: *Nelson textbook of pediatrics,* 17e, Philadelphia, 2004, Saunders.

Fig. 3-8. Seidel H, Ball J, Dains J, Benedict GW: *Mosby's guide to physical examination,* 5e, St. Louis, 2003, Mosby.

Chapter Four

Figs. 4-3, 4-4, 4-7, 4-8, 4-9, 4-12. Chapleau W: *Emergency medical technician: making the difference,* St. Louis, 2007, Mosby.

Fig. 4-5. Aehlert B: *Mosby's comprehensive pediatric emergency care,* St. Louis, 2006, Mosby.

Fig. 4-6. Sanders M: *Mosby's paramedic textbook,* 4e, St. Louis, 2012, Mosby.

Figs. 4-10, 4-18, 4-19. Price D: *Pediatric nursing: an introductory text,* 10e, Philadelphia, 2007, Saunders.

Figs. 4-11, 4-17, 4-24. Aehlert B: *Paramedic practice today: above and beyond,* revised 1e, St. Louis, 2011, Mosby.

Figs. 4-13A, 4-15. American College of Emergency Physicians (Kohmer, editor): *EMT-basic field care: a case-based approach,* St. Louis, 1999, Mosby.

Figs. 4-13B, 4-14, 4-16, 4-27, 4-28, 4-31. McSwain N, Paturas J: *The basic EMT: comprehensive prehospital patient care,* 2e, St. Louis, 2003, Mosby.

Figs. 4-20, 4-21. EMSC Slide Set (CD-ROM). 1996. Courtesy of the Emergency Medical Services for Children Program, administered by the U.S. Department of Health and Human Service's Health Resources and Services Administration, Maternal and Child Health Bureau.

Fig. 4-22. Hockenberry M, Wilson D: *Wong's nursing care of infants and children,* 9e, St. Louis, 2010, Mosby.

Figs. 4-25, 4-30. Mack D: *Mosby's comprehensive EMT-B refresher and review,* St. Louis, 2002, Mosby.

Figs. 4-26, 4-29. Henry M, Stapleton E: *EMT prehospital care,* 3e, St. Louis, 2004, Mosby.

Figs. 4-33, 4-36. Thibodeau G, Patton K: *Anatomy and physiology,* 5e, St. Louis, 2003, Mosby.

Figs. 4-34, 4-35. Shade BR: *Mosby's EMT-intermediate textbook,* St. Louis, 2002, Mosby.

Figs. 4-36, 4-37. Dieckmann R, Fiser D, Selbst S: *Illustrated textbook of pediatric emergency and critical care procedures,* 1e, St. Louis, 1997, Mosby.

Chapter Five

Fig. 5-1. Herlihy B, Maebius N: *The human body in health and illness,* 2e, St. Louis, 2003, Saunders.

Figs. 5-2, 5-3, 5-4, 5-5, 5-6, 5-9, 5-10, 5-13, 5-16, 5-17, 5-19, 5-20, 5-21. Aehlert B: *ECGs made easy study cards,* 2e, St. Louis, 2004, Mosby.

Figs. 5-7, 5-11. Park MK, Guntheroth WG: *How to read pediatric ECGs,* 3e, St. Louis, Mosby, 1992.

Figs. 5-8, 5-12, 5-15, 5-18. Aehlert B: *ECGs made easy,* 4e, St. Louis, 2009, Mosby.

Fig. 5-14. Aehlert B: *ACLS Quick Review Study Guide,* 2e, St. Louis, 2002, Mosby.

Chapter Six

Figs. 6-3, 6-12, 6-13, 6-15A, 6-17, 6-18, 6-19. Dieckmann R, Fiser D, Selbst S: *Illustrated textbook of pediatric emergency and critical care procedures,* 1e, St. Louis, 1997, Mosby.

Fig. 6-4. Hockenberry M, Wilson D, Winkelstein M, Kline N: *Wong's nursing care of infants and children,* 7e, St. Louis, 2002, Mosby.

Figs. 6-5B&C, 6-15B, 6-16, 6-23A. EMSC Slide Set (CD-ROM). 1996. Courtesy of the Emergency Medical Services for Children Program, administered by the U.S. Department of Health and Human Service's Health Resources and Services Administration, Maternal and Child Health Bureau.

Fig. 6-7. Sanders M: *Mosby's paramedic textbook,* 4e, St. Louis, 2012, Mosby.

Figs. 6-9, 6-10. Sanders M: *Mosby's paramedic textbook,* revised 3e, St. Louis, 2007, Mosby.

Fig. 6-20A-E. Roberts J, Hedges J: *Clinical procedures in emergency medicine,* 3e, Philadelphia, 1998, Saunders.

Figs. 6-21, 6-22A&B. Courtesy Medtronic, Inc.

Fig. 6-24. American College of Emergency Physicians (Pons P, Carson D, editors): *Paramedic field care: a complaint-based approach,* St. Louis, 1997, Mosby.

Fig. 6-25A&B. Images provided courtesy of Philips Medical Systems.

Figs. 6-26, 6-27. Aehlert B: *ECGs made easy,* 4e, St. Louis, 2009, Mosby.

Chapter 6: Quiz Question 6. Aehlert B: *ECGs made easy,* 4e, St. Louis, 2009, Mosby.

Chapter 6: Quiz Question 18. Aehlert B: *ACLS quick review study guide,* 2e, St. Louis, 2002, Mosby.

Chapter Seven

Figs. 7-1, 7-2. Hockenberry M, Wilson D, Winkelstein M, Kline N: *Wong's nursing care of infants and children,* 7e, St. Louis, 2002, Mosby.

Figs. 7-3, 7-4. Dieckmann R, Fiser D, Selbst S: *Illustrated textbook of pediatric emergency and critical care procedures,* 1e, St. Louis, 1997, Mosby.

Figs. 7-5, 7-7. Hockenberry M, Wilson D, Winkelstein M, Kline N: *Wong's nursing care of infants and children,* 7e, St. Louis, 2002, Mosby.

Fig. 7-6. From Wong DL, Hockenberry M, Wilson D, Winkelstein M, Schwartz P: *Wong's essentials of pediatric nursing*, 6e, St. Louis, 2001, Mosby.

Chapter Eight

Figs. 8-1, 8-2, 8-3, 8-18. From McSwain N, Paturas J: *The basic EMT: comprehensive prehospital patient care*, 2e, St. Louis, 2003, Mosby.

Figs. 8-4, 8-5, 8-6. Prehospital Trauma Life Support Committee of the NAEMT: *PHTLS: basic and advanced prehospital trauma life support*, 5e, St. Louis, 2003, Mosby.

Figs. 8-7, 8-8, 8-9. Zitelli B, Davis H: *Atlas of pediatric physical diagnosis*, 4e, St. Louis, 2002, Mosby.

Fig. 8-10. Sheehy S: *Emergency nursing*, 3e, St. Louis, 1992, Mosby.

Figs. 8-11, 8-16, 8-17. Gould B: *Pathophysiology for the health professions*, 2e, Philadelphia, 2002, Saunders.

Figs. 8-12A-C, 8-13A&B, 8-14A-D. Shade B, Rothenberg M, Wertz E, Jones S, Collins T: *Mosby's EMT-intermediate textbook*, 2e, St. Louis, 2002, Mosby.

Fig. 8-15. Courtesy Kristen Burke.

Chapter Nine

Fig. 9-1. McSwain N, Paturas J: *The basic EMT: comprehensive prehospital patient care*, 2e, St. Louis, 2003, Mosby.

Figs. 9-1, 9-2, 9-3. Henry M, Stapleton E: *EMT prehospital care*, 3e, St. Louis, 2004, Mosby.

Chapter Eleven

Fig. 11-1. Zitelli B, Davis H: *Atlas of pediatric physical diagnosis*, 4e, St. Louis, 2002, Mosby.

Figs. 11-2, 11-6. Chaudhry B, Harvey D: *Mosby's color atlas and text of pediatrics and child health*, London, 2001, Mosby.

Fig. 11-3A&B. Sanders M: *Mosby's paramedic textbook*, revised 2e, St. Louis, 2001, Mosby.

Fig. 11-7A. Sanders M: *Mosby's paramedic textbook*, 4e, St. Louis, 2012, Mosby.

Fig. 11-4. American College of Emergency Physicians (Pons P, Carson D, editors): *Paramedic field care: a complaint-based approach*, St. Louis, 1997, Mosby.

Figs. 11-5, 11-12. Henry M, Stapleton E: *EMT prehospital care*, 3e, St. Louis, 2004, Mosby.

Figs. 11-7B, 11-15, 11-16. Hockenberry M, Wilson D, Winkelstein M, Kline N: *Wong's nursing care of infants and children,* 7e, St. Louis, 2002, Mosby.

Fig. 11-8A-C. Courtesy Smiths Medical.

Figs. 11-9, 11-11. Courtesy Nellcor.

Fig. 11-10. Roberts J, Hedges J: *Clinical procedures in emergency medicine,* 3e, Philadelphia, 1998, Saunders.

Figs. 11-13, 11-14. Dieckmann R, Fiser D, Selbst S: *Illustrated textbook of pediatric emergency and critical care procedures,* 1e, St. Louis, 1997, Mosby.

Fig. 11-17. Courtesy Cooke Incorporated, Bloomington, Indiana.

Chapter Twelve

Fig. 12-1. McSwain N, Paturas J: *The basic EMT: comprehensive prehospital patient care,* 2e, St. Louis, 2003, Mosby.

Figs. 12-2, 12-3, 12-6, 12-7, 12-8, 12-9. Al-Azzawi F: *Color atlas of childbirth and obstetrics,* London, 1995, Mosby-Wolfe.

Figs. 12-4, 12-5. Stoy W: *Mosby's EMT-basic textbook,* 1e, St. Louis, 1996, Mosby.

Fig. 12-11. Sanders M: *Mosby's paramedic textbook,* 4e, St. Louis, 2012, Mosby.

Fig. 12-16. Sanders M: *Mosby's paramedic textbook,* revised 3e, St. Louis, 2007, Mosby.

Fig. 12-10. Reproduced with permission, PALS Provider Manual © 2002, American Heart Association.

Figure on page 445. Reprinted with permission *2010 American Heart Association Guidelines for Cardiopulmonary Resuscitation and Emergency Cardiovascular Care,* Part 15: Neonatal Resuscitation Circulation. 2010;122[suppl 3]: S909-S919. Copyright © 2010 American Heart Association, Inc.

Fig. 12-12. Chaudhry B, Harvey D: *Mosby's color atlas and text of pediatrics and child health,* London, 2001, Mosby.

Fig. 12-13. Courtesy Marjorie M Pyle.

Figs. 12-14, 12-15. Dieckmann R, Fiser D, Selbst S: *Illustrated textbook of pediatric emergency and critical care procedures,* 1e, St. Louis, 1997, Mosby.

Glossary

Adrenergic having the characteristics of the sympathetic division of the autonomic nervous system

Afterload the pressure or resistance against which the ventricles must pump to eject blood

Agonist a drug or substance that produces a predictable response (stimulates action)

ALTE apparent life-threatening event, a nonfatal condition characterized by apnea continuing for more than 20 seconds, especially when accompanied by cyanosis, atony, or unresponsiveness

Amnesia lack of memory about events occurring during a particular period

Analgesia absence of pain in response to stimulation that would normally be painful

Anaphylaxis a severe allergic response to a foreign substance with which the patient has had prior contact

Anemia a condition in which oxygen-transporting material in the blood (such as erythrocytes) is abnormally low

Anesthesia a state of unconsciousness

Antagonist an agent that exerts an opposite action to another (blocks action)

Antepartum the maternal period before delivery

Anticholinergic antagonistic to the action of parasympathetic (cholinergic) nerve fibers

Antidote a substance that neutralizes a poison

Anxiolysis relief of apprehension and uneasiness without alteration of awareness

Arrhythmia term often used interchangeably with "dysrhythmia"; any disturbance or abnormality in a normal rhythmic pattern; any cardiac rhythm other than a sinus rhythm

Artifact distortion of an ECG tracing by electrical activity that is noncardiac in origin (e.g., electrical interference, poor electrical conduction, patient movement)

Assistive technology a term used to describe devices that are used by children and adults with a disability to compensate for functional limitations and to enhance and increase learning, independence, mobility, communication, environmental control, and choice

Asystole absence of cardiac electrical activity viewed as a straight (isoelectric) line on the ECG

Atelectasis the absence of air in part or the entire lung; may be chronic or acute; may be caused by secretions, obstruction by foreign bodies or compression

Atony lack of muscle tone; flaccidity

Bacteremia the presence of viable bacteria in the blood

Baroreceptors specialized nerve tissue (sensors) located in the internal carotid arteries and the aortic arch that detect changes in blood pressure and cause a reflex response in either the sympathetic or the parasympathetic division of the autonomic nervous system; pressoreceptors

Barotrauma lung damage due to excessive ventilatory pressure

bpm abbreviation for beats per minute. The abbreviation bpm usually refers to an intrinsic heart rate, while pulses per minute (ppm) usually refers to a paced rate.

BiPAP   bilevel positive airway pressure; a form of noninvasive, positive-pressure mechanical ventilation

Blood pressure   the force exerted by the blood on the inner walls of the blood vessels

Blunt trauma   any mechanism of injury that occurs without actual penetration of the body; typically results from motor vehicle crashes, falls, or assaults with a blunt object

Bronchiole   a small air passage in the lower airway

Bronchiolitis   inflammation of the bronchioles

Bronchomalacia   degeneration of elastic and connective tissue of the bronchi and trachea, causing collapse and relative upper airway obstruction during inhalation

Bronchopulmonary dysplasia   a chronic lung disease characterized by persistent respiratory distress

Bronchospasm   an abnormal contraction of the smooth muscle of the bronchi, resulting in acute narrowing and obstruction

Capacitor   a device for storing an electrical charge

Capnography   the continuous analysis and recording of carbon dioxide concentrations in respiratory gases

Capnometer   a device that measures the concentration of carbon dioxide at the end of exhalation

Capnometry   the measurement of CO_2 concentrations without a continuous written record or waveform

Carboxyhemoglobin   the resultant product when the oxygen in hemoglobin is displaced by carbon monoxide so that red blood cells cannot transport oxygen from the lungs to the tissues

Cardiac arrest   the cessation of cardiac mechanical activity, confirmed by the absence of a detectable pulse, unresponsiveness, and apnea or agonal, gasping respiration

Cardiac output   the amount of blood pumped into the aorta each minute by the heart. It is calculated as the stroke volume (amount of blood ejected from a ventricle with each heart beat) times the heart rate.

Cardiomyopathy   a disease of the heart muscle that affects the heart's pumping ability

Carina   the point where the trachea bifurcates into the right and left mainstem bronchi (approximately the level of the 5th or 6th thoracic vertebra)

Caustic   capable of burning or destroying tissue by chemical action

Cerebral resuscitation   a term used to emphasize the need to preserve the cerebral viability of the cardiac arrest victim

Chance fracture   a horizontal fracture of the thoracic or lumbar spine caused by hyperflexion injuries with little or no compression of the vertebral body; also called a seatbelt fracture, since they are commonly associated with the wearing of lap-type seatbelts

Chelation   use of a chemical compound that combines with a heavy metal for rapid, safe excretion

Chronotrope   a substance that affects heart rate

Clonic   rhythmic muscle contraction and relaxation

Cognitive disability   an impairment that affects an individual's awareness, memory, and ability to learn, process information, communicate, and make decisions

Compensated shock   inadequate tissue perfusion without hypotension (i.e., shock with a "normal" blood pressure)

Compliance   the resistance of the patient's lung tissue to ventilation

Continuous Positive Airway Pressure (CPAP)   the delivery of a steady, gentle flow of air by means of a medical device through a soft mask worn over the nose or over the mouth and nose

Costochondritis   an inflammation of the cartilage that connects the inner end of each rib to the sternum

Crackles   high-pitched breath sounds (formerly referred to as rales) that indicate lower airway pathology, such as pneumonia or asthma

Crepitation   a fine crackling sound resembling that of a hair rubbed between the fingers or a grating sensation felt over a fracture or an area of subcutaneous air

Cricoid pressure   the use of gentle, continuous downward pressure on the cricoid cartilage of the larynx; intended to aid in protection from aspiration by compressing the larynx against the esophagus

Cricothyroid membrane   a fibrous membrane located between the cricoid and thyroid cartilage; site for surgical and alternative airway placement

Croup   respiratory distress caused by narrowing below the glottis characterized by hoarseness, inspiratory stridor, and a bark-like cough

Crowing   abnormal respiratory sound that suggests narrowing of the tracheal opening and laryngeal spasm

Cullen's sign   a bluish discoloration around the umbilicus that may indicate intra-abdominal or retro-peritoneal hemorrhage

Cushing's triad   hypertension, bradycardia, and abnormal respirations resulting from increased intra-cranial pressure

Cystic fibrosis   a hereditary disease of the exocrine glands characterized by production of viscous mucus that obstructs the bronchi

Decannulation   the removal of a cannula; in the case of a child with a tracheostomy, the removal of the tracheostomy tube

Decannulation cap   a cap located in the outer cannula of a fenestrated tracheostomy tube that blocks airflow through the stoma

Decompensated shock   a clinical state of tissue perfusion that is inadequate to meet the body's metabolic demands, accompanied by hypotension; also called progressive or late shock

Defasciculation agent   a medication that is given to inhibit muscle twitching

Defibrillation   the therapeutic delivery of unsynchronized electrical current through the myocardium over a very brief period to terminate a cardiac dysrhythmia

Defibrillation threshold   the least amount of energy in joules or volts delivered to the heart that reproducibly converts ventricular fibrillation to a perfusing rhythm

Defibrillator   a device used to administer an electrical shock at a preset voltage to terminate a cardiac dysrhythmia

Diaphoresis   profuse sweating

Distraction   in pain management, the strategy of focusing one's attention on stimuli other than pain or the accompanying negative emotions

Diuretic   a medication that increases urine output; used to treat hypertension, congestive heart failure, and edema

Dromotrope   a substance that affects atrioventricular (AV) conduction velocity

Drowning   death from suffocation in a liquid

Drug   any chemical compound that produces an effect on a living organism

Dyspnea   difficulty breathing; shortness of breath

Endocarditis   an infection of the heart valves and the inner lining of the heart muscle

Endotracheal   within or through the trachea

Endotracheal intubation   an advanced airway procedure in which a tube is placed directly into the trachea

Epiglottis   a small, leaf-shaped cartilage located at the top of the larynx that prevents food from entering the respiratory tract during swallowing

Epiglottitis   a bacterial infection of the epiglottis and supraglottic structures; also called acute supra-glottitis

Epithelium   the cellular, avascular layer covering tissue surfaces

ET   endotracheal

ETT   endotracheal tube

Extravasation   the actual (unintentional) escape or leakage of an agent that is irritating and causes blistering (a vesicant) from a vessel into the surrounding tissue

Fasciculations   involuntary muscle twitches

Gasp   inhaling and exhaling with quick, difficult breaths

Gastrostomy   a surgically created passageway between the skin and the stomach through which a tube is placed to provide nutrients or medication

General anesthesia   a controlled state of unconsciousness accompanied by partial or complete loss of protective reflexes, including inability to maintain an airway independently and inability to respond purposefully to physical stimulation or verbal command

Glottis   the true vocal cords and the space between them

Gravida   refers to the number of a woman's current and past pregnancies

Grey-Turner's sign   bruising of the flanks that may indicate intra-abdominal hemorrhage, often splenic (retroperitoneal) in origin

Grunting   a short, low-pitched sound heard at the end of exhalation that represents an attempt to generate positive end-expiratory pressure (PEEP) by exhaling against a closed glottis, prolonging the period of oxygen and carbon dioxide exchange across the alveolar-capillary membrane; a compensatory mechanism to help maintain patency of small airways and prevent atelectasis

Gurgling   abnormal respiratory sound associated with collection of liquid or semi-solid material in the patient's upper airway

Hard palate   the bony portion of the roof of the mouth that forms the floor of the nasal cavity

Head bobbing   indicator of increased work of breathing in infants; the head falls forward with exhalation and comes up with expansion of the chest on inhalation

Hemoglobin   the red oxygen-binding protein of erythrocytes

Hemoptysis   expectoration of blood that originates in the lungs or bronchi

Hemorrhage   an acute loss of circulating blood

Herniation   protrusion of a structure through tissues normally containing it

His-Purkinje system   the portion of the conduction system consisting of the bundle of His, bundle branches, and Purkinje fibers

Hypoperfusion   the inadequate circulation of blood through an organ or a part of the body; shock

Hypotonia   decreased muscle tone

Hypoxemia   in adults, children, and infants older than 28 days, hypoxemia is defined as an arterial oxygen tension (PaO2) of less than 60 torr or arterial oxygen saturation (SaO2) of less than 90% in an individual breathing room air or with a PaO2 and/or SaO2 below the desirable range for a specific clinical situation

Hypoxia   a deficiency of oxygen reaching the tissues of the body

Hyperpnea   abnormally deep breathing

Iatrogenic   a response to a medical or surgical treatment induced by the treatment itself

Immersion syndrome   death following submersion in extremely cold water

Impedance   resistance to the flow of current. Transthoracic impedance (resistance) refers to the resistance of the chest wall to current.

Induction   the use of pharmacologic agents, whether it be intravenous solutions or inhaled gases, that act on the brain to quickly move from consciousness to unconsciousness; to create a plane or level of anesthesia

Infiltration   the intentional or unintentional process in which a substance enters or infuses into another substance or a surrounding area

Inherent   natural, intrinsic

Inotrope   a substance affects myocardial contractility

Inotropic effect   refers to a change in myocardial contractility

Interval   a waveform and a segment; in pacing, the period, measured in milliseconds, between any two designated cardiac events

Intraosseous infusion (IOI)   the infusion of fluids, medications, or blood directly into the bone marrow cavity

Intravenous cannulation   the placement of a catheter into a vein to gain access to the body's venous circulation

Intrinsic rate   rate at which a pacemaker of the heart normally generates impulses

Intubation   passing a tube into a body opening; when used alone, the term implies endotracheal intubation (placement of a tube into the trachea)

Ischemia   a decreased supply of oxygenated blood to a body part or organ

Isoelectric line   an absence of electrical activity observed on the ECG as a straight line

J point   the point where the QRS complex and ST segment meet

Joule   the basic unit of energy; equivalent to watt-seconds

Kawasaki disease   an inflammation of the walls of small and medium-sized arteries throughout the body; the leading cause of acquired heart disease in children

Kehr's sign   left upper quadrant pain with radiation to the left shoulder suggests injury to the spleen or liver (pain occurs because of blood or bile irritating the diaphragm)

Kinematics   the process of predicting injury patterns

KVO   abbreviation meaning, "keep the vein open." Also known as TKO, "to keep open."

Laryngoscope   an instrument used to examine the interior of the larynx. During endotracheal intubation, the device is used to visualize the glottic opening.

Laryngotracheobronchitis   croup

Lead   an electrical connection attached to the body to record electrical activity

Learning disability   a general term that refers to a group of disorders manifested by significant difficulties in the acquisition and use of listening, spelling, reading, writing, reasoning, or mathematical skills

Ligation   tying

Medication   drugs used in the practice of medicine as a remedy

Membrane potential   a difference in electrical charge across the cell membrane

Mental impairment   any mental or psychological disorder, such as mental retardation, organic brain syndrome, emotional or mental illness, and specific learning disabilities

Milliampere (mA)   the unit of measure of electrical current needed to elicit depolarization of the myocardium

Minute volume   the amount of air moved in and out of the lungs in one minute; determined by multiplying the tidal volume by the respiratory rate.

Monomorphic   having the same shape

Moro reflex   (also called startle response, startle reflex, embrace reflex) a primitive reflex present at birth and typically disappears by the age of about four to six months. When an infant is startled by a loud noise or sudden movement, the arms are thrown apart with the palms up and the thumbs flexed, the legs extend, and the head is thrown back. As the reflex ends the infant draws the arms back to the body, elbows flexed, and then relaxes. The reflex should be brisk and symmetrical. Absence of this reflex in an infant is abnormal. Presence of a Moro reflex in an older infant, child, or adult is also abnormal. Absence of this reflex on one side suggests a fractured clavicle or injury to the brachial plexus, possibly due to birth trauma. Two-sided absence of this reflex suggests damage to the brain or spinal cord.

Multiple organ dysfunction syndrome (MODS)   the progressive failure of two or more organ systems after a very severe illness or injury

mV   abbreviation for millivolt

Myocardial cells   working cells of the myocardium that contain contractile filaments and form the muscular layer of the atrial walls and the thicker muscular layer of the ventricular walls

Myocarditis   inflammation of the heart muscle with or without involvement of the endocardium or pericardium

Myocardium   the middle and thickest layer of the heart; contains the cardiac muscle fibers that cause contraction of the heart and contains the conduction system

Myoclonus   shock-like contraction of a muscle

Nasal flaring   widening of the nostrils on inhalation; an attempt to increase the size of the airway and increase the amount of available oxygen

Near-drowning   survival, at least temporarily, after suffocation in a liquid

Needle thoracostomy   insertion of an over-the-needle catheter into the chest to relieve a tension pneumothorax

Neglect   failure to provide for a child's basic needs. Neglect can be physical, educational, or emotional

Neurogenic shock   a type of shock that occurs as a result of a spinal cord injury that disrupts sympathetic control of vascular tone

Neuromuscular relaxing agent   a medication that produces chemical paralysis of skeletal muscle; also called paralytic agent, neuromuscular blocker

Neurotransmitter   a chemical responsible for transmission of an impulse across a synapse

Oliguria   scanty urine production

Orthopnea   difficulty breathing brought on or aggravated by lying flat; changing to a sitting or standing position typically permits deeper and more comfortable breathing

Orthostatic hypotension   an inappropriate fall in blood pressure on assumption of an upright posture

Pacemaker cells   specialized cells of the heart's electrical conduction system capable of spontaneously generating and conducting electrical impulses

Pain   an unpleasant sensory and emotional experience associated with actual or potential tissue damage, or described in terms of such damage

Pain tolerance level   the greatest level of pain that a subject is prepared to tolerate

Pain threshold   the least experience of pain that a subject can recognize

Para   refers to the number of a woman's past pregnancies that have remained viable to delivery; a woman who is pregnant for the first time is gravida 1, para 0; para can be further divided into **four categories** number of term infants, number of premature infants, number of abortions/miscarriages, number of living children

Paradoxical irritability   irritable when held and lethargic when left alone; may be seen in infants and small children with neurologic infections

Partial seizure   a seizure confined to one area of the brain

Patent ductus arteriosus   a heart defect that occurs when the ductus arteriosus, a blood vessel present during fetal development that connects the pulmonary artery to the descending aorta, fails to close after birth

Penetrating trauma   any mechanism of injury that causes a cut or piercing of skin

Perfusion   the circulation of blood through an organ or a part of the body

Pericardium   a double-walled sac that encloses the heart and helps to anchor the heart in place, preventing excessive movement of the heart in the chest when body position changes, and protect it from trauma and infection

Pericarditis   inflammation of the pericardium that results in an increase in the volume of pericardial fluid that surrounds the heart

Perinatal   occurring at or near the time of birth

Peripheral vascular resistance   resistance to the flow of blood determined by blood vessel diameter and the tone of the vascular musculature

Petechiae   reddish-purple nonblanchable discolorations in the skin less than 0.5 cm in diameter

Pocket mask   a transparent semi-rigid mask designed for mouth-to-mask ventilation of an adult, child, or infant

Poison   a substance that, on ingestion, inhalation, absorption, application, injection, or development within the body in relatively small amounts, may cause structural damage or functional disturbance

Poisoning   exposure to a substance that is harmful in any dosage

Polarized state   period of time following repolarization of a myocardial cell (also called the "resting state") when the outside of the cell is positive and the interior of the cell is negative

Polymorphic   varying in shape

Preload   the force exerted by the blood on the walls of the ventricles at the end of diastole

Prenatal   existing or occurring before birth

Preoxygenate   the administration of oxygen to a patient before attempting a procedure (e.g., intubation)

Presyncope   an episode in which the patient experiences signs and symptoms that precede actual syncope; presyncope does not include loss of consciousness

Primary apnea   the newly born's initial response to hypoxemia consisting of initial tachypnea, then apnea, bradycardia, and a slight increase in blood pressure; if stimulated, responds with resumption of breathing

Primary bradycardia   bradycardia caused by structural heart disease

Primipara   a woman who has given birth only once

Prodrome   symptoms that precede the patient's present chief complaint

Prolonged QT syndrome cardiac disorder in which the interval between the QRS complex and the T wave is unusually long

Pulse oximetry the use of the light absorption characteristics of oxygenated and deoxygenated hemoglobin to display an indirect measurement of the percentage of hemoglobin saturated with oxygen

Pulse pressure the difference between the systolic and diastolic blood pressure; an indicator of stroke volume

Pulseless electrical activity (PEA) organized electrical activity observed on a cardiac monitor (other than VT or VF) without a palpable pulse

Purkinje fibers an elaborate web of fibers distributed throughout the ventricular myocardium

Purpura red-purple nonblanchable discolorations greater than 0.5 cm in diameter. Large purpura are called ecchymoses.

PVC abbreviation for premature ventricular complex

R wave On an EGG, the first positive deflection in the QRS complex, representing ventricular depolarization

Rapid sequence intubation the use of medications to sedate and paralyze a patient to rapidly achieve tracheal intubation

Reentry the propagation of an impulse through tissue already activated by that same impulse

Refractoriness the extent to which a cell is able to respond to a stimulus.

Repolarization movement of ions across a cell membrane in which the inside of the cell is restored to its negative charge

Respiratory distress increased work of breathing (respiratory effort)

Respiratory failure a clinical condition in which there is inadequate blood oxygenation and/or ventilation to meet the metabolic demands of body tissues

Retractions sinking in of the soft tissues above the sternum or clavicle, or between or below the ribs during inhalation

Retrograde moving backward; moving in the opposite direction to that which is considered normal

Seat-belt sign abdominal contusion consisting of ecchymosis and bruising in a band that corresponds to the position of the seat belt across the abdomen

Secondary apnea when asphyxia is prolonged, a period of deep, gasping respirations with a concomitant fall in blood pressure and heart rate; gasping becomes weaker and slower and then ceases

Secondary bradycardia a slow heart rate due to a non-cardiac cause

Secondary drowning death occurring longer than 24 hours after submersion secondary to severe respiratory decompensation (e.g., acute respiratory distress syndrome, pulmonary edema)

Sedation depression of an individual's awareness of the environment and reduction of his or her responsiveness to external stimulation

Seizure a temporary alteration in behavior or consciousness caused by abnormal electrical activity of one or more groups of neurons in the brain

Sellick maneuver technique used to compress the cricoid cartilage causing occlusion of the esophagus, thereby reducing the risk of aspiration; also called cricoid pressure

Sequence of survival a concept that represents the ideal sequence of events that should take place immediately following the recognition of an injury or the onset of sudden illness; early access to care, early CPR, early defibrillation, and early advanced care

Sepsis the systemic response to an infection

Septicemia   an infection of the blood

Septic shock   sepsis with hypotension, despite adequate fluid resuscitation, along with the presence of perfusion abnormalities that may include, but are not limited to, lactic acidosis, oliguria, or an acute alteration in mental status

Severe sepsis   sepsis associated with organ dysfunction, hypoperfusion, or hypotension

Shock   a clinical syndrome resulting from the failure of the cardiovascular system to deliver sufficient oxygen and nutrients to sustain vital organ function

Sniffing position   In this position, the neck is flexed at the 5th and 6th cervical vertebrae, and the head is extended at the 1st and 2nd cervical vertebrae. This position aligns the axes of the mouth, pharynx, and trachea, opening the airway and increasing airflow.

Snoring   noisy breathing through the mouth and nose during sleep, caused by air passing through a narrowed upper airway

Soft palate   composed of mucous membrane, muscular fibers, and mucous glands and is suspended from the posterior border of the hard palate, forming the roof of the mouth

ST-segment   the portion of the ECG representing the end of ventricular depolarization (end of the R wave) and the beginning of ventricular repolarization (T wave).

Status epilepticus   a single seizure lasting longer than 30 minutes or repeated seizures without full recovery of responsiveness between seizures and lasting longer than 30 minutes

Stridor   a harsh, high-pitched sound heard on inspiration associated with upper airway obstruction. It is frequently described as a high-pitched crowing or "seal-bark" sound.

Stroke volume   the amount of blood ejected by either ventricle during one contraction; can be calculated as cardiac output divided by heart rate

Stylet   a malleable plastic-covered wire used for molding and maintaining the shape of an endotracheal tube

Synchronized cardioversion   the delivery of a shock to the heart to terminate a rapid dysrhythmia that is timed to avoid the vulnerable period during the cardiac cycle

Syncope   a brief loss of consciousness caused by transient cerebral hypoxia

Systemic inflammatory response syndrome (SIRS)   a response to infection manifested by derangement in two or more of the following: temperature, heart rate, respiratory rate, and white blood cell count

Tachycardia   in adults, a heart rate > 100 beats/min. In the pediatric patient, the term is used to describe a significant and persistent increase in heart rate. In infants, a tachycardia is a heart rate of more than 200 beats/min. In a child over 5 years of age, a tachycardia is a heart rate of more than 160 beats/min.

Tachypnea   abnormally rapid breathing

Therapeutic effect   a beneficial action of a drug that corrects a bodily dysfunction

Tidal volume   the amount of air exchanged with each breath

TKO   abbreviation meaning "to keep open." Also known as KVO, "keep the vein open."

Toxidrome   a constellation of signs and symptoms useful for recognizing a specific class of poisoning

Toxin   a poisonous substance of plant or animal origin

Tracheitis   inflammation of the mucous membrane of the trachea

Tracheobronchial   pertaining to the trachea and bronchi

Tracheomalacia   degeneration of the elastic and connective tissue of the trachea

Tragus   a tongue-like projection of cartilage anterior to the external opening of the ear

Transthoracic impedance (resistance)   the resistance of the chest wall to current

Tripod position   position used to maintain airway patency, sitting upright and leaning forward with the neck slightly extended, chin projected, and mouth open and supported by their arms

Turgor   elasticity

Vagal maneuver   methods used to stimulate the vagus nerve in an attempt to slow conduction through the AV node, resulting in slowing of the heart rate

Vallecula   the space (or "pocket") between the base of the tongue and the epiglottis; an important landmark when performing endotracheal intubation with a curved laryngoscope blade

Vascular resistance   the amount of opposition that blood vessels give to the flow of blood

Venous return   the amount of blood flowing into the right atrium each minute from the systemic circulation

Waddell's triad   the injury pattern experienced by a child involved in a pedestrian injury; extremity trauma, thoracic and abdominal trauma, and head trauma

Watt-second   a unit of energy equivalent to the joule

Waveform   movement away from the baseline in either a positive or a negative direction

Wheezes   high-pitched "whistling" sounds produced by air moving through narrowed airway passages

Index